Approved Abbreviations for Medications

Abbreviation	Meaning	Abbreviation	Meaning
ā	before	ml or mL	milliliter
ac	before meals	NG, NGT	nasogastric tube
ad lib	as desired; freely	NKA	no known allergies
ADE	adverse drug event	NKDA	no known drug allergies
A.M., a.m., AM, am	in the morning; before noon	NPO	nothing by mouth
amp	ampule	NS	normal saline
aq	water	oz	ounce
bid	twice a day	OTC	over the counter
BSA	body surface area	p̄	after
C	Celsius	pc	after meals
c̄	with	PCA	patient-controlled analgesia
cap or caps	capsule	per	through, by (route)
CD*	controlled dose	per	each (math term)
comp	compound	PO, po	by mouth
dil.	dilute	P.M., p.m., PM, pm	afternoon; evening
DS	double strength	prn	as needed; when necessary
elix	elixir	q	each, every
ext	external; extract	q2h, q4h, etc.	every 2 hours, every 4 hours, etc.
F	Fahrenheit	qs	as much as needed; quantity sufficient
fl. or fld	fluid	rep.	repeat
g	gram	Rx	give, treatment, prescription
gt, gtt	drop, drops	s̄	without
h, hr	hour	SL, subl	sublingual (under the tongue)
ID	intradermal(ly)	sol. or soln.	solution
IM	intramuscular(ly)	stat	immediately, at once
inj	injection	subcut	subcutaneous(ly)
IV	intravenous(ly)	supp	suppository
IVPB	intravenous piggyback	susp.	suspension
kg	kilogram	Syr	syrup
KVO	keep vein open	tab	tablet
L	liter	tbs., tbsp, or T	tablespoon
lb	pound	tid	three times a day
liq.	liquid	tinct	tincture
m	meter	TKO	to keep open
m²	square meter	tsp	teaspoon
mcg	microgram	ung	ointment
mEq	milliequivalent	vag	vaginal
mg	milligram		
Write out	milliunit		

⚠ CLINICAL ALERT!

*The manufacturer acronyms that follow medication names have caused confusion and errors. CD, CR, DR, E-R, LA, SA, SR, TR, XL, XR, XT all refer to various timed-release forms of the drug. They cannot be used interchangeably. Some need to be taken more than once a day; some tablets can be cut, others cannot. Double check the order and the acronym with a current drug reference and the patient medication history to protect the patient from a medication type or dose error.

Do NOT confuse DS—double strength—with other acronyms. DS pertains *only* to strength, not timing of release.

The Joint Commission's Official "Do Not Use" List

Official "Do Not Use" List[1]

Do Not Use	Potential Problem	Use Instead
U (unit)	Mistaken for "0" (zero), the number "4" (four) or "cc"	Write "unit"
IU (International Unit)	Mistaken for IV (intravenous) or the number 10 (ten)	Write "International Unit"
Q.D., QD, q.d., qd (daily)	Mistaken for each other	Write "daily"
Q.O.D., QOD, q.o.d, qod (every other day)	Period after the Q mistaken for "I" and the "O" mistaken for "I"	Write "every other day"
Trailing zero (X.0 mg)* Lack of leading zero (.X mg)	Decimal point is missed	Write X mg Write 0.X mg
MS	Can mean morphine sulfate or magnesium sulfate	Write "morphine sulfate" Write "magnesium sulfate"
MSO_4 and $MgSO_4$	Confused for one another	

[1] Applies to all orders and all medication-related documentation that is handwritten (including free-text computer entry) or on preprinted forms.

*Exception: A "trailing zero" may be used only where required to demonstrate the level of precision of the value being reported, such as for laboratory results, imaging studies that report size of lesions, or catheter/tube sizes. It may not be used in medication orders or other medication-related documentation.

Additional Abbreviations, Acronyms and Symbols
(For possible future inclusion in the Official "Do Not Use" List)

Do Not Use	Potential Problem	Use Instead
> (greater than) < (less than)	Misinterpreted as the number "7" (seven) or the letter "L" Confused for one another	Write "greater than" Write "less than"
Abbreviations for drug names	Misinterpreted due to similar abbreviations for multiple drugs	Write drug names in full
Apothecary units	Unfamiliar to many practitioners Confused with metric units	Use metric units
@	Mistaken for the number "2" (two)	Write "at"
cc	Mistaken for U (units) when poorly written	Write "mL" or "ml" or "milliliters" ("mL" is preferred)
µg	Mistaken for mg (milligrams) resulting in one thousand-fold overdose	Write "mcg" or "micrograms"

© The Joint Commission, 2010. Reprinted with permission.

Institute for Safe Medication Practices (ISMP) Dangerous Abbreviations and Notations

Abbreviation	Write	Abbreviation	Write
AD, AS, or AU	right ear, left ear, or both ears	X 3d	for 3 days
OD, OS, or OU	right eye, left eye, or both eyes	SC, SQ, or sub q	subcut or subcutaneous(ly)
BT	bedtime	ss	one half
cc	mL for milliliters	SSI	sliding scale (insulin)
HS	bedtime	µg	mcg
qhs	nightly	 >	less than greater than
qid	4 times a day	+	plus or and
qn	nightly	@	at

Please note: This is a partial list. For a more complete list, refer to www.ISMP.org.
© ISMP, 2013. Reprinted with permission.

TENTH EDITION

Drug Calculations

Ratio and Proportion Problems for Clinical Practice

META BROWN SELTZER, MEd, RN

RN, Mountainside Hospital
Glen Ridge, New Jersey;
BA, Nursing and Health Education
New Jersey City University
Jersey City, New Jersey;
MEd, Nursing Education
Arizona State University
Phoenix, Arizona;
Former Captain, USAF Reserve
41st Strategic Air Command
Luke AFB, Arizona;
Retired Colonel, US Army
Combat Hospital;
Former Director, Division of Nursing
Gateway Community College
Phoenix, Arizona

JOYCE M. MULHOLLAND, MS, RN, ANP, MA

Nursing Education Consultant
Tucson, Arizona;
MS, Nursing, California State University,
Long Beach, California;
MA, Education, Arizona State University,
Tempe, Arizona;
BS, Fairleigh Dickinson College,
Rutherford, New Jersey;
Former Captain, USAF Reserve,
41st Casualty Staging Unit
Luke AFB, Arizona

ELSEVIER

DRUG CALCULATIONS: RATIO AND PROPORTION
PROBLEMS FOR CLINICAL PRACTICE, Tenth Edition

ISBN: 978-0-323-31659-0

Copyright © 2016 by Elsevier Inc. All rights reserved.

No part of this publication may be reproduced or transmitted in any form or by any means, electronic or mechanical, including photocopying, recording, or any information storage and retrieval system, without permission in writing from the publisher. Details on how to seek permission, further information about the Publisher's permissions policies and our arrangements with organizations such as the Copyright Clearance Center and the Copyright Licensing Agency, can be found at our website: www.elsevier.com/permissions.

This book and the individual contributions contained in it are protected under copyright by the Publisher (other than as may be noted herein).

> **Notices**
>
> Knowledge and best practice in this field are constantly changing. As new research and experience broaden our understanding, changes in research methods, professional practices, or medical treatment may become necessary.
>
> Practitioners and researchers must always rely on their own experience and knowledge in evaluating and using any information, methods, compounds, or experiments described herein. In using such information or methods they should be mindful of their own safety and the safety of others, including parties for whom they have a professional responsibility.
>
> With respect to any drug or pharmaceutical products identified, readers are advised to check the most current information provided (i) on procedures featured or (ii) by the manufacturer of each product to be administered, to verify the recommended dose or formula, the method and duration of administration, and contraindications. It is the responsibility of practitioners, relying on their own experience and knowledge of their patients, to make diagnoses, to determine dosages and the best treatment for each individual patient, and to take all appropriate safety precautions.
>
> To the fullest extent of the law, neither the Publisher nor the authors, contributors, or editors, assume any liability for any injury and/or damage to persons or property as a matter of products liability, negligence or otherwise, or from any use or operation of any methods, products, instructions, or ideas contained in the material herein.

Previous editions copyrighted 2012, 2008, 2000, 1996, 1992, 1988, 1984, 1979

International Standard Book Number: 978-0-323-31659-0

Senior Content Strategist: Yvonne Alexopoulos
Content Development Manager: Jean Sims Fornango
Senior Content Development Specialist: Danielle M. Frazier
Publishing Services Manager: Julie Eddy
Senior Project Manager: Mary Stueck
Design Direction: Amy Buxton

Printed in Canada

Last digit is the print number: 9 8 7 6 5 4 3 2 1

Reviewers

Bret Alan Barker, MSN, RN, CCRN, PHN
    Nursing Instructor
    Allied Health Department
    Gavilan College
    Gilroy, California;
    ICU/CCU Staff Nurse
    Salinas Valley Memorial Hospital
    Salinas, California

Jessica Gonzales ARNP, MSN, RN
    Nursing Instructor
    Lake Washington Institute of Technology
    Redmond, Washington

Preface to Instructors

Drug Calculations was originally designed in the late 1970s as a basic practical resource for nursing students and faculty in classrooms and clinical areas. Additional content was added over the years to be current with the increased roles and responsibilities of the nurse and to be useful for refresher courses, nurses practicing in specialty areas, distance-learning nursing students, and nursing students who must master the material independently.

The current text has been updated to reflect feedback from reviewers, colleagues, and students, and student needs related to current trends in nursing education and practice.

Continuing in This Edition

Ratio and proportion calculations are presented in the second chapter following a math review so that the student has the method reinforced throughout the rest of the text for maximum competence. *As with earlier editions, the text presents one calculation method—ratio and proportion—to maximize the teaching and learning time for reinforcement, practice, and mastery within the brief time the student has to devote to this critical subject.*

The material is sequential with logical steps and ample practice problems to facilitate mastery of the concepts.

The quizzes and tests are brief and can be completed in one sitting. Answers are worked out.

Each medication problem has a frequently encountered diagnosis attached to make the problem more realistic and help the student assimilate clinical relevance.

A high-alert red flag is attached to the Institute for Safe Medication Practices (ISMP)–identified medication labels to call attention to these medications.

The sample hand-off communication report in Appendix D has highlighted medication-related inclusions.

The Joint Commission (TJC) and ISMP abbreviations and QSEN patient safety recommendations are emphasized.

Clinical relevance and patient safety measures are included for the benefit of students who are studying independently as well as those in the classroom.

New to This Edition

- The fraction cross product multiplication setup of ratio and proportion calculations is presented as an optional alternative to the colon setup because it is a familiar method taught in most elementary schools and high schools.
- Emphasis on *ISMP latest safety recommendations, QSEN patient safety goals,* and several additional clinically relevant concepts tie the math to the clinical setting and patient safety related to preparation and administration of medications.
- Content has been arranged for improved sequencing.
- Many updated labels, photographs, and illustrations have been provided to help visualize the application of the math.
- Additional clinically relevant anecdotes are included to increase the understanding of application and safety measures related to the nurse's role.
- A new appendix, "Sample Medication Errors and Potential Clinical Implications," emphasizes the need to reduce medication errors.
- The answer keys are conveniently placed at the end of each chapter.
- Vocabulary at the beginning of each chapter is a useful reference as students proceed through each chapter.

Acknowledgments

We extend our thanks to all the reviewers, editors, production, and marketing teams who contributed to this edition. We included as many of their recommendations as permitted by space, content, and text design.

Meta Seltzer wishes to thank Sarah Severs for her contribution to the chapter on diabetes management.

Joyce Mulholland is very appreciative of the assistance of Marty Mulholland, who kept her computer functioning; Susan Mulholland, NCIDQ; Shari Robinson, MSN, RN; April Perkins, FNP, RN; and the clinical pharmacy professionals who provided information for this edition.

Meta Brown Seltzer
Joyce M. Mulholland

Preface to Students

Drug Calculations: Ratio and Proportion for Clinical Practice provides all the information, explanation and practice you need to competently and confidently calculate drug dosages.

A General Mathematics Self-Assessment is provided as a refresher to identify areas needed for further study. Chapter 1 provides a basic review of all the arithmetic needed to calculate medication dosages. The Ratio and Proportion method of calculating dosages is used throughout the text. Chapter 2 introduces two Ratio and Proportion setups: Using colons and the Fraction Cross-Product (Multiplication). You may use whichever R and P method you prefer. Be sure that you have complete mastery of Chapter 1 and 2 before proceeding with the rest of the text.

Each chapter has a series of quizzes with a Multiple-Choice and Final test at the end of each chapter. Each of the quizzes and tests can be completed in one sitting. Answers with proofs are worked out in the Answer Key at the end of each chapter.

- Clinical Alerts in red will point out potential errors that can occur in the clinical setting.
- Clinical Relevance information is provided to help you connect math to the safe application in the clinical setting.
- A high-alert medication icon flag is a visual reminder of high-risk drugs identified by the Institute for Safe Medication Practices (ISMP).

Samples of look-alike medications (ISMP) that have caused medication errors are included. Pay close attention to all of the icons and textbox notes. They relate to actual safe and unsafe practice. Tall Man letters distinguish differences between similar names.

Critical Thinking Exercises at the end of each chapter help you understand how medication errors occur and how they might have been prevented. Discuss the exercises with other nursing students to elicit various ways to avoid medication errors.

Multiple-Choice and Comprehensive Finals test your knowledge on all of the chapters studied. Spend extra review time in the text on any questions that you cannot answer correctly.

NEW VERSION! ***Drug Calculations Companion, version 5.*** This is a completely updated, interactive student tutorial that includes an extensive menu of various topic areas within drug calculations, such as oral, parenteral, pediatric, and intravenous calculations. It contains over 600 practice problems covering ratio and proportion, formula, and dimensional analysis methods.

evolve Look for this icon at the end of the chapters. It will refer you to ***Drug Calculations Companion, version 5*** for additional practice problems and content information.

Contents

General Mathematics Self-Assessment, 1

1. General Mathematics, 5
2. Ratio and Proportion, 41
3. Safe Medication Administration, 57
4. Medication Measurements and Oral Dose Calculations, 99
5. Injectable Medication Calculations, 145
6. Reconstitution of Medications From Powders and Crystals: Oral and Intramuscular, 179
7. Basic Intravenous Therapy Calculations, 229
8. Advanced Intravenous Calculations, 273
9. Insulin Administration and Type 2 Diabetes Medications, 305
10. Parenteral Nutrition, 353
11. Anticoagulants, 379
12. Children's Dosages, 415

Multiple-Choice Final, 449

Comprehensive Final, 459

Appendixes

A. ISMP List of High-Alert Medications in Acute Care Settings, 477
B. ISMP's List of Error-Prone Abbreviations, Symbols, and Dose Designations, 479
C. Sample Medication Administration Errors With Potential Clinical Outcomes, 481
D. 5-Minute Sample Verbal Communication From Nurses to Subsequent Caregivers, 483

Index, 485

General Mathematics Self-Assessment

The accurate calculation of medication dosages, a skill that is central to patient safety, builds on a knowledge of fundamental mathematics. Competency and skill in using the basic principles of arithmetic are essential for safe medication administration. To progress in the *Drug Calculations* text, students must know how to solve problems using addition, subtraction, multiplication, division, fractions, decimals, and percentages. Use the problems provided in the following self-assessment to gauge current knowledge. Answers are on page 4. Chapter 1, General Mathematics, provides a refresher for each type of problem in the self-assessment. Consult a text for general mathematics as needed.

Fractions

Change to whole or mixed numbers.

1. $\dfrac{9}{2}$
2. $\dfrac{26}{5}$

Change to improper fractions.

3. $8\dfrac{1}{3}$
4. $5\dfrac{2}{5}$

Find the lowest common denominator.

5. $\dfrac{4}{11}$ and $\dfrac{1}{8}$
6. $\dfrac{2}{5}$ and $\dfrac{5}{9}$

Add.

7. $\dfrac{1}{5}$, $\dfrac{1}{6}$, and $\dfrac{2}{3}$
8. $1\dfrac{1}{2} + 3\dfrac{1}{8} + 2\dfrac{1}{6}$

Subtract.

9. $\dfrac{5}{7} - \dfrac{1}{3}$
10. $8\dfrac{1}{4} - 3\dfrac{3}{8}$

Multiply and reduce to lowest terms.

11. $\dfrac{1}{6} \times \dfrac{1}{3}$
12. $\dfrac{2}{8} \times 1\dfrac{1}{3}$

Divide and reduce to lowest terms.

13. $\dfrac{1}{3} \div \dfrac{2}{5}$
14. $1\dfrac{1}{8} \div 2\dfrac{1}{2}$

Reduce to lowest terms (numbers).

15. $\dfrac{4}{120}$ **16.** $\dfrac{3}{7}$

Decimals

Write as decimals.

17. Twelve hundredths   **18.** Three and sixteen thousandths

Add.

19. 3.04 + 1.864   **20.** 25.7 + 3.008

Subtract.

21. 3 − 0.04   **22.** 0.96 − 0.1359

Multiply.

23. 0.05 × 2   **24.** 3 × 0.4

Divide and carry to the third decimal place.

25. 500 ÷ 15   **26.** 20.6 ÷ 0.21

Change to decimals and carry to the third decimal place.

27. $\dfrac{24}{44}$ **28.** $9\dfrac{1}{8}$

Percentages

Find the percentages.

29. 25% of 300   **30.** 1% of 50

Change the decimals to fractions and reduce to lowest terms.

31. 0.005   **32.** 0.05

Change the fractions to a decimal and a percentage.

33. $\dfrac{3}{4}$ **34.** $\dfrac{1}{8}$

Rounding

Round the decimals (35–39) in the chart below.

	Decimal	Nearest Whole Number	Nearest Hundredth	Nearest Tenth
35.	0.8734			0.9
36.	0.842			0.8
37.	0.553			
38.	0.689			
39.	2.75			

Answer the questions.

40. What is 25% of 2?   Ans: fraction _____   Ans: decimal _____

41. What is $\frac{1}{4}$ of 2?   Ans: fraction _____   Ans: decimal _____

42. What is 75% of 2?   Ans: fraction _____   Ans: decimal _____

43. Divide 0.5 by 0.25:

44. Divide 0.2 by 0.1:

45. Divide $\frac{1}{100}$ by $\frac{1}{200}$:

Answer Key

General Mathematics Self-Assessment (page 1)

1. $4\frac{1}{2}$
2. $5\frac{1}{5}$
3. $\frac{25}{3}$
4. $\frac{27}{5}$
5. 88
6. 45
7. $1\frac{1}{30}$
8. $6\frac{19}{24}$
9. $\frac{8}{21}$
10. $4\frac{7}{8}$
11. $\frac{1}{18}$
12. $\frac{1}{3}$
13. $\frac{5}{6}$
14. $\frac{9}{20}$
15. $\frac{1}{30}$
16. $\frac{3}{7}$
17. 0.12
18. 3.016
19. 4.904
20. 28.708
21. 2.96
22. 0.8241
23. 0.1
24. 1.2
25. 33.333
26. 98.095
27. 0.545
28. 9.125
29. 75
30. 0.5
31. $\frac{5}{1000} = \frac{1}{200}$
32. $\frac{5}{100} = \frac{1}{20}$
33. 0.75   75%
34. 0.125 $12\frac{1}{2}$%

	Decimal	Nearest Whole Number	Nearest Hundredth	Nearest Tenth
35.	0.8734	1	0.87	0.9
36.	0.842	1	0.84	0.8
37.	0.553	1	0.55	0.6
38.	0.689	1	0.69	0.7
39.	2.75	3	2.75	2.8

40. $\frac{1}{2}$ (0.5)
41. $\frac{1}{2}$ (0.5)
42. $1\frac{1}{2}$ (1.5)
43. 2
44. 2
45. 2

General Mathematics

Objectives
- Add, subtract, multiply, and divide fractions and mixed numbers.
- Convert improper fractions and mixed numbers.
- Reduce fractions to lowest terms.
- Create equivalent fractions and compare values.
- Add, subtract, multiply, and divide decimals.
- Compare decimal values.
- Round decimals.
- Convert decimals, fractions, and percentages.

Introduction This chapter provides a thorough and easy-to-follow review of the arithmetic needed for accurate medication dose calculations. Many examples, practice problems, and answers related to fractions, decimals, rounding, and percentages are offered. Your ability to avoid medication errors and solve medication dose-related problems starts with competence in basic arithmetic. If you need further review, refer to a basic mathematics text. Mastery of these concepts is essential before you proceed to the following chapters and medication-related calculations.

Fractions

A fraction is part of a whole number. The fraction $\frac{6}{8}$ means that there are 8 parts to the whole number (bottom number, or denominator), but you want to measure only 6 of those parts (top number, or numerator).

The fraction $\frac{6}{8}$ can be reduced by dividing both the numbers by 2.

$$\frac{6 \div 2}{8 \div 2} = \frac{3}{4} \quad \begin{array}{l}\text{numerator}\\ \text{denominator}\end{array}$$

The fraction $\frac{3}{9}$ means that there are 9 parts to the whole number.

Example The fraction $\frac{3}{9}$ can be reduced by dividing both numbers by the same number.

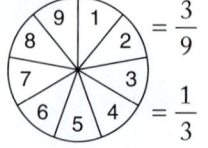

$\begin{array}{l}3 \div 3 = 1 \\ 9 \div 3 = 3\end{array}$ numerator
denominator

remember The whole number of the fraction is always the denominator.

Value of Fractions

RULE The denominator determines the number of parts into which the whole number is divided. The smaller the denominator of a fraction, the greater the fraction's value if the numerators are the same.

Example Which would you rather have, $\frac{1}{6}$ or $\frac{1}{9}$ of your favorite candy bar? $\frac{1}{6}$ is greater than $\frac{1}{9}$. It represents a larger part of the whole unit.

$\frac{1}{6}$	$\frac{1}{6}$	$\frac{1}{6}$	$\frac{1}{6}$	$\frac{1}{6}$	$\frac{1}{6}$

= 6 parts   Each $\frac{1}{6}$ part is **larger** than the $\frac{1}{9}$ part.

$\frac{1}{9}$	$\frac{1}{9}$	$\frac{1}{9}$	$\frac{1}{9}$	$\frac{1}{9}$	$\frac{1}{9}$	$\frac{1}{9}$	$\frac{1}{9}$	$\frac{1}{9}$

= 9 parts   Each $\frac{1}{9}$ part is **smaller** than the $\frac{1}{6}$ part.

Answers on page 32

WORKSHEET 1A | Value of Fractions

Answer the following questions by circling the correct answer.

1. Would you rather own $\frac{1}{10}$ or $\frac{1}{20}$ of a lottery ticket?

2. Would you rather have 2 out of 7 or 2 out of 14 days off?

3. If you had a choice of a bonus of $\frac{1}{20}$ or $\frac{1}{30}$ of your annual salary, which would you prefer?

4. Which would be the *greater* incidence of a disease, 1 out of approximately every 100,000 people $\left(\frac{1}{100,000}\right)$ or 1 out of approximately 250,000 people $\left(\frac{1}{250,000}\right)$?

5. If a tablet was ordered for a patient at grain $\frac{1}{4}$ and you had tablets labeled grain $\frac{1}{8}$, would you need to give *more* or *less* than what is on hand?

6. Which is **greater**? $\frac{1}{5}$ or $\frac{1}{8}$

7. Which is **smaller**? $\frac{1}{100}$ or $\frac{1}{150}$

8. Which is **greater**? $\frac{1}{250}$ or $\frac{1}{300}$

9. Which is **smaller**? $\frac{1}{7}$ or $\frac{1}{9}$

10. Which is **smaller**? $\frac{1}{50}$ or $\frac{1}{200}$

Changing Improper Fractions to Whole or Mixed Numbers

An improper fraction has a numerator that is larger than the denominator, as in $\frac{8}{4}$.

> ### Steps for Changing Improper Fractions to Whole or Mixed Numbers
> 1. When the top number (numerator) is larger than the bottom number (denominator), divide the bottom number (denominator) into the top number (numerator).
> 2. Write the remainder as a fraction and reduce to lowest terms.

Examples

$\frac{8}{4} = 8 \div 4 = 2$ *This is a whole number.*

$\frac{16}{6} = 16 \div 6 = 2\frac{4}{6} = 2\frac{2}{3}$ *This is a mixed number because it has a whole number plus a fraction.*

Answers on page 32

WORKSHEET 1B | Changing Improper Fractions to Whole or Mixed Numbers

Change the following to whole numbers or mixed fractions and reduce to lowest terms.

1. $\frac{6}{6} =$
2. $\frac{10}{2} =$
3. $\frac{13}{4} =$

4. $\frac{14}{9} =$
5. $\frac{34}{6} =$
6. $\frac{100}{20} =$

7. $\frac{9}{4} =$
8. $\frac{120}{64} =$
9. $\frac{18}{3} =$

10. $\frac{41}{6} =$

Changing Mixed Numbers to Improper Fractions

> ### Steps for Changing Mixed Numbers to Improper Fractions
> 1. Multiply the whole number by the denominator of the fraction.
> 2. Add this to the numerator of the fraction.
> 3. Write the sum as the numerator of the fraction; the denominator of the fraction remains the same.

Examples

$2\frac{3}{8} = \frac{8 \times 2 + 3}{8} = \frac{19}{8}$ Numerator / Denominator

$4\frac{2}{5} = \frac{5 \times 4 + 2}{5} = \frac{22}{5}$ Numerator / Denominator

CHAPTER 1 General Mathematics

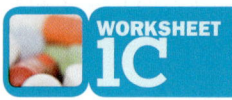

Answers on page 32

WORKSHEET 1C | Changing Mixed Numbers to Improper Fractions

Change the following to improper fractions.

1. $3\dfrac{1}{2} =$ 　　　　2. $1\dfrac{1}{6} =$ 　　　　3. $4\dfrac{1}{8} =$

4. $3\dfrac{7}{12} =$ 　　　5. $13\dfrac{3}{5} =$ 　　　6. $16\dfrac{1}{3} =$

7. $3\dfrac{5}{6} =$ 　　　　8. $2\dfrac{5}{8} =$ 　　　　9. $10\dfrac{3}{6} =$

10. $125\dfrac{2}{3} =$

Finding a Common Denominator for Two or More Fractions

To add and subtract fractions, the denominators must be the *same*.

Example Fractions with same denominators

$$\dfrac{5}{16} - \dfrac{2}{16} \quad \text{or} \quad \dfrac{3}{8} + \dfrac{1}{8} \quad \text{or} \quad \dfrac{3}{4} + \dfrac{1}{4}$$

These fractions can be added and subtracted. Each set's value is also easier to compare because of the common denominators.

Example Different denominators in fractions with the same value as the fractions in example A:

$$\dfrac{5}{16} - \dfrac{1}{8} \quad \text{or} \quad \dfrac{3}{8} + \dfrac{2}{16} \quad \text{or} \quad \dfrac{3}{4} + \dfrac{2}{8}$$

These fractions cannot be added or subtracted until they are converted to *equivalent* fractions with a *common* denominator. The relative value of each set is harder to compare until they are converted to equivalent fractions. A *common* denominator is a number that can be divided evenly by *all* the denominators in the problem. It is easier to add or subtract fractions if the lowest common denominator is used.

> ### Steps for Finding a Common Denominator for Two or More Fractions
>
> 1. Examine the largest denominator in the group to determine whether the other denominators will divide *evenly* into it.
> 2. If any of the denominators will not divide evenly into the largest denominator, begin multiplying the largest denominator by 2. If the other denominators cannot be divided by 2 evenly, then proceed to multiply the denominator by 3, 4, 5, 6, and so on until all denominators can be divided into the number equally. This becomes the common denominator.

Example $\dfrac{5}{16}$ and $\dfrac{1}{8}$: the largest denominator, 16, can be divided by 8 without a remainder. Therefore 16 is the common denominator.

8　Drug Calculations: *Ratio and Proportion Problems for Clinical Practice*

Example $\frac{2}{8}$ and $\frac{3}{4}$ and $\frac{1}{2}$: the largest denominator, 8, can be divided by 4 and by 2 without a remainder. Therefore 8 is the common denominator.

Example $\frac{1}{7}, \frac{1}{6},$ and $\frac{1}{3}$
3 and 6 will *not* divide evenly into 7.

Multiples of 7: 14, 21, 28, 35, and 42.
42 is the lowest number that can be divided evenly by 6 and 3. Therefore **42** is a common denominator, the lowest common denominator.

Changing Fractions to Equivalent Fractions

RULE To maintain equivalence, the numerator and the denominator must be divided (or multiplied) by the *same* number.

Whatever you do to the denominator (multiply or divide by a number), you must do the *same* to the numerator so that the value does not change.

> **Steps for Changing Fractions to Equivalent Fractions**
> 1. Find the common denominator—in this case 24.
> 2. Multiply each *numerator* by the *same* number used to obtain the common denominator for that fraction.

Example $\frac{3}{8}$ and $\frac{2}{3}$ and $\frac{1}{4}$: 3 will *not* divide evenly into 8.

The largest denominator in the group is **8**.
$8 \times 2 = 16$ 3 will *not* divide evenly into 16.
$8 \times 3 = 24$ Both 3 and 4 will divide evenly into **24**.
$8 \times 4 = 32$ 3 will *not* divide evenly into 32.
$8 \times 5 = 40$ 3 will *not* divide evenly into 40.
$8 \times 6 = 48$ Both 3 and 4 will divide evenly into **48**.

Therefore 24 and 48 are common denominators for $\frac{3}{8}$ and $\frac{2}{3}$ and $\frac{1}{4}$, but 24 is the *lowest* common denominator for the three numbers.

Examples

Proving Fractions Are Equivalent by Using the Cross Fraction Product Method

$\frac{3}{8}_{(\times 3)} = \frac{?}{24}$ $3 \times 3 = 9$ Therefore $\frac{3}{8} \times \frac{9}{24} = $ $3 \times 24 = 72$
$9 \times 8 = 72$

$\frac{2}{3}_{(\times 8)} = \frac{?}{24}$ $2 \times 8 = 16$ Therefore $\frac{2}{3} \times \frac{16}{24} = $ $2 \times 24 = 48$
$3 \times 16 = 48$

$\frac{1}{4}_{(\times 6)} = \frac{?}{24}$ $1 \times 6 = 6$ Therefore $\frac{1}{4} \times \frac{6}{24} = $ $1 \times 24 = 24$
$4 \times 6 = 24$

Reducing Fractions to Lowest Terms

A fraction is in lowest terms when the numerator and denominator cannot be divided by any other number except one.

RULE To reduce a fraction to *lowest* terms, *divide* the numerator and denominator by the *largest* same whole number that will divide evenly into both. When there are no whole numbers that can be used except one, the fraction is in lowest terms.

The fraction $\frac{6}{8}$ is not in lowest terms because it can be reduced by dividing both the numerator and the denominator by 2, a common denominator. $\frac{3}{4}$ is expressed in lowest terms.

Example $\frac{6 \div 2 = 3}{8 \div 2 = 4}$ Note that both 6 and 8 are divided by 2.

Example $\frac{10 \div 5 = 2}{15 \div 5 = 3}$ Note that both 10 and 15 are divided by 5.

Example $\frac{4 \div 4 = 1}{24 \div 4 = 6}$ Note that both 4 and 24 are divided by 4.

$\frac{3}{4}$ and $\frac{2}{3}$ and $\frac{1}{6}$ cannot be further reduced. No other number than one will divide evenly into both the numerator and denominator. They are now in their simplest or *lowest* terms.

Changing to Equivalent Fractions Using Higher Terms

RULE To change a fraction to *higher* terms and maintain equivalence, *multiply* both the numerator and the denominator by the *same* number.

Example $\frac{6 \times 2 = 12}{8 \times 2 = 16}$ $\frac{6}{8} = \frac{12}{16}$

The value has not changed because the multiplier 2 is used for both the numerator and the denominator, and $\frac{2}{2} = 1$.

Multiplying or dividing numbers by one does *not* change the value. Equivalence is maintained.

Addition of Fractions and Mixed Numbers

RULE If fractions have the same denominator, add the numerators, and place the result over the denominator and reduce.

Example

$$\frac{1}{5} + \frac{2}{5} = \frac{3}{5}$$

$$\frac{2}{6} + \frac{1}{6} = \frac{3}{6} = \frac{1}{2}$$

RULE If fractions have different denominators, convert each fraction to an equivalent fraction using the lowest common denominator and then add the numerators.

Example

$$\frac{3}{5} = \frac{9}{15}$$
$$+\frac{2}{3} = +\frac{10}{15}$$
$$\frac{19}{15} = 19 \div 15 = 1\frac{4}{15}$$

$$\frac{3(\times 3)}{5(\times 3)} = \frac{9}{15}$$
$$\frac{2(\times 5)}{3(\times 5)} = \frac{10}{15}$$

RULE To add mixed numbers, first add the fractions by converting to a common denominator and then add this to the sum of the whole numbers.

Example

$$9\frac{5}{8} = 9\frac{15}{24}$$
$$+6\frac{1}{6} = +6\frac{4}{24}$$
$$15\frac{19}{24}$$

$$\frac{5(\times 3)}{8(\times 3)} = \frac{15}{24}$$
$$\frac{1(\times 4)}{6(\times 4)} = \frac{4}{24}$$

Answers on page 32

WORKSHEET 1D | Addition of Fractions and Mixed Numbers

Add the following fractions and mixed numbers, using the common denominator, and reduce to lowest terms.

1. $\frac{2}{5}$
   $+\frac{2}{5}$

2. $\frac{4}{5}$
   $+\frac{2}{3}$

3. $6\frac{1}{6}$
   $+9\frac{5}{8}$

4. $2\frac{1}{4}$
   $+3\frac{1}{8}$

5. $1\frac{3}{4}$
   $+9\frac{9}{10}$

6. $\frac{1}{8}$
   $\frac{1}{4}$
   $+\frac{3}{9}$

7. $\frac{7}{9}$
   $\frac{4}{5}$
   $+\frac{9}{10}$

8. $3\frac{1}{4}$
   $+9\frac{3}{4}$

9. $8\frac{2}{5}$
   $14\frac{7}{10}$
   $+9\frac{9}{10}$

10. $2\frac{1}{3}$
    $+4\frac{1}{6}$

CHAPTER 1 General Mathematics   11

Subtraction of Fractions and Mixed Numbers

RULE If fractions have the same denominator, find the difference between the numerators and write it over the common denominator. Reduce the fraction if necessary.

Example
$$\frac{27}{32} - \frac{18}{32} = \frac{9}{32}$$

The difference between the numerators (27 minus 18) equals 9. The denominator is 32.

RULE If fractions have different denominators, find the lowest common denominator and proceed as above.

Example
$$\frac{7}{8} = \frac{21}{24}$$
$$-\frac{2}{3} = \frac{16}{24}$$
$$\frac{5}{24}$$

The difference between the numerators (21 minus 16) equals 5. The lowest common denominator is 24.

RULE To subtract mixed numbers, first subtract the fractions and then find the difference in the whole numbers. If the lower fraction is larger than the upper fraction, you cannot subtract it. *You must borrow from the whole number before subtracting the fraction.*

Example
$$21\frac{7}{16}$$
$$-7\frac{12}{16}$$

You cannot subtract 12 from 7 because 12 is larger than 7. Therefore you must borrow a whole number (1) from the 21, make a fraction out of $1\left(\frac{16}{16}\right)$, and add the 7.

$$\frac{16}{16} + \frac{7}{16} = \frac{23}{16}$$

Because you added a whole number to the fraction, you must take a whole number away from 21 and make it 20. The problem is now set up as follows:

$$21\frac{7}{16} = 20\frac{16}{16} + \frac{7}{16} = 20\frac{23}{16}$$
$$-7\frac{12}{16}$$
$$13\frac{11}{16}$$

RULE Reduce your answer to lowest terms.

Answers on page 33

WORKSHEET 1E | Subtraction of Fractions and Mixed Numbers

Subtract fractions and mixed numbers, and reduce the answers to lowest terms.

1. $\dfrac{2}{3} - \dfrac{1}{2}$

2. $\dfrac{27}{32} - \dfrac{18}{32}$

3. $10\dfrac{2}{5} - 6\dfrac{1}{4}$

4. $7\dfrac{16}{24} - 3\dfrac{1}{8}$

5. $6\dfrac{3}{10} - 2\dfrac{1}{5}$

6. $\dfrac{7}{8} - \dfrac{1}{3}$

7. $3\dfrac{5}{8} - 1\dfrac{3}{8}$

8. $5\dfrac{3}{7} - 1\dfrac{6}{7}$

9. $7 - 1\dfrac{3}{4}$

10. $2\dfrac{7}{8} - \dfrac{3}{4}$

Multiplication of Fractions and Mixed Numbers

Steps for Multiplication of Fractions and Mixed Numbers

1. Change the mixed number to an improper fraction if necessary.
2. Cancel, if possible, by dividing the numerators and denominators by the largest common divisor contained in each.
3. Multiply the remaining numerators to find a result, or product.
4. Multiply the denominators to find a result, or product.
5. Reduce the answer to lowest terms.

Example

$\dfrac{4}{5} \times \dfrac{15}{16} = \dfrac{\cancel{4}^{1}}{\cancel{5}_{1}} \times \dfrac{\cancel{15}^{3}}{\cancel{16}_{4}} = \dfrac{3}{4}$

$4\dfrac{1}{2} \times 2\dfrac{1}{4} = \dfrac{9}{2} \times \dfrac{9}{4} = \dfrac{81}{8} = 10\dfrac{1}{8}$

$6 \times \dfrac{3}{8} = \dfrac{6}{1} \times \dfrac{3}{8} = \dfrac{\cancel{6}^{3}}{1} \times \dfrac{3}{\cancel{8}_{4}} = \dfrac{9}{4} = 2\dfrac{1}{4}$

CHAPTER 1 General Mathematics 13

Answers on page 33

WORKSHEET 1F | Multiplication of Fractions and Mixed Numbers

Multiply the following fractions and mixed numbers, and reduce the answers to lowest terms.

1. $\dfrac{1}{5} \times \dfrac{2}{4} =$

2. $\dfrac{1}{5} \times \dfrac{1}{6} =$

3. $\dfrac{3}{5} \times \dfrac{5}{8} =$

4. $4 \times 3\dfrac{1}{3} =$

5. $\dfrac{2}{4} \times 2\dfrac{1}{6} =$

6. $5\dfrac{1}{2} \times 3\dfrac{1}{8} =$

7. $1\dfrac{3}{4} \times 3\dfrac{1}{7} =$

8. $\dfrac{5}{6} \times 1\dfrac{9}{16} =$

9. $\dfrac{5}{100} \times 900 =$

10. $2\dfrac{1}{10} \times 4\dfrac{1}{3} =$

Division of Fractions and Mixed Numbers

Steps for Division of Fractions and Mixed Numbers

1. Change mixed numbers to improper fractions if necessary.
2. Invert the number after the ÷ (division) sign.
3. Follow the steps for multiplication, and reduce any fractions.

Examples

$$\dfrac{1}{2} \div \dfrac{1}{3} = \dfrac{1}{2} \times \dfrac{3}{1} = \dfrac{3}{2} = 1\dfrac{1}{2}$$

$$8\dfrac{3}{4} \div 15 = \dfrac{\cancel{35}^{7}}{4} \times \dfrac{1}{\cancel{15}_{3}} = \dfrac{7}{12} \text{ *}$$

Answers on page 34

WORKSHEET 1G | Division of Fractions and Mixed Numbers

Divide the following fractions and mixed numbers, and reduce the answers to lowest terms.

1. $\dfrac{1}{5} \div \dfrac{1}{8} =$

2. $\dfrac{1}{3} \div \dfrac{1}{2} =$

3. $\dfrac{3}{4} \div \dfrac{1}{8} =$

4. $\dfrac{1}{16} \div \dfrac{1}{4} =$

5. $8\dfrac{3}{4} \div 15 =$

6. $\dfrac{3}{4} \div 6 =$

7. $2 \div \dfrac{1}{5} =$

8. $3\dfrac{3}{8} \div 4\dfrac{1}{2} =$

9. $\dfrac{3}{5} \div \dfrac{3}{8} =$

10. $4 \div 2\dfrac{1}{8} =$

---

*Reducing fractions to $\left(\dfrac{7}{4} \times \dfrac{1}{3}\right)$ makes the math easier and reduces errors.

14   Drug Calculations: *Ratio and Proportion Problems for Clinical Practice*

Value of Decimals

A decimal fraction is a fraction whose denominator (bottom number) is 10, 100, 1000, 10,000, and so on. It differs from a common fraction in that the denominator is *not* written but is expressed by the proper placement of the decimal point.

Observe the scale below. All whole numbers are to the left of the decimal point; all decimal fractions are to the right.

RULE All whole numbers are to the left of the decimal; all decimal fractions are to the right of the decimal point.

To read a decimal fraction, read the number to the right of the decimal and use the name that applies to "place value" of the *last* figure other than zero. Decimal fractions read with a *ths* on the end.

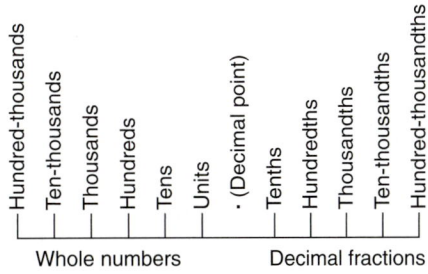

Examples
- 0.2 = Two Ten*ths*
- 0.25 = Twenty-five hundred*ths*
- 0.257 = Two hundred fifty-seven thousand*ths*
- 0.2057 = Two thousand fifty-seven ten-thousand*ths*
- 0.20057 = Twenty thousand fifty-seven hundred-thousand*ths*

RULE For a whole number and a fraction, read the decimal point as an **and**.

Example 327.006 = Three hundred twenty-seven *and* six thousand*ths*

Comparison of Decimals

To determine which decimal is larger or smaller, compare the decimals from left to right, starting with the tenths place value, then the hundredths if needed, and so on.

Examples

0.4 and 0.5	5 is greater than 4, and 0.5 is greater than 0.4.
0.123 and 0.234	2 is greater than 1 in the tenths place, so 0.234 is greater than 0.123.
0.189 and 0.194	Both have 1 in the tenths column, but comparing the hundredths column reveals that the 9 is greater than 8. Therefore 0.194 is greater than 0.189.
0.34 and 0.269	Avoid distraction because of the length of the numbers. Compare the tenths place value first: 3 is greater than 2. Therefore 0.34 is greater than 0.269.

CHAPTER 1 General Mathematics

Rounding Decimals

> **Steps for Rounding Decimals**
> 1. Calculate *one* decimal place beyond the desired place.
> 2. If the final digit is **4** or less, make no adjustment. If the final digit is **5** or more, *increase* the prior digit by one number.
> 3. Drop the final digit.

Examples
- Round 2.7 to the nearest whole number. Examine the tenths column.
- Because 7 is greater than 5, the answer is 3 and 0.7 is dropped.

- Round 2.55 to the nearest tenth.
  Examine the second decimal place (hundredths column).
  Because the hundredths column is 5, the 2.5 is rounded up to 2.6 and the final 0.05 (hundredths) is dropped.
- Round 3.762 to the nearest hundredth.
  Examine the third decimal place (thousandths column).
  Because 2 is less than 5, no adjustment will be made in the hundredths column and the 2 is dropped. 3.76 is the answer.

	Nearest Whole Number	Nearest Tenth	Nearest Hundredth
3.689	4	3.7	3.69
204.534	205	204.5	204.53
7.87	8	7.9	7.87
3.366	3	3.4	3.37
0.845*	1	0.8	0.85

*To reduce reading errors, develop the habit of placing a zero (0) in front of the decimal when a whole number is absent.

⊖ CLINICAL ALERT!

Do **not** round dosages of oral medication or injections to the nearest whole number because this could result in an overdose. Syringes are calibrated in tenths and hundredths of a milliliter; therefore rounding to a whole number could result in an overdose. For instructions on how to round medication doses, refer to Chapter 4.

Answers on page 34

WORKSHEET 1HA | Rounding Decimals

Round the decimal to the nearest whole number, the nearest tenth, and the nearest hundredth.

	Nearest Whole Number	Nearest Tenth	Nearest Hundredth
1. 93.489	_____	_____	_____
2. 25.43	_____	_____	_____

16 Drug Calculations: *Ratio and Proportion Problems for Clinical Practice*

	Nearest Whole Number	Nearest Tenth	Nearest Hundredth
3. 38.2	_____	_____	_____
4. 57.8888	_____	_____	_____
5. 0.0092	_____	_____	_____
6. 3.144	_____	_____	_____
7. 8.999	_____	_____	_____
8. 77.788	_____	_____	_____
9. 12.959	_____	_____	_____
10. 5.7703	_____	_____	_____

Answers on page 34

WORKSHEET 1HB | Value of Decimals

Read the following decimals and write them out in words.

1. 0.06 _____

2. 0.096 _____

3. 0.005 _____

4. 100.01 _____

5. 0.9 _____

Write the following as decimals.

6. Thirty-four hundredths   _____

7. Four thousandths   _____

8. Two and seventeen thousandths   _____

9. Nine and two ten-thousandths   _____

10. Thirty-four and one tenth   _____

⊖ CLINICAL ALERT!

Make it your habit to always insert a zero (0) in front of a decimal fraction when a whole number is absent. This draws attention to the decimal and avoids two potentially critical errors: missing the decimal or mistaking it for a number "1."

CHAPTER 1   General Mathematics   17

Answers on page 34

WORKSHEET 1IA | Rounding Decimals

Round to tenths 0.0

1. 0.297 _____
2. 4.435 _____
3. 2.754 _____
4. 0.845 _____
5. 6.766 _____

Round to hundredths 0.00

6. 0.297 _____
7. 4.435 _____
8. 2.754 _____
9. 0.845 _____
10. 6.766 _____

Round to thousandths 0.000

11. 8.9374 _____
12. 5.6256 _____
13. 10.8976 _____
14. 4.6255 _____
15. 3.7386 _____

Round to ten-thousandths 0.0000

16. 8.93749 _____
17. 5.62568 _____
18. 10.89763 _____
19. 4.62557 _____
20. 3.73869 _____

Answers on page 35

WORKSHEET 1IB | Rounding Decimals

One of the keys to avoiding decimal errors when calculating medication doses is to know at a glance whether the amount you will give is *more* or *less* than the amount provided. Refer to page 16 for a review.

Which is *smaller*? Circle the correct answer.

1. 0.2 or 0.3
2. 0.5 or 0.25
3. 0.125 or 0.25
4. 2.309 or 2.07
5. 1.465 or 1.29

Which is *larger*? Circle the correct answer.

6. 0.9 or 0.1
7. 0.07 or 0.7
8. 0.58 or 0.09
9. 0.25 or 0.05
10. 0.001 or 0.1

18   Drug Calculations: *Ratio and Proportion Problems for Clinical Practice*

Addition of Decimals

Steps for Adding Decimals

1. Write decimals in a column, keeping the decimal points under each other (A).
2. Add as in whole numbers, from right to left.
3. Place the decimal point in the answer directly under the decimal points in the numbers to be added.
4. Insert zeros as placeholders if desired within the problem after the last number (B).

Examples

A	B	C
0.8	1.64	2.42
+ 0.5	+ 2.10	+ 1.08
1.3	3.74	3.5̸0̸

remember Line up the decimal points.
Remove trailing zeros from the final answer (C).

Answers on page 35

WORKSHEET 1J | Addition of Decimals

Add the following decimals.

1. 0.4 + 0.7 =

2. 5.03 + 2.999 =

3. 2.27 + 0.07 + 4 =

4. 15.6 + 0.19 + 500 =

5. 210.79 + 2 + 68.41 =

Subtraction of Decimals

Steps for Subtracting Decimals

1. Write decimals in a column, keeping the decimal points under each other.
2. Subtract as in whole numbers, from right to left.
3. Place the decimal point in the answer directly under the decimal points in the numbers to be subtracted (zeros can be added *after* the decimal point without changing the value).

Examples

0.604	0.500
− 0.524	− 0.123
0.08̸0̸	0.377

remember Line up the decimal points.
Remove trailing zeros from the final answer.

Answers on page 35

WORKSHEET 1K | Subtraction of Decimals

Subtract the following decimals.

1. 2.5 − 1.25 =

2. 0.5 − 0.25 =

3. 0.45 − 0.367 =

4. 108.56 − 5.4 =

5. 1.25 − 0.75 =

Multiplication of Decimals

Steps for Multiplying Decimals

1. Multiply as with whole numbers.
2. Count the total number of decimal places in the multiplier and in the number to be multiplied.
3. Start from the right and count off the same number of places in the answer.
4. If the answer does not have enough places, supply as many zeros as needed, counting from right to left as illustrated on the following page. Eliminate trailing zeros in the answer.

Example 2.5 × 0.0002 =

```
      2.5      (1 decimal place)
  × 0.0002     (4 decimal places)
  ────────
   0.00050     (5 decimal places from right to left in the answer
                before the trailing zero is deleted)
```

Answers on page 35

WORKSHEET 1L | Multiplication of Decimals

Multiply the following decimals.

1. 100 × 0.5 =

2. 0.25 × 2 =

3. 3.14 × 0.072 =

4. 2.14 × 0.03 =

5. 58.7 × 70.1 =

Division of Decimals

Examine the divisor—the number you are dividing by. Is it a *whole* number or a *decimal*?

 RULE If the divisor is a *whole* number, the dividend decimal place is unchanged. Immediately place the decimal point prominently on the answer line directly *above* the decimal point in the dividend. Use zeros in the answer to hold places until you can divide. Prove your answer.

Example 1.20 ÷ 15

```
              0.08    ← Answer
Divisor → 15)1.20    ← Dividend
              1 20
```

PROOF	(Divisor × answer = dividend)
	0.08
	× 15
	1.20

20 Drug Calculations: *Ratio and Proportion Problems for Clinical Practice*

Example 3.15 ÷ 7

```
      0.45
    ┌─────
  7 ) 3.15
      2 8
      ───
        35
        35
        ──
```

PROOF   0.45
       ×   7
       ──────
         3.15

RULE If the divisor has a *decimal*, you must make it a whole number by moving the decimal point to the right. Move the decimal point in the dividend the same number of places to the right and immediately place the decimal point directly above on the answer line. Then divide as with whole numbers. Prove your answer.

Example 10 ÷ 4.4

```
        2.27
      ┌────────
  4.4)10.0 00
      8 8
      ────
      1 20
        88
      ────
        3 20
        3 08
        ────
          12   Remainder
```

PROOF
  2.27   (2 decimal places)
× 4.4   (1 decimal place)
──────
  908
  908
──────
 9988
+ 12   Remainder
──────
10.000   Move decimal 3 places.

Example 30 ÷ 5.2

```
         5.7
      ┌──────
  5.2)30.0 0
      26 0
      ────
       4 0 0
       3 6 4
       ─────
         3 6   Remainder
```

PROOF
  5.2   (1 decimal place)
× 5.7   (1 decimal place)
──────
  36 4
  260
──────
  296 4
+ 3 6   Remainder
──────
30.00   Move decimal 2 places

Note that, as with whole division, a remainder is not just added to the answer in decimal division. Additional division will allow the remainder to be converted to a decimal fraction.

Example 2.6 ÷ 4

```
      0.6                0.65
    ┌─────             ┌──────
  4 ) 2.6            4 ) 2.60
      2 4                2 4
      ───                ───
        2 Remainder        20
                           20
                           ──
```

remember Keep all the decimal points dark for accuracy.

Answers on page 36

WORKSHEET 1M — Division of Decimals

In the following problems, the divisor is a whole number. Place the decimal point on the answer line as illustrated in red in #1. Do NOT do the math in these problems.

1. 60)1.35

2. 20)15.6

3. 19)10.14

4. 7)60.5

5. 25)35.9

In the following problems, the divisor has a decimal. Make the divisor a whole number, move the decimal place an equal number of places in the dividend, and place the decimal point on the answer line as illustrated in red in #6. Calculate the answer to the *nearest tenth*. Add zeros to the dividend as necessary.

6. $0.25\overline{)0.50}$

7. $0.1\overline{)0.5}$

8. $4.8\overline{)2.04}$

9. $0.5\overline{)0.25}$

10. $0.12\overline{)0.44}$

Answers on page 36

WORKSHEET 1N | More Division of Decimals

Divide the following and carry to the *third* decimal place if necessary. Prove the answers.

1. 200 ÷ 6 =

2. 15.06 ÷ 6 =

3. 79.4 ÷ 0.87 =

4. 158.4 ÷ 48 =

5. 670.8 ÷ 0.78 =

Changing Decimals to Fractions

RULE The numbers to the *right* of the decimal can be written as a fraction because they are only part of the whole number.

remember The first number past the decimal to the *right* is ten*ths*, the second is hundred*ths*, the third is thousand*ths*, the fourth is ten-thousand*ths*, and so on.

So if your problem has 3 numbers to the *right* of the decimal, just remove the decimal and put the number over 1000.

Example 0.376 has 3 numbers to the *right* of the decimal. To make a fraction out of 0.376 and also get rid of the decimal, place it over 1000.

0.376 written as a fraction is $\frac{376}{1000}$.

Example It's easy to remember: 3 numbers on top and 3 zeros on the bottom.

0.95 written as a fraction is $\frac{95}{100}$.

The idea is the same as above: 2 numbers on top and 2 zeros on the bottom. The fraction $\frac{90}{100}$ can be reduced to $\frac{9}{10}$ by dividing the numerator and the denominator by 10.

Drug Calculations: *Ratio and Proportion Problems for Clinical Practice*

Answers on page 37

WORKSHEET 1O — Changing Decimals to Fractions

Change the following decimals to fractions, and reduce to lowest terms.

1. 0.8 =
2. 0.4 =
3. 0.25 =
4. 1.32 =
5. 4.08 =
6. 0.5 =
7. 0.75 =
8. 0.2 =
9. 0.65 =
10. 0.7 =

Changing Common Fractions to Decimals

RULE To change a common fraction to a decimal, divide the numerator by the denominator and place the decimal point in the proper position on the answer line.

Examples

$$\frac{2}{5} = 5\overline{)2.0} \quad \begin{array}{r} 0.4 \\ \underline{2\,0} \end{array}$$

$$\frac{1}{8} = 8\overline{)1.000} \quad \begin{array}{r} 0.125 \\ \underline{8} \\ 20 \\ \underline{16} \\ 40 \\ \underline{40} \end{array}$$

Answers on page 37

WORKSHEET 1P — Changing Common Fractions to Decimals

Carry out the following division problems to the *third* decimal place as needed.

1. $\frac{1}{5} =$
2. $\frac{2}{3} =$
3. $\frac{1}{2} =$
4. $\frac{1}{12} =$
5. $\frac{6}{8} =$

Percentages, Decimals, and Fractions

The term "percent" and its symbol (%) mean parts per hundred. A percent number is a fraction whose numerator is already known and whose denominator is always understood to be 100. 25% means 25 parts per hundred.

CHAPTER 1 General Mathematics

Changing a Percentage to a Decimal

RULE To change a percentage to a decimal, divide the percentage by 100, moving the decimal point two places to the *left*. Remove the percent sign. (Remember that an implied decimal point immediately follows a whole number.)

Examples 5% ÷ 100 = 0.05 (5% has an implied decimal point after the 5)

0.5% = 0.005

10% = 0.1 (10% has an implied decimal point after the 10)

Changing a Percentage to a Fraction

RULE To change the percentage to a fraction, *first* change the percentage to a decimal by dividing the percentage by 100, moving the decimal point two places to the *left*. Write the decimal as a fraction.

Example 5% (÷100) = 0.05 = $\frac{5}{100}$

The fraction can then be further reduced to $\frac{1}{20}$

0.1% = 0.001 = $\frac{1}{1000}$

10% = 0.1 = $\frac{10}{100}$ = $\frac{1}{10}$

Converting a Decimal to a Percentage

RULE To change a decimal to a percentage, multiply the decimal by 100 by moving the decimal point 2 places to the *right*. Then add the percent sign.

Examples 0.1 (× 100) = 10%

0.01 = 1%

0.5 = 50%

Answers on page 37

WORKSHEET 1Q | Percentages, Decimals, and Fractions

Fill in the following blanks with the appropriate equivalents.

	Fraction	Decimal	Percentage
1.	$\frac{1}{2}$		
2.			50%
3.		0.05	
4.	$\frac{1}{12}$		
5.	$\frac{3}{1000}$		
6.		0.10	
7.			250%

24   Drug Calculations: *Ratio and Proportion Problems for Clinical Practice*

8. _____ 0.35 _____

9. _____ $\frac{4}{5}$ _____

10. _____ _____ 75%

Steps for Finding the Percentage

1. Change the percentage to a decimal or common fraction.
2. *Multiply* the number by this decimal.

Examples 50% of 120 = 0.5 × 120 = 60 or $\frac{1}{2}$ × 120 = 60

10% of 120 = 0.1 × 120 = 12 or $\frac{1}{10}$ × 120 = 12

Answers on page 37

WORKSHEET 1R — Finding the Percentage

Solve the following problems.

1. 2% of 1500 =
2. 114% of 240 =
3. 28% of 50 =
4. 9% of 200 =
5. $\frac{1}{2}$% of 9328 =
6. $\frac{1}{3}$% of 930 =
7. 120% of 400 =
8. 5% of 105.80 =
9. 10% of 520 =
10. 3% of 40.80 =

Answers on page 38

WORKSHEET 1S — Using Fractions to Percentages to Make Solutions

In the hospital, you might be asked to prepare a baby formula diluted to 50% ($\frac{1}{2}$) strength from a full-strength formula. If the baby was to receive 120 mL (4 oz) at each feeding, the nurse would multiply 0.5 (or $\frac{1}{2}$) × 120 for a result of 60 mL. 60 mL of full-strength formula would be measured and 60 mL of water added (120 mL − 60) for the total 120 mL to make a 50%-strength formula.

For 10% strength, the nurse would multiply 0.1 × 120 for a result of 12 mL full-strength formula. The nurse would measure 12 mL of full-strength formula and add 108 mL of water (120 mL total − 12 mL formula = 108 mL) for the total of 120 mL of 10%-strength formula.

Another way to do the math would be by ratio and proportion. This method will be introduced in Chapter 2. It is simpler to convert percentages, decimals, and fractions using basic arithmetic.

10 mL : 100 mL = x mL : 120 mL   Multiply the two inside numbers (the means).
         100 x = 10 × 120   Then multiply the two outside numbers (the
             x = 12 mL of full-strength formula   extremes). Divide the x number 100 into the
    120 − 12 = 108 mL of water to be added   product of 10 × 120 = 1200. The answer is
                                          the amount of formula needed.

CHAPTER 1 General Mathematics

Make 150 mL of a 50% Betadine solution using normal saline (NS). 50% can be written as 50 : 100 or 1 : 2. The Betadine solution is the active solution and the NS is the solvent.

1 mL : 2 mL = x mL : 150 mL.

Multiply the two inside numbers (means) and then the 2 outside numbers (extremes). Always divide the x number into the number on the right to get the answer. The resulting answer is the amount of solvent (Betadine) needed to make a 50% solution. The formula is called a ratio and proportion:

1 mL : 2 mL = x mL : 150 mL

Example
$2x = 1 \times 150 = 150$
$2x = 150$
$x = 75$ mL Betadine + 75 mL of NS = 150 mL of a 50% solution.

Make the following solutions using Betadine solution as the active ingredient and NS as the diluent.

1. Make 450 mL yielding a $\frac{2}{3}$ strength solution.
2. Make 6 oz of a $\frac{1}{3}$ strength solution.
3. Make a $\frac{1}{4}$ strength solution for a total of 500 mL.
4. Make 800 mL yielding a $\frac{3}{4}$ strength solution.
5. Make a $\frac{2}{5}$ ratio solution for a total of 120 mL.

Answers on page 38

WORKSHEET 1T | Multiple-Choice Practice

Solve the following problems and select the correct answer. Estimate the correct answer before working the problem.

1. $\frac{30}{9}$ can be converted to which whole and mixed number?

   a. $3\frac{3}{9} = 3\frac{1}{3}$ c. $2\frac{1}{8}$

   b. $2\frac{1}{30}$ d. $4\frac{2}{9}$

2. Select the *fraction* equivalent for $3\frac{5}{6}$.

   a. $\frac{15}{6}$ c. $4\frac{1}{6}$

   b. $\frac{23}{6}$ d. $\frac{8}{6}$

3. $\frac{7}{8}$ and $\frac{3}{5}$ have which lowest common denominator?

   a. 8   c. 13
   b. 10   d. 40

4. $5\frac{1}{8} + 1\frac{1}{4} + 4\frac{1}{2} =$

   a. $10\frac{7}{8}$ c. $12\frac{1}{2}$

   b. $9\frac{1}{6}$ d. $10\frac{3}{4}$

5. $6\frac{3}{4} - 5\frac{1}{3} =$

   a. $\frac{1}{2}$ c. $1\frac{5}{12}$

   b. $1\frac{1}{2}$ d. $1\frac{5}{8}$

6. $\frac{5}{6} \times \frac{2}{8} =$

   a. $\frac{1}{12}$ c. $\frac{7}{14}$

   b. $\frac{5}{24}$ d. $\frac{10}{44}$

7. Divide the following fraction and reduce to the lowest term: $\frac{1}{6} \div \frac{1}{3}$

   a. $\frac{2}{12}$ c. $\frac{1}{6}$

   b. $\frac{1}{2}$ d. $\frac{1}{3}$

8. Divide the following fraction and reduce to the lowest term: $\frac{5}{6} \div \frac{1}{3}$

   a. $\frac{1}{6}$ c. $1\frac{1}{6}$

   b. $\frac{5}{18}$ d. $2\frac{1}{2}$

9. Two and eighteen thousandths can be written in decimal form as:
   a. 2.0018   c. 2.18
   b. 2.018   d. 2.118

10. $0.41 - 0.2538 =$
    a. 0.1562   c. 0.4138
    b. 0.2503   d. 0.6638

11. $5 \times 0.9 =$
    a. 0.45   c. 5.09
    b. 4.5   d. 45

12. $79.4 \div 0.87 =$
    a. 12.024   c. 80.276
    b. 21.084   d. 91.264

13. Change $\frac{1}{6}$ to a decimal and round the answer to the nearest *hundredth*.
- **a.** 0.02
- **b.** 0.0625
- **c.** 0.167
- **d.** 0.17

14. 20% of 450 =
- **a.** 90
- **b.** 135
- **c.** 150
- **d.** 185

15. $6\frac{1}{4}$% of 9328 =
- **a.** 0.56
- **b.** 540
- **c.** 583
- **d.** 5596

16. Change 0.285 to a fraction.
- **a.** $\frac{285}{1000}$
- **b.** $\frac{28}{100}$
- **c.** $\frac{285}{100}$
- **d.** $\frac{29}{1000}$

17. Change $\frac{2}{5}$ to a decimal to the nearest *tenth*.
- **a.** 0.4
- **b.** 0.25
- **c.** 0.04
- **d.** 0.025

18. Change $\frac{1}{8}$ to a decimal to the nearest *hundredth*.
- **a.** 0.13
- **b.** 0.12
- **c.** 0.17
- **d.** 0.125

19. Round 58.09 to the nearest *tenth*.
- **a.** 58
- **b.** 58.07
- **c.** 58.1
- **d.** 58.7

20. Change 4% to a decimal.
- **a.** 0.4
- **b.** 0.04
- **c.** 0.25
- **d.** 0.2

CHAPTER 1 Final

Change to whole or mixed numbers.

1. $\dfrac{25}{4}$ ✓ $\boxed{6\frac{1}{4}}$

2. $\dfrac{48}{6}$ ✓ $\boxed{8}$

Change to an improper fraction.

3. $10\dfrac{1}{5}$ ✓ $\boxed{\dfrac{51}{5}}$

4. $3\dfrac{5}{6}$ ✓ $\boxed{\dfrac{23}{6}}$

Find the lowest common denominator in the following pairs of fractions.

5. $\dfrac{17}{20}$ and $\dfrac{4}{5}$ ✓ $\boxed{20}$

6. $\dfrac{7}{8}$ and $\dfrac{3}{5}$ ✓ $\boxed{40}$

Add the following.

7. $\dfrac{2}{18} + \dfrac{1}{4} + \dfrac{2}{9}$ ✓   (work: 4, 9, 8; 36) $\boxed{\dfrac{21}{36} = \dfrac{7}{12}}$

8. $5\dfrac{1}{8} + 1\dfrac{1}{4} + 4\dfrac{1}{2}$ ✓ (work: 41, 10, 36 over 8) $\dfrac{87}{8}$ or $\boxed{10\dfrac{7}{8}}$

Subtract the following.

9. $\dfrac{7}{8} - \dfrac{2}{3}$ ✓   (21 − 16 over 24) $\boxed{\dfrac{5}{24}}$

10. $6\dfrac{2}{4} - 5\dfrac{1}{2}$ ✓ $\boxed{1}$

Multiply the following.

11. $\dfrac{5}{6} \times \dfrac{2}{8}$ ✓ $\dfrac{10}{48} = \boxed{\dfrac{5}{24}}$

12. $\dfrac{1}{5} \times \dfrac{1}{6}$ ✓ $\boxed{\dfrac{1}{30}}$

Divide the following.

13. $\dfrac{3}{4} \div \dfrac{1}{8}$ ✓ $\boxed{6}$

14. $3\dfrac{3}{8} \div 4\dfrac{1}{2}$ (27/8 ÷ 36/8) $\boxed{\dfrac{27}{36}}$ or $\boxed{\dfrac{3}{4}}$

Reduce the following fractions to lowest terms (numbers).

15. $\dfrac{2}{500}$ ✓ $\boxed{\dfrac{1}{250}}$

16. $\dfrac{9}{27}$ ✓ $\boxed{\dfrac{1}{3}}$

Write the following as decimals.

17. Five hundredths ✓ $\boxed{0.05}$

18. Two and seventeen thousandths ✓ $\boxed{2.017}$

Add the following.

19. $5.01 + 2.999$ ✓ $\boxed{8.009}$

20. $36.87 + 8.26 + 15.84$ ✓

```
  36.87
   8.26
  15.84
```
$\boxed{60.97}$

CHAPTER 1 General Mathematics

Subtract the following.

21. 4 − 0.176   **3.824**

22. 0.53 − 0.2538   **0.2762**

Multiply the following.

23. 0.0005 × 0.02   **0.00001**

24. 5 × 0.7   **3.5**

Divide the following and carry to the third decimal place.

25. 158.4 ÷ 48   **3.3**

26. 79.4 ÷ 0.87   **91.264**

Change the following to decimals.

27. $\frac{57}{48}$ **1.19**

28. $8\frac{1}{16}$ **8.06**

Find the following percentages.

29. 24% of 52   **12.48**

30. $6\frac{1}{4}$% of 9328   **583**

$\frac{9328}{100} \quad \frac{x}{6.25}$

Change the following decimals to fractions.

31. 0.4   **2/5**

32. 0.285   **57/200**

$\frac{0.285}{1} \times \frac{1000}{1000}$

$\frac{285}{1000}$

Fill in the following blanks with the appropriate equivalents.

	Fraction	Decimal to Nearest Tenth	Decimal to Nearest Hundredth	Percentage
33.	$\frac{1}{3}$	0.3	0.33	33%
34.	$\frac{1}{20}$	0.1	0.05	5%
35.	$\frac{2}{5}$	0.4	0.40	40%
36.	$\frac{11}{50}$	0.2	0.22	22%
37.	$\frac{1}{8}$	0.1	0.13	12.5% 13%?
38.	$\frac{1}{10}$	0.1	0.10	10%
39.	$\frac{1}{12}$	0.1	0.08	8%
40.	$\frac{1}{1000}$	0.0	0.01	$\frac{1}{2}$%
41.	$\frac{5}{16}$	0.3	0.31	31%
42.	$\frac{3}{20}$	0.2	0.15	15%
43.	$\frac{1}{4}$	0.3	0.25	25%
44.	$\frac{3}{25}$	0.1	0.12	12%
45.	$\frac{1}{100}$	0.0	0.01	1%
46.	$\frac{4}{5}$	0.8	0.80	80%
47.	$\frac{1}{200}$	0.0	0.01	$\frac{1}{2}$% 0.5%
48.	$\frac{1}{3}$	0.3	0.33	33%
49.	$\frac{1}{250}$	0.0	0.00	0.4%
50.	$\frac{3}{4}$	0.8	0.75	75%

evolve Refer to the Mathematics Review section of Drug Calculations Companion, version 5 on Evolve for additional practice problems.

Answer Key

1 General Mathematics

WORKSHEET 1A (page 6)

1. $\dfrac{1}{10}$
2. $\dfrac{2}{7}$
3. $\dfrac{1}{20}$
4. $\dfrac{1}{100{,}000}$
5. More
6. $\dfrac{1}{5}$
7. $\dfrac{1}{150}$
8. $\dfrac{1}{250}$
9. $\dfrac{1}{9}$
10. $\dfrac{1}{200}$

WORKSHEET 1B (page 7)

1. 1
2. 5
3. $3\dfrac{1}{4}$
4. $1\dfrac{5}{9}$
5. $5\dfrac{2}{3}$
6. 5
7. $2\dfrac{1}{4}$
8. $1\dfrac{7}{8}$
9. 6
10. $6\dfrac{5}{6}$

WORKSHEET 1C (page 8)

1. $\dfrac{7}{2}$
2. $\dfrac{7}{6}$
3. $\dfrac{33}{8}$
4. $\dfrac{43}{12}$
5. $\dfrac{68}{5}$
6. $\dfrac{49}{3}$
7. $\dfrac{23}{6}$
8. $\dfrac{21}{8}$
9. $\dfrac{63}{6}$
10. $\dfrac{377}{3}$

WORKSHEET 1D (page 11)

1. $\begin{array}{r}\dfrac{2}{5}\\[2pt]+\dfrac{2}{5}\\ \hline \dfrac{4}{5}\end{array}$

2. $\begin{array}{r}\dfrac{4}{5}=\dfrac{12}{15}\\[2pt]+\dfrac{2}{3}=\dfrac{10}{15}\\ \hline \dfrac{22}{15}=1\dfrac{7}{15}\end{array}$

3. $\begin{array}{r}6\dfrac{1}{6}=6\dfrac{4}{24}\\[2pt]+9\dfrac{5}{8}=9\dfrac{15}{24}\\ \hline 15\dfrac{19}{24}\end{array}$

4. $\begin{array}{r}2\dfrac{1}{4}=2\dfrac{2}{8}\\[2pt]+3\dfrac{1}{8}=3\dfrac{1}{8}\\ \hline 5\dfrac{3}{8}\end{array}$

5. $\begin{array}{r}1\dfrac{3}{4}=1\dfrac{30}{40}\\[2pt]+9\dfrac{9}{10}=9\dfrac{36}{40}\\ \hline 10\dfrac{66}{40}=11\dfrac{13}{20}\end{array}$

6. $\begin{array}{r}\dfrac{1}{8}=\dfrac{9}{72}\\[2pt]\dfrac{1}{4}=\dfrac{18}{72}\\[2pt]+\dfrac{3}{9}=\dfrac{24}{72}\\ \hline \dfrac{51}{72}\end{array}$

7. $\begin{array}{r}\dfrac{7}{9}=\dfrac{70}{90}\\[2pt]\dfrac{4}{5}=\dfrac{72}{90}\\[2pt]+\dfrac{9}{10}=\dfrac{81}{90}\\ \hline \dfrac{223}{90}=2\dfrac{43}{90}\end{array}$

8. $\begin{array}{r}3\dfrac{1}{4}\\[2pt]+9\dfrac{3}{4}\\ \hline 12\dfrac{4}{4}=13\end{array}$

$$8\frac{2}{5} = 8\frac{4}{10}$$
$$14\frac{7}{10} = 14\frac{7}{10}$$
$$+9\frac{9}{10} = 9\frac{9}{10}$$

9. $31\frac{20}{10} = 33$

10. $2\frac{1}{3} = 2\frac{2}{6}$
$+4\frac{1}{6} = 4\frac{1}{6}$
$6\frac{3}{6} = 6\frac{1}{2}$

WORKSHEET 1E (page 13)

1. $\frac{2}{3} = \frac{4}{6}$; $-\frac{1}{2} = \frac{3}{6}$; $\frac{1}{6}$

2. $\frac{27}{32}$; $-\frac{18}{32}$; $\frac{9}{32}$

3. $10\frac{2}{5} = 10\frac{8}{20}$; $-6\frac{1}{4} = 6\frac{5}{20}$; $4\frac{3}{20}$

4. $7\frac{16}{24} = 7\frac{16}{24}$; $-3\frac{1}{8} = 3\frac{3}{24}$; $4\frac{13}{24}$

(Must borrow from the whole number.)

5. $6\frac{3}{10} = 6\frac{3}{10}$; $-2\frac{1}{5} = 2\frac{2}{10}$; $4\frac{1}{10}$

6. $\frac{7}{8} = \frac{21}{24}$; $-\frac{1}{3} = \frac{8}{24}$; $\frac{13}{24}$

7. $3\frac{5}{8}$; $-1\frac{3}{8}$; $2\frac{2}{8} = 2\frac{1}{4}$

8. $5\frac{3}{7} = 4\frac{10}{7}$; $-1\frac{6}{7} = 1\frac{6}{7}$; $3\frac{4}{7}$

(Must borrow from the whole number.)

9. $7 = 6\frac{4}{4}$; $-1\frac{3}{4} = 1\frac{3}{4}$; $5\frac{1}{4}$

10. $2\frac{7}{8} = 2\frac{7}{8}$; $-\frac{3}{4} = \frac{6}{8}$; $2\frac{1}{8}$

(Must borrow from the whole number.)

WORKSHEET 1F (page 14)

1. $\frac{1}{5} \times \frac{2}{4} = \frac{2}{20} = \frac{1}{10}$

2. $\frac{1}{5} \times \frac{1}{6} = \frac{1}{30}$

3. $\frac{3}{5} \times \frac{5}{8} = \frac{15}{40} = \frac{3}{8}$

4. $4 \times 3\frac{1}{3} = 4 \times \frac{10}{3} = \frac{40}{3} = 13\frac{1}{3}$

5. $\frac{2}{4} = 2\frac{1}{6} = \frac{\cancel{2}^1}{4} \times \frac{13}{\cancel{6}_3} = \frac{13}{12} = 1\frac{1}{12}$

6. $5\frac{1}{2} \times 3\frac{1}{8} = \frac{11}{2} \times \frac{25}{8} = \frac{275}{16} = 275 \div 16 = 17\frac{3}{16}$

7. $1\frac{3}{4} \times 3\frac{1}{7} = \frac{\cancel{7}^1}{4} \times \frac{22}{\cancel{7}_1} = \frac{22}{4} = 22 \div 4 = 5\frac{1}{2}$

8. $\frac{5}{6} \times 1\frac{9}{16} = \frac{5}{6} \times \frac{25}{16} = \frac{125}{96} = 125 \div 96 = 1\frac{29}{96}$

9. $\frac{5}{100} \times 900 = \frac{5}{\cancel{100}_1} \times \frac{\cancel{900}^9}{1} = 45$

10. $2\frac{1}{10} \times 4\frac{1}{3} = \frac{21}{10} \times \frac{13}{\cancel{3}_1}^{\cancel{7}} = \frac{91}{10} = 9\frac{1}{10}$

Answer Key 33

WORKSHEET 1G (page 14)

1. $\dfrac{1}{5} \div \dfrac{1}{8} = \dfrac{1}{5} \times \dfrac{8}{1} = \dfrac{8}{5} = 1\dfrac{3}{5}$

2. $\dfrac{1}{3} \div \dfrac{1}{2} = \dfrac{1}{3} \times \dfrac{2}{1} = \dfrac{2}{3}$

3. $\dfrac{3}{4} \div \dfrac{1}{8} = \dfrac{3}{\cancel{4}_1} \times \dfrac{\cancel{8}^2}{1} = 6$

4. $\dfrac{1}{16} \div \dfrac{1}{4} = \dfrac{1}{\cancel{16}_4} \times \dfrac{\cancel{4}^1}{1} = \dfrac{1}{4}$

5. $8\dfrac{3}{4} \div 15 = \dfrac{\cancel{35}^7}{4} \times \dfrac{1}{\cancel{15}_3} = \dfrac{7}{12}$

6. $\dfrac{3}{4} \div 6 = \dfrac{\cancel{3}^1}{4} \times \dfrac{1}{\cancel{6}_2} = \dfrac{1}{8}$

7. $2 \div \dfrac{1}{5} = \dfrac{2}{1} \times \dfrac{5}{1} = 10$

8. $3\dfrac{3}{8} \div 4\dfrac{1}{2} = \dfrac{27}{8} \div \dfrac{9}{2} = \dfrac{\cancel{27}^3}{\cancel{8}_4} \times \dfrac{\cancel{2}^1}{\cancel{9}_1} = \dfrac{3}{4}$

9. $\dfrac{3}{5} \div \dfrac{3}{8} = \dfrac{\cancel{3}^1}{5} \times \dfrac{8}{\cancel{3}_1} = \dfrac{8}{5} = 1\dfrac{3}{5}$

10. $4 \div 2\dfrac{1}{8} = \dfrac{4}{1} \times \dfrac{8}{17} = \dfrac{32}{17} = 1\dfrac{15}{17}$

WORKSHEET 1HA (page 16)

	Nearest Whole Number	Nearest Tenth	Nearest Hundredth
1. 93.489	93	93.5	93.49
2. 25.43	25	25.4	25.43
3. 38.2	38	38.2	38.20
4. 57.8888	58	57.9	57.89
5. 0.0092	0	0	0.01
6. 3.144	3	3.1	3.14
7. 8.999	9	9.0	9.00
8. 77.788	78	77.8	77.79
9. 12.959	13	13.0	12.96
10. 5.7703	6	5.8	5.77

WORKSHEET 1HB (page 17)

1. Six hundredths
2. Ninety-six thousandths
3. Five thousandths
4. One hundred and one hundredth
5. Nine tenths
6. 0.34
7. 0.004
8. 2.017
9. 9.0002
10. 34.1

WORKSHEET 1IA (page 18)

Round to tenths
1. 0.3
2. 4.4
3. 2.8
4. 0.8
5. 6.8

Round to hundredths
6. 0.30
7. 4.44
8. 2.75
9. 0.84
10. 6.77

Round to thousandths
11. 8.937
12. 5.626
13. 10.9
14. 4.626
15. 3.739

Round to ten-thousandths
16. 8.9375
17. 5.6257
18. 10.8976
19. 4.6256
20. 3.7387

34 Answer Key

WORKSHEET 1IB (page 18)

Smaller:
1. 0.2
2. 0.25
3. 0.125
4. 2.07
5. 1.29

Larger:
6. 0.9
7. 0.7
8. 0.58
9. 0.25
10. 0.1

WORKSHEET 1J (page 19)

1. 0.4
   + 0.7
   ─────
    1.1

2. 5.030
   + 2.999
   ──────
    8.029

3. 2.27
    0.17
   + 4.00
   ─────
    6.34

4. 15.60
    0.19
   + 500.00
   ───────
    515.79

5. 210.79
    2.00
   + 68.41
   ──────
    281.20*

WORKSHEET 1K (page 20)

1. 2.50
   − 1.25
   ─────
    1.25

2. 0.50
   − 0.25
   ─────
    0.25

3. 0.450
   − 0.367
   ──────
    0.083

4. 108.56
   − 5.40
   ──────
    103.16

5. 1.25
   − 0.75
   ─────
    0.50*

WORKSHEET 1L (page 20)

1. 100
   × 0.5
   ─────
    50.0   Count 1 decimal place in from the right.

2. 0.25
   × 2
   ─────
    0.50   Count 2 decimal places in from the right.

3. 3.14
   × 0.072
   ──────
    0.22608   You do not have to multiply zeros. Count 5 decimal places in from the right, adding zeros where needed.

4. 2.14
   × 0.03
   ─────
    0.0642   Count 4 decimal places in from the right, adding zeros as needed.

5. 58.7
   × 70.1
   ─────
    58.7
    41090
   ──────
    4114.87

---

*Trailing zeros must be removed from answers.

WORKSHEET 1M (page 21)

1. 60)1.35̇

2. 20)15.6̇

3. 19)10.1̇4

4. 7)60.5̇

5. 25)35.9̇

6.
```
       2.
0.25)0.50    ANSWER: 2
     50
      0
```

7.
```
      5.
0.1)0.5    ANSWER: 5
```

8.
```
       0.40
4.8)2.0 40    ANSWER: 0.425
    1 9 2
       20
```

9.
```
      0.5
0.5)0.2 5    ANSWER: 0.5
     2 5
```

10.
```
         3.66    ANSWER: 3.7
0.12)0.44 00
     36
     8 0
     7 2
       80
       72
        8
```

WORKSHEET 1N (page 22)

1.
```
        3 3.333                  PROOF
6)200.0 000                       33.333
  180                          ×     60
   20 0                         1999.980
   18 0
    2 0 0
    1 8 0
      2 00
      1 80
        200
        180
```

2.
```
      2.51              PROOF
6)15.06                  2.51
  12                   ×    6
   30                   15.06
   30
    06
     6
```

3.
```
         91.264              PROOF
0.87)79.40 000                91.264
     78 30                  ×     87
      1 10                    638 848
        87                   7301 12
        23 0                 7939.968
        17 4
         5 60
         5 22
           380
           348
```

4.
```
        3.3            PROOF
48)158.4                 48
   144                ×  3.3
    14 4               14 4
    14 4               144
                       158.4
```

5.
```
        860.           PROOF
0.78)670.80             860
     624              × 78
      46 8            6880
      46 8            6020
                      67080
```

36   Answer Key

WORKSHEET 1O (page 23)

1. $\dfrac{8}{10} = \dfrac{4}{5}$
2. $\dfrac{4}{10} = \dfrac{2}{5}$
3. $\dfrac{25}{100} = \dfrac{1}{4}$
4. $1\dfrac{32}{100} = 1\dfrac{8}{25}$
5. $4\dfrac{8}{100} = 4\dfrac{2}{25}$
6. $\dfrac{5}{10} = \dfrac{1}{2}$
7. $\dfrac{75}{100} = \dfrac{3}{4}$
8. $\dfrac{2}{10} = \dfrac{1}{5}$
9. $\dfrac{65}{100} = \dfrac{13}{20}$
10. $\dfrac{7}{10}$

WORKSHEET 1P (page 23)

1.
```
    0.2
5)1.0
    1 0
    ___
```

2.
```
    0.666
3)2.000
  1 8
  ___
    20
    18
    ___
     20
     18
     ___
```

3.
```
    0.5
2)1.0
  1 0
  ___
```

4.
```
     0.083
12)1.000
   96
   ___
    40
    36
    ___
```

5.
```
    0.75
8)6.00
  5 6
  ___
    40
    40
    ___
```

WORKSHEET 1Q (page 24)

1. Decimal: 0.5
   Percentage: 50%
2. Fraction: $\dfrac{1}{2}$
   Decimal: 0.5
3. Fraction: $\dfrac{5}{100} = \dfrac{1}{20}$
   Percentage: 5%
4. Decimal: 0.083
   Percentage: 8.33%
5. Decimal: 0.003
   Percentage: 0.3%
6. Fraction: $\dfrac{1}{10}$
   Percentage: 10%
7. Fraction: $\dfrac{250}{100} = \dfrac{5}{2}$
   Decimal: 2.5
8. Fraction: $\dfrac{7}{20}$
   Percentage: 35%
9. Decimal: 0.8
   Percentage: 80%
10. Fraction: $\dfrac{75}{100} = \dfrac{3}{4}$
    Decimal: 0.75

WORKSHEET 1R (page 25)

1.
```
  1500
× 0.02
_____
 30.00*
```

2.
```
   240
× 1.14
_____
   960
   240
   240
_____
273.60*
```

3.
```
    50
× 0.28
_____
   400
   100
_____
 14.00*
```

4.
```
   200
× 0.09
_____
 18.00*
```

5. $\dfrac{\frac{1}{2}}{100} = \dfrac{1}{2} \div \dfrac{100}{1} = \dfrac{1}{2} \times \dfrac{1}{100} = \dfrac{1}{200} = 200)\overline{1.000}$ → 0.005

```
  9328
× 0.005
_____
46.640*
```

6. $\dfrac{\frac{1}{3}}{100} = \dfrac{1}{3} \div \dfrac{100}{1} = \dfrac{1}{3} \times \dfrac{1}{100} = \dfrac{1}{300} = 300)\overline{1.000}$ → 0.003
```
   900
   ___
   100
```

```
   930
× 0.003
_____
 2.790*
```

7. 400	8. 105.80	9. 520	10. 40.80
× 1.20	× 0.05	× 0.10	× 0.03
8000	5.2900 *	52.00 *	1.2240 *
400			
480.00 *			

WORKSHEET 1S (page 25)

1. 2 : 3 = x : 450
   3x = 2 × 450 = 900
   x = 300 mL of Betadine + 150 mL NS = $\frac{2}{3}$ strength solution

2. 1 : 3 = x : 6
   3x = 6
   x = 2 oz of Betadine + 4 oz of NS = 6 oz of $\frac{1}{3}$ strength solution

3. 1 : 4 = x : 500
   4x = 500
   x = 125 mL Betadine + 375 mL NS = 500 mL $\frac{1}{4}$ strength solution

4. 3 : 4 = x : 800
   4x = 3 × 800 = 2400
   x = 600 mL Betadine + 200 mL NS = 800 mL $\frac{3}{4}$ strength solution

5. 2 : 5 = x : 120
   5x = 2 × 120 = 240
   x = 48 mL Betadine + 72 mL NS = 120 mL $\frac{2}{5}$ strength solution

WORKSHEET 1T (page 26)

1. a The other responses can be eliminated quickly because only **a** offers 3 as the whole number.
2. b
3. d
4. a
5. c
6. b
7. b
8. d
9. b
10. a
11. b
12. d
13. c
14. a
15. c
16. a
17. a
18. a
19. c
20. b

CHAPTER 1 FINAL: GENERAL MATHEMATICS (page 29)

1. $6\frac{1}{4}$
2. 8
3. $\frac{51}{5}$
4. $\frac{23}{6}$
5. 20
6. 40
7. $\frac{21}{36}$
8. $10\frac{7}{8}$
9. $\frac{5}{24}$
10. 1
11. $\frac{10}{48} = \frac{5}{24}$
12. $\frac{1}{30}$
13. $\frac{24}{4} = 6$
14. $\frac{3}{4}$
15. $\frac{1}{250}$
16. $\frac{1}{3}$

---

*Trailing zeros must be removed from answers.

17. 0.05
18. 2.017
19. 8.009
20. 60.97
21. 3.824
22. 0.2762
23. 0.000010*
24. 3.5
25. 3.3*
26. 91.264
27. 1.1875
28. 8.0625
29. 12.48
30. 583
31. $\dfrac{2}{5}$
32. $\dfrac{57}{200}$

Fraction	Decimal to Nearest Tenth	Decimal to Nearest Hundredth	Percentage
33. $\dfrac{1}{3}$	0.3	0.33	33%
34. $\dfrac{5}{100} = \left(\dfrac{1}{20}\right)$	0.1	0.05	5%
35. $\dfrac{2}{5}$	0.4	0.40	40%
36. $\dfrac{22}{100} = \left(\dfrac{11}{50}\right)$	0.2	0.22	22%
37. $\dfrac{1}{8}$	0.1	0.13	12.5%
38. $\dfrac{10}{100} = \left(\dfrac{1}{10}\right)$	0.1	0.10	10%
39. $\dfrac{1}{12}$	0.1	0.08	8%
40. $\dfrac{1}{200}$	0.0	0.01	$\dfrac{1}{2}$%
41. $\dfrac{5}{16}$	0.3	0.31	31%
42. $\dfrac{15}{100} = \left(\dfrac{3}{20}\right)$	0.2	0.15	15%
43. $\dfrac{1}{4}$	0.3	0.25	25%
44. $\dfrac{12}{100} = \left(\dfrac{3}{25}\right)$	0.1	0.12	12%
45. $\dfrac{1}{100}$	0.0	0.01	1%
46. $\dfrac{80}{100} = \left(\dfrac{4}{5}\right)$	0.8	0.80	80%
47. $\dfrac{1}{200}$	0.0	0.01	0.5%
48. $\dfrac{33}{100}$	0.3	0.33	33%
49. $\dfrac{1}{250}$	0.0	0.00	$\dfrac{2}{5}$%
50. $\dfrac{75}{100} = \left(\dfrac{3}{4}\right)$	0.8	0.75	75%

*Trailing zeros must be removed from answers.

Ratio and Proportion

Objectives
- Identify the differences between ratio and proportion.
- Express ratios in lowest terms.
- Solve proportion problems for a missing quantity (x).
- Set up one-step ratio and proportion problems from a word problem.
- Estimate, solve, and prove answers.

Introduction

Ratio and proportion is a simple, provable method for solving medication dose problems. The ample examples and practice in this chapter are provided to enable you to solve more complex dose problems in later chapters.

Ratio

A ratio is a comparison of two quantities. Two ways to express a ratio are with a colon (:), as in 2 : 3, or as a fraction $\left(\frac{2}{3}\right)$. A colon is read as the word "to" or "is to."

Examples one to three $\left(1 : 3 \text{ or } \frac{1}{3}\right)$ three to five $\left(3 : 5 \text{ or } \frac{3}{5}\right)$

2 scoops coffee to 1 cup water $\left(\text{two to one, } 2 : 1, \text{ or } \frac{2}{1}\right)$

Ratios, like fractions, can be expressed in lowest terms to simplify problem recognition and the arithmetic.

Examples 2 : 8 reduced to 1 : 4   50 : 100 reduced to 1 : 2

Answers on page 51

WORKSHEET 2A — Expressing Ratios in Lowest Terms

Express the following ratios in lowest whole-number terms. Reading and writing them as fractions may be helpful (see Chapter 1, page 22).

Example 70 : 100 = 7 : 10 $\left(\dfrac{70}{100} = \dfrac{7}{10}\right)$

1. 2 : 4
2. 250 : 125
3. 2 : 5
4. 0.5 : 1
5. 2 : 3
6. 0.5 : 0.25
7. 100 : 10
8. 0.1 : 1
9. 0.1 : 0.2
10. 0.2 : 0.05

Proportion

A proportion is a statement that shows the relationship between *two equal* ratios. We calculate proportions when we alter quantities on hand but want to maintain the same ratio. You may use a colon or fraction setup. The quantities and numbers must be in the correct sequence.

Examples

Using Colons

1 chicken : 3 guests = 3 chickens : 9 guests

(1 : 3 = 3 : 9)

1 qt paint : 100 sq. ft = 4 qt paint : 400 sq. ft

(1 : 100 = 4 : 400)

Using Fractions

$\dfrac{1 \text{ chicken}}{3 \text{ guests}} = \dfrac{3 \text{ chickens}}{9 \text{ guests}}$

$\left(\dfrac{1}{3} = \dfrac{3}{9}\right)$

$\dfrac{1 \text{ qt paint}}{100 \text{ sq. ft}} = \dfrac{4 \text{ qt paint}}{400 \text{ sq. ft}}$

$\left(\dfrac{1}{100} = \dfrac{4}{400}\right)$

Steps to Prove a Proportion Is Correct

Example

Using colons 1 : 5 = 5 : 25
multiply

Using Fractions
Cross product

Extremes / Means
$\dfrac{1}{5} = \dfrac{5}{25}$
Means / Extremes

1. Multiply the *means* (two middle numbers)   5 × 5 = 25.
2. Multiply the *extremes* (two end numbers)   1 × 25 = 25.
3. Compare the two products. If the ratios are equal, the products of the means and extremes will be equal. The proportion will be correct.

Example 3 : 5 = 6 : 10 $\dfrac{3}{5} = \dfrac{6}{10}$
multiply

Multiply the means: 5 × 6 = 30.
Multiply the extremes: 3 × 10 = 30.

Solving Proportion Problems When One of the Numbers Is *Unknown,* or *x*

Example $2 : 8 = x : 24$

Multiply the means.

$8 \times x = 8x$

Multiply the extremes.

$2 \times 24 = 48$

Move the *x* product to the **left** side of the equation. It will look like this:

$8x = 48$

Now you must get *x* to stand alone.

RULE To solve for the value of *x*, *divide* both sides of the equation by the number *next* to *x*. Those numbers will cancel each other. The result will be that *x* will stand alone.

What you do to one side of the equation, you must do to the other to keep the sides equal.

Example $\dfrac{8}{8}x = \dfrac{48}{8}$

$x = 6$

Example KNOW   WANT TO KNOW
$2 : 3 = 6 : x$

$2x = 3 \times 6$
$2x = 18$ Keep the *x* product on the left side of the equation.
$\dfrac{2x}{2} = \dfrac{18}{2}$ Divide both sides of the equation by the number next to *x*.
$x = 9$
$2 : 3 = 6 : 9$

Example KNOW   WANT TO KNOW
$10 : 5 = x : 3$
$5x = 30$
$\dfrac{5x}{5} = \dfrac{30}{5}$
$x = 6$

Proof $10 : 5 = 6 : 3$

CHAPTER 2   Ratio and Proportion

RULE To check your answer and prove the proportion is correct, substitute the answer for *x* in the original problem. Multiply the means and extremes. The products must be equal.

Steps
1. *Substitute the answer (6) for x.*
2. *Multiply the means. Multiply the extremes.* The products must be equal.

KNOW WANT TO KNOW

$2 : 8 = x : 24$ $\dfrac{2}{8} = \dfrac{x}{24}$
(multiply means and extremes)

$2 : 8 = 6 : 24$ $\dfrac{2}{8} = \dfrac{6}{24}$

Proof $8 \times 6 = 48$ product of means $= 2 \times 24 = 48$ product of extremes

The ratios are equal. The proportion is correct.

Answers on page 51

WORKSHEET 2B | Solving Proportion Practice Problems for the Value of *x*

Use the colon or fraction cross-product method to multiply the means and extremes, then move the *x* product to the left side of the equation. Solve for *x*. Prove the answer.

1. $5 : 100 = 9 : x$ $\left(\dfrac{5}{100} = \dfrac{9}{x}\right)$

2. $9 : 27 = 300 : x$ $\left(\dfrac{9}{27} = \dfrac{300}{x}\right)$

3. $1 : 8 = \dfrac{1}{2} : x$ $\left(\dfrac{1}{8} = \dfrac{\frac{1}{2}}{x}\right)$

4. $4 : 120 = x : 600$ $\left(\dfrac{4}{120} = \dfrac{x}{600}\right)$

5. $0.7 : 70 = x : 1000$ $\left(\dfrac{0.7}{70} = \dfrac{x}{1000}\right)$

Answers on page 52

WORKSHEET 2C | Solving Proportion Practice Problems for the Value of *x*

Use the colon or fraction cross-product method to estimate, solve the following proportions for *x*, and prove the answer.

1. $15 : 30 = x : 12$

2. $5 : 10 = 15 : x$

3. $6 : 12 = 0.25 : x$

4. $7.5 : 12 = x : 28$

5. $0.4 : 12 = 10 : x$

44 Drug Calculations: *Ratio and Proportion Problems for Clinical Practice*

Setting Up Ratios and Proportions from Given Information

1. Read the problem and identify the unknown wanted quantity (*x*).
2. Estimate the size of the *x* (wanted) quantity.
3. Always enter the ratio of what you already *know* or already *have* on the *left* side of the equal sign.
4. On the *right* side, enter your *x* ratio—what you want to know.
5. Solve for *x* and prove the proportion. Check your estimate with the answer.

Each of the two ratios must be set up in the *same sequence for the answer to be correct.*

Apples : Pears = Apple : *x* Pears Sugar : Tea = Sugar : Tea

Example You are making coffee for a group meeting. The label says 2 scoops per cup. You will need 20 cups. How many scoops will you use?

Estimate The *x* unknown is scoops. You will need many more than 2 scoops. (Make the estimate *before* the setup and math.)

Correct Setup

KNOW WANT TO KNOW
2 scoops : 1 coffee = *x* scoops : 20 coffees

$\left(\dfrac{2}{1} = \dfrac{x}{20}\right)$

$x = 20 \times 2$
$x = 40$ scoops.
2 : 1 = 40 : 20 Estimate is correct. 40 is many more than 2

PROOF $1 \times 40 = 40$
$2 \times 20 = 40$

Example of Incorrect Setup

2 : 20 = *x* : 2
20*x* = 4

$\dfrac{20}{20}x = \dfrac{4}{20}$

$x = \dfrac{1}{5}$ cup

remember The math can be correct and the proportion can be correct, but if the setup is wrong, the answer to the problem will be wrong.

$20 \times \dfrac{1}{5} = 4$
$2 \times 2 = 4$

remember Placements, labels, estimates, and proofs are important to reduce errors. Estimates provide a rough guide to the approximate size of the answer. Estimates *are not* a substitute for proofs. They may protect from major math errors if the setup is correct. Recheck the setup, numbers, and placements if the estimate and/or the proof is incorrect.

Example You wish to make a floral bouquet of 6 daffodils for every 4 roses. How many daffodils will you use for 30 roses?

Estimate: x daffodils will be many more than 6 daffodils.

KNOW　　　　　　　　WANT TO KNOW

6 daffodils : 4 roses = x daffodils : 30 roses
———————multiply———————

$$\frac{6}{4} = \frac{x}{30}$$

$4x = 6 \times 30$

$\frac{4}{4}x = \frac{180}{4}$

$x = 45$ daffodils

My estimate is correct.　　6 : 4 = 45 : 30

PROOF $4 \times 45 = 180$
$6 \times 30 = 180$

The product of the means = the product of the extremes.

Example Make a necklace that has 19 blue beads for every yellow bead. How many blue beads are needed if you have 8 yellow beads?

Estimate: x blue beads will be many more than 19 blue beads (8 times more).

KNOW　　　　　　　　WANT TO KNOW

19 blue beads : 1 yellow bead = x blue beads : 8 yellow beads
———————multiply———————

$x = 19 \times 8$
$x = 152$ blue beads needed
My estimate is correct.

PROOF $19 \times 8 = 152$
$1 \times 152 = 152$

Answers on page 52

WORKSHEET 2D | Setting Up and Solving Ratios and Proportions

Set up a proportion for each of the following problems. Estimate the value of x, label, and prove your answers. Use the colon or fraction cross-product method.

1. You have to make a fruit basket with 6 bananas for every 9 apples. How many bananas will there be for 72 apples?

2. You are making coffee, and 7 scoops make 8 cups. How many scoops make 40 cups?

3. You have a recipe for cocoa: 4 scoops make 6 cups of cocoa. You want to make 18 cups for a party. How many scoops of cocoa are needed? Set up a proportion.

4. Ordered: 2 tablets each day. The patient will be taking the medication for 21 days. How many tablets will the patient need for discharge?

5. You wish to plant 8 bushes for every 2 trees in your yard. How many bushes will there be if there are 36 trees?

6. Ordered: 2 cups of green tea every day. How many days would it take to consume 24 cups of green tea?

7. It takes 4 cups of flour to make 3 loaves of bread. How many loaves of bread can be made from 24 cups of flour?

8. Your recipe for punch calls for 3 cups of soda for every $\frac{1}{2}$ cup of fruit juice. How many cups of soda will be needed for 2 cups of fruit juice?

9. You need 4 tablespoons of sugar for every glass of lemonade you prepare. How many tablespoons of sugar will be needed for 6 glasses of lemonade?

10. Ordered: 4 capsules every day. How many capsules would be needed for 14 days?

Answers on page 54

WORKSHEET 2E | Ratio and Proportion Practice

Use ratio and proportion to set up and solve the following problems, estimate, label, and prove your answers. Use the colon or fraction cross-product method.

1. The office needs 4000 envelopes. The boxes on hand contain 200 envelopes per box. How many boxes will you send to the office?

2. The order is for 300 operating room gowns. The packages on hand contain 10 gowns per package. How many packages will you send?

3. If one computer is allocated for every 18 students, how many computers will be needed for an enrollment of 1260 students?

4. Your doctor tells you to drink 3 glasses of water and eat 2 apples every day. How many apples will you have eaten when you have drunk 24 glasses of water?

5. If all the teachers were to receive 6 pens for every 8 pencils, how many pens would you give them if the teachers have 72 pencils?

6. The nurse is assigned 6 patients per shift. How many nurses will be needed for 36 patients?

7. If baby formula calls for 4 tablespoons of powdered formula for every 8 ounces of water, how many tablespoons of powdered formula would be needed for 56 ounces of water?

8. The hospital requires 2 nurses for every unit for each 12-hour shift. How many nurses are needed for each unit for 72 hours?

9. If a patient takes 3 aspirin tablets per day, how many aspirin tablets will the patient need for a 2-week vacation?

10. If a multidose liquid medication contains 100 mL and the patient takes 5 mL (1 teaspoon) per day, how many days will the medication last?

Answers on page 55

WORKSHEET 2F — Multiple-Choice Practice

Use ratio and proportion to solve the following problems. Label, estimate, and prove your answers.

1. If you need 10 diapers a day, how many days will a package of 50 diapers last?
   - **a.** 5 days
   - **b.** 10 days
   - **c.** 15 days
   - **d.** 20 days

2. Ordered: 120 insulin syringes. They are delivered in units of 10 per package. How many packages will you receive?
   - **a.** 10 packages
   - **b.** 12 packages
   - **c.** 15 packages
   - **d.** 20 packages

3. You have to take 4 teaspoons of medicine every day. The bottle contains 80 teaspoons. How many days will the bottle last?
   - **a.** 2 days
   - **b.** 5 days
   - **c.** 10 days
   - **d.** 20 days

4. Ordered: 3 capsules per day. How many capsules will the patient need for 21 days?
   - **a.** 12 capsules
   - **b.** 20 capsules
   - **c.** 31 capsules
   - **d.** 63 capsules

5. You have a vial holding 30 mL of liquid. If the average dose given is 5 mL, how many doses are available?
   - **a.** 5 doses
   - **b.** 6 doses
   - **c.** 8 doses
   - **d.** 10 doses

6. The hospital has allotted 120 days of inservice for 15 departments. How many days of inservice can each department use?
   - **a.** 4 days
   - **b.** 8 days
   - **c.** 12 days
   - **d.** 15 days

7. The hospital staffs every 8 patients with one RN. How many RNs will be needed when the census is 240?
   - **a.** 30 RNs
   - **b.** 60 RNs
   - **c.** 90 RNs
   - **d.** 120 RNs

8. The directions state that for every $\frac{1}{2}$ cup portion of baby cereal you will need 4 ounces of milk. How many ounces of milk will you need to prepare 20 portions?
   - **a.** 20 ounces
   - **b.** 40 ounces
   - **c.** 80 ounces
   - **d.** 100 ounces

9. If you receive $15 an hour in overtime pay, how many hours would you need to work overtime to receive $450 in overtime earnings?
   - **a.** 3 hours
   - **b.** 15 hours
   - **c.** 30 hours
   - **d.** 45 hours

10. If a patient is to receive 3 liters of an intravenous fluid every 8 hours, how many liters would be needed for 72 hours?
    - **a.** 9 liters
    - **b.** 18 liters
    - **c.** 27 liters
    - **d.** 36 liters

CHAPTER 2 Final

Solve each problem using ratio and proportion. Label, estimate, and prove your answers.

1. The hospital assigns 5 nursing supervisors per shift. How many supervisors are needed for 3 shifts? **15 supervisors**

2. Each nurse is assigned 6 patients. How many nurses are needed for 150 patients in a hospital? 150/6 = **25 nurses**

3. The hospital laundry provides 4 sheets per bed per day. How many sheets are needed per day for a 200-bed hospital? 200 × 4 = **800 sheets**

4. The average number of discharges is 32 patients per day. How many patients are discharged each week? 32 × 7 = **224 patients**

5. A nurse earns $20 an hour in extra pay for overtime hours. How much extra pay will the nurse earn for 24 hours of overtime in a pay period? **$480**

6. A CNA is hired for every 12 beds in the hospital. How many CNAs would be hired for a 360-bed hospital? **30 CNAs**

7. There is 1 administrator for every 50 beds. How many administrators would be needed for a 200-bed hospital? **4 administrators**   *CROSS MULTIPLY!*

8. The hospital spends $750 a day for portable oxygen canister rentals. How much will a 4-week supply of canisters cost? **$21,000**

9. Approximately 1 resident and 2 interns are assigned for every 20 patients. How many interns are needed for 210 patients? $\frac{2}{20} = \frac{21}{210}$ **21 interns**

10. Some studies show that approximately 1 of every 6 medications given involves an error. Approximately how many medication errors would occur for every 240 medications given? **40 errors** $\frac{1 \text{ errors}}{6 \text{ med}} = \frac{x}{240}$

11. If a patient has to take 1 antiinflammatory tablet every 6 hours, how many tablets will he or she need for 3 days? **12 tablets**

12. If a staff member is allotted 1.5 PTO (personal time off) days per month, how many PTO days will be accumulated in 6 months? **9 days**

13. Ordered: 2 tablets, 3 times daily. How many days will a bottle of 60 tablets last? Hint: You need to enter total tablets per day in the equation. 6 tabl/day **10 days**   *CROSS MULTIPLY!*

14. The patient is to drink 4 ounces of water every $\frac{1}{2}$ hour. How much water should the patient have consumed in 8 hours? 8 oz/hr **64 oz**

15. The budget permits 48 inservice days per year. There are 12 units. How many inservice days could each unit receive for a year? **4 inservice days**

16. A multidose vial contains 20 mL. If each dose is 2.5 mL, how many doses are in the vial? **8 doses**

17. If the average adult weight is 150 pounds and the elevator can hold 1800 pounds, how many people, on average, can the elevator safely carry at one time? **12 people**

18. If each orientation for an RN costs approximately $3000, how many RNs can the hospital plan to hire with an annual orientation budget of $96,000? **32 RNs**

19. If a guest speaker is paid a $50 honorarium, how many guest speakers can be invited if the budget is $600? **12 speakers**

20. If a patient needs a 30-day supply of tablets and takes 2 tablets four times a day, how many tablets will the patient need at discharge? **8 tab/day** **240 tablets**

evolve Refer to the Mathematics Review section of Drug Calculations Companion, version 5 on Evolve for additional practice problems.

Answer Key

2 Ratio and Proportion

WORKSHEET 2A (page 42)

1. $2 : 4 = 1 : 2 \quad \left(\dfrac{2}{4} = \dfrac{1}{2}\right)$

2. $250 : 125 = 2 : 1 \quad \left(\dfrac{250}{125} = \dfrac{2}{1}\right)$

3. $2 : 5 = 2 : 5 \quad \left(\dfrac{2}{5} = \dfrac{2}{5}\right)$

4. $0.5 : 1 = 1 : 2 \quad \left(\dfrac{0.5}{1} = \dfrac{1}{2}\right)$

5. $2 : 3 = 2 : 3 \quad \left(\dfrac{2}{3} = \dfrac{2}{3}\right)$

6. $0.5 : 0.25 = 2 : 1 \quad \left(\dfrac{0.5}{0.25} = \dfrac{2}{1}\right)$

7. $100 : 10 = 10 : 1 \quad \left(\dfrac{100}{10} = \dfrac{10}{1}\right)$

8. $0.1 : 1 = 1 : 10 \quad \left(\dfrac{0.1}{1} = \dfrac{1}{10}\right)$

9. $0.1 : 0.2 = 1 : 2 \quad \left(\dfrac{0.1}{0.2} = \dfrac{1}{2}\right)$

10. $0.2 : 0.05 = 4 : 1 \quad \left(\dfrac{0.2}{0.05} = \dfrac{4}{1}\right)$

WORKSHEET 2B (page 44)

1. $5 : 100 = 9 : x$
   $5x = 9 \times 100$
   $5x = 900$
   $\dfrac{\cancel{5}}{\cancel{5}}x = \dfrac{900}{5} = 900 \div 5$
   $x = 180$
   PROOF
   $180 \times 5 = 900$
   $9 \times 100 = 900$

2. $9 : 27 = 300 : x$
   $9x = 27 \times 300 = 8100$
   $\dfrac{\cancel{9}}{\cancel{9}}x = \dfrac{8100}{9} = 8100 \div 9$
   $x = 900$
   PROOF
   $27 \times 300 = 8100$
   $9 \times 900 = 8100$

3. $1 : 8 = \dfrac{1}{2} : x$
   $x = \dfrac{8}{1} \times \dfrac{1}{2}$
   $x = \dfrac{8}{2}$
   $x = 4$
   PROOF
   $4 \times 1 = 4$
   $\dfrac{1}{2} \times 8 = 4$

4. $4 : 120 = x : 600$
   $120x = 4 \times 600 = 2400$
   $\dfrac{\cancel{120}}{\cancel{120}}x = \dfrac{\cancel{2400}}{120} = 240 \div 12$
   $x = 20$
   PROOF
   $600 \times 4 = 2400$
   $20 \times 120 = 2400$

5. $0.7 : 70 = x : 1000$
   $70x = 0.7 \times 1000 = 700$
   $\dfrac{\cancel{70}}{\cancel{70}}x = \dfrac{\cancel{700}}{\cancel{70}} = 70 \div 7$
   $x = 10$
   PROOF
   $70 \times 10 = 700$
   $0.7 \times 1000 = 700$

WORKSHEET 2C (page 44)

1. $15 : 30 = x : 12$
$30x = 15 \times 12$
$30x = 180$
$\dfrac{\cancel{30}}{\cancel{30}} x = \dfrac{\cancel{180}}{\cancel{30}} = 180 \div 30$
$x = 6$
PROOF
$30 \times 6 = 180$
$15 \times 12 = 180$

2. $5 : 10 = 15 : x$
$\dfrac{\cancel{5}x}{\cancel{5}} = \dfrac{150}{5}$
$x = 30$
PROOF
$10 \times 15 = 150$
$5 \times 30 = 150$

3. $6 : 12 = 0.25 : x$
$6x = 12 \times 0.25 = 3$
$\dfrac{\cancel{6}}{\cancel{6}} x = \dfrac{3}{6} = 3 \div 6$
$x = 0.5$
PROOF
$12 \times 0.25 = 3$
$6 \times 0.5 = 3$

4. $7.5 : 12 = x : 28$
$12x = 7.5 \times 28 = 210$
$\dfrac{\cancel{12}}{\cancel{12}} x = \dfrac{210}{12} = 210 \div 12$
$x = 17.5$
PROOF
$7.5 \times 28 = 210$
$12 \times 17.5 = 210$

5. $0.4 : 12 = 10 : x$
$0.4x = 10 \times 12 = 120$
$\dfrac{\cancel{0.4}}{\cancel{0.4}} x = \dfrac{120}{0.4} = 120 \div 0.4$
$x = 300$
PROOF
$10 \times 12 = 120$
$300 \times 0.4 = 120$

WORKSHEET 2D (page 46)

1. KNOW   WANT TO KNOW
Bananas : Apples = x Bananas : Apples
$6 : 9 = x : 72$
$9x = 6 \times 72 = 432$
$\dfrac{\cancel{9}}{\cancel{9}} x = \dfrac{432}{9}$
$x = 48$ bananas
PROOF
$6 : 9 = 48 : 72$
$9 \times 48 = 432$
$6 \times 72 = 432$

2. KNOW   WANT TO KNOW
Scoops : Cups = x Scoops : Cups
$7 : 8 = x : 40$
$8x = 40 \times 7 = 280$
$\dfrac{\cancel{8}}{\cancel{8}} x = \dfrac{280}{8}$
$x = 35$ scoops
PROOF
$7 : 8 = 35 : 40$
$8 \times 35 = 280$
$7 \times 40 = 280$

remember   Scoops : Cups = Scoops : Cups
Apples : Bananas = Apples : Bananas
Miles : Gallons = Miles : Gallons

3. KNOW   WANT TO KNOW
Scoops : Cups = x Scoops : Cups
$4 : 6 = x : 18$
$6x = 72$
$\dfrac{\cancel{6}}{\cancel{6}}x = \dfrac{72}{6}$
$x = 12$ scoops of cocoa
PROOF
$4 : 6 = 12 : 18$
$6 \times 12 = 72$
$4 \times 18 = 72$

4. KNOW   WANT TO KNOW
2 tablets : 1 day = x tablets : 21 days
$x = 2 \times 21$
$x = 42$ tablets
PROOF
$2 : 1 = 42 : 21$
$2 \times 21 = 42$
$1 \times 42 = 42$

5. KNOW   WANT TO KNOW
Bushes : Trees = x Bushes : Trees
$8 : 2 = x : 36$
$2x = 8 \times 36 = 288$
$\dfrac{\cancel{2}}{\cancel{2}}x = \dfrac{288}{2}$
$x = 144$ bushes
PROOF
$8 : 2 = 144 : 36$
$8 \times 36 = 288$
$2 \times 144 = 288$

6. KNOW   WANT TO KNOW
Cups : Day = Cups : x Days
$2 : 1 = 24 : x$
$2x = 24$
$\dfrac{\cancel{2}}{\cancel{2}}x = \dfrac{24}{2}$
$x = 12$ days
PROOF
$2 : 1 = 24 : 12$
$1 \times 24 = 24$
$2 \times 12 = 24$

7. KNOW   WANT TO KNOW
Cups : Loaves = Cups : x Loaves
$4 : 3 = 24 : x$
$4x = 24 \times 3 = 72$
$\dfrac{\cancel{4}}{\cancel{4}}x = \dfrac{72}{4}$
$x = 18$ loaves
PROOF
$4 : 3 = 24 : 18$
$4 \times 18 = 72$
$3 \times 24 = 72$

8. KNOW   WANT TO KNOW
3 soda : $\dfrac{1}{2}$ fruit juice = x soda : 2 fruit juice
$\dfrac{1}{2}x = 3 \times 2$
$\dfrac{\cancel{\frac{1}{2}}}{\cancel{\frac{1}{2}}}x = \dfrac{6}{\frac{1}{2}} = 6 \div \dfrac{1}{2} = 6 \times \dfrac{2}{1}$
$x = 12$ cups soda
PROOF
$3 : \dfrac{1}{2} = 12 : 2$
$3 \times 2 = 6$
$\dfrac{1}{2} \times 12 = 6$

9. KNOW   WANT TO KNOW
4 Tbsp sugar : 1 glass = x Tbsp sugar : 6 glasses
$x = 6 \times 4$
$x = 24$ Tbsp sugar
PROOF
$4 : 1 = 24 : 6$
$4 \times 6 = 24$
$1 \times 24 = 24$

10. KNOW   WANT TO KNOW
4 capsules : 1 day = x capsules : 14 days
$x = 4 \times 14$
$x = 56$ capsules
PROOF
$4 : 1 = 56 : 14$
$4 \times 14 = 56$
$1 \times 56 = 56$

WORKSHEET 2E (page 47)

1. KNOW	WANT TO KNOW
200 envelopes : 1 box = 4000 envelopes : x boxes
$200x = 4000$
$\dfrac{200}{200}x = \dfrac{4000}{200}$
$x = 20$ boxes
PROOF
$200 \times 20 = 4000$
$1 \times 4000 = 4000$

2. KNOW	WANT TO KNOW
10 gowns : 1 package = 300 gowns : x packages
$10x = 300$
$\dfrac{10}{10}x = \dfrac{300}{10}$
$x = 30$ packages of gowns
PROOF
$10 \times 30 = 300$
$1 \times 300 = 300$

3. KNOW	WANT TO KNOW
1 computer : 18 students = x computers : 1260 students
$18x = 1260$
$\dfrac{18}{18}x = \dfrac{1260}{18}$
$x = 70$ computers
PROOF
$1 \times 1260 = 1260$
$18 \times 70 = 1260$

4. KNOW	WANT TO KNOW
3 glasses : 2 apples = 24 glasses : x apples
$3x = 48$
$\dfrac{3}{3}x = \dfrac{48}{3}$
$x = 16$ apples
PROOF
$3 \times 16 = 48$
$2 \times 24 = 48$

5. KNOW	WANT TO KNOW
6 pens : 8 pencils = x pens : 72 pencils
$8x = 432$
$\dfrac{8}{8}x = \dfrac{432}{8}$
$x = 54$ pens
PROOF
$6 \times 72 = 432$
$8 \times 54 = 432$

6. KNOW	WANT TO KNOW
1 nurse : 6 patients = x nurses : 36 patients
$6x = 36$
$\dfrac{6}{6}x = \dfrac{36}{6}$
$x = 6$ nurses
PROOF
$1 \times 36 = 36$
$6 \times 6 = 36$

7. KNOW	WANT TO KNOW
4 Tbsp : 8 oz water = x Tbsp : 56 oz water
$8x = 4 \times 56 = 224$
$\dfrac{8}{8}x = \dfrac{224}{8}$
$x = 28$ Tbsp formula
PROOF
$4 \times 56 = 224$
$8 \times 28 = 224$

8. KNOW	WANT TO KNOW
2 nurses : 12 hr = x nurses : 72 hr
$12x = 144$
$\dfrac{12}{12}x = \dfrac{144}{12}$
$x = 12$ nurses needed
PROOF
$12 \times 12 = 144$
$2 \times 72 = 144$

9. KNOW	WANT TO KNOW
3 aspirin : 1 day = x aspirin : 14 days
$x = 3 \times 14$
$x = 42$ aspirin tablets
PROOF
$3 \times 14 = 42$
$1 \times 42 = 42$

10. KNOW	WANT TO KNOW
5 mL : 1 day = 100 mL : x days
$\dfrac{5}{5}x = \dfrac{100}{5}$
$x = 20$ days
PROOF
$5 \times 20 = 100$
$1 \times 100 = 100$

WORKSHEET 2F (page 48)

1. a. KNOW　　　WANT TO KNOW
10 diapers : 1 day = 50 diapers : x days
$$\frac{\cancel{10}}{\cancel{10}}x = \frac{50}{10}$$
x = 5 days
PROOF
$10 \times 5 = 50$
$1 \times 50 = 50$

3. d. KNOW　　　WANT TO KNOW
4 tsp : 1 day = 80 tsp : x days
$$\frac{\cancel{4}}{\cancel{4}}x = \frac{80}{4}$$
x = 20 days
PROOF
$4 \times 20 = 80$
$1 \times 80 = 80$

5. b. KNOW　　　WANT TO KNOW
5 mL : 1 dose = 30 mL : x doses
$$\frac{\cancel{5}}{\cancel{5}}x = \frac{30}{5}$$
x = 6 doses
PROOF
$5 \times 6 = 30$
$1 \times 30 = 30$

7. a. KNOW　　　WANT TO KNOW
8 patients : 1 RN = 240 patients : x RNs
$$\frac{\cancel{8}}{\cancel{8}}x = \frac{240}{8}$$
x = 30 RNs
PROOF
$8 \times 30 = 240$
$1 \times 240 = 240$

9. c. KNOW　　　WANT TO KNOW
$15 : 1 hr = $450 : x hr
$$\frac{\cancel{15}}{\cancel{15}}x = \frac{450}{15}$$
x = 30 hr
PROOF
$15 \times 30 = 450$
$1 \times 450 = 450$

2. b. KNOW　　　WANT TO KNOW
10 syringes : 1 package = 120 syringes : x packages
$$\frac{\cancel{10}}{\cancel{10}}x = \frac{120}{10}$$
x = 12 packages
PROOF
$10 \times 12 = 120$
$1 \times 120 = 120$

4. d. KNOW　　　WANT TO KNOW
3 capsules : 1 day = x capsules : 21 days
$x = 3 \times 21$
x = 63 capsules
PROOF
$3 \times 21 = 63$
$1 \times 63 = 63$

6. b. KNOW　　　WANT TO KNOW
120 days : 15 depts = x days : 1 dept
$$\frac{\cancel{15}}{\cancel{15}}x = \frac{120}{15}$$
x = 8 days
PROOF
$120 \times 1 = 120$
$15 \times 8 = 120$

8. c. KNOW　　　WANT TO KNOW
4 oz : 1 portion = x oz : 20 portions
$x = 4 \times 20$
x = 80 oz
PROOF
$4 \times 20 = 80$
$1 \times 80 = 80$

10. c. KNOW　　　WANT TO KNOW
3 liters : 8 h = x liters : 72 h
$8x = 3 \times 72$
$$\frac{\cancel{8}}{\cancel{8}}x = \frac{216}{8}$$
x = 27 liters
PROOF
$3 \times 72 = 216$
$8 \times 27 = 216$

Answer Key　55

CHAPTER 2 FINAL: RATIO AND PROPORTION (page 49)

1. 15 supervisors
2. 25 nurses
3. 800 sheets
4. 224 patient discharges
5. $480
6. 30 CNAs
7. 4 administrators
8. $21,000 for 4 weeks
9. 21 interns
10. approximately 40 medication errors
11. 12 tablets
12. 9 PTO (personal time off) days
13. 10 days
14. 64 oz
15. 4 inservice days
16. 8 doses
17. 12 people
18. 32 RNs
19. 12 guest speakers
20. 240 tablets

Safe Medication Administration

Objectives
- State seven medication-related patient rights.
- Use The Joint Commission (TJC)– and Institute for Safe Medication Practices (ISMP)– approved abbreviations.
- Distinguish forms of oral medications.
- Convert 12-hour clock time to 24-hour clock time (military time).
- Interpret medication labels, prescriber orders, and medication administration records.
- Identify abbreviations and prescriber orders that require clarification.
- State recommended patient-safety practices related to medication administration.
- State the need for medication-related incident reports.
- Analyze medication errors using critical thinking.

Introduction Safe medication administration involves more than accurate dose measurement and calculations. Before calculation, the nurse must be able to interpret a variety of medication-related documents. Interpretation requires knowledge of medical terminology and abbreviations, as well as familiarity with drug label information and current drug references. Attention to detail and observance of patient medication-related rights are key elements of patient safety.

Vocabulary **Adverse Drug Event (ADE):** A medication-related occurrence that causes harm to a patient.

Drug Concentration (strength): The ratio of medication amount to a specific amount of liquid or solid (e.g., the amount of drug, such as 50 milligrams) per tablet or metric-calibrated teaspoon, or the amount of drug in the total quantity or weight supplied (e.g., 1 gram per 500-milliliter container).

Food and Drug Administration (FDA): The federal agency responsible for ensuring the safety, efficacy, and security of drugs, biological products such as vaccines, medical devices, and more. FDA approves medications for specific uses and sale in the United States.

Generic Drug: Drug product that is comparable to a brand-name drug product in dosage form, strength, route of administration, quality and performance characteristics, and intended use.

High-Alert Medication: ⚑ Medication identified by ISMP as capable of causing significant harm to patients if used in error. The red flag icon is placed next to high-alert medications in the text as a visual reminder to help the reader become familiar with some of these drugs.

Institute for Safe Medication Practices (ISMP): A nonprofit, voluntary agency dedicated to educating the health care community and consumers about safe medication practices (http://www.ismp.org).

Patent: A license giving the original manufacturer exclusive rights to manufacture the approved new product for a period of about 20 years from the time the patent was filed. When the patent expires, other companies may manufacture a generic copy of the product (e.g., drug).

Sentinel Event: The Joint Commission definition is an unexpected occurrence involving death or serious physical or psychological injury or the risk thereof. Serious injury specifically includes the loss of limb or function.

The Joint Commission (TJC): A national nonprofit, independent agency that provides accreditation and certification to health care organizations, with an emphasis on high standards and patient safety, including medication administration safety (http://www.jointcommission.org).

Unit-Dose Packaging: Non-reusable packaged and labeled single serving of drug dose ordered for the patient; usually used in health care institutions. May contain more than one unit of the drug, depending on the order (e.g., 2 tablets per serving). Keeps the medication free from contaminants, is opened just before using, and reduces the need for measurement and calculations, thus reducing the chance of dosage errors.

Usual Dose: The average dose ordered for the desired therapeutic effect for the target population (e.g., usual dose for children age 5 to 12 years: 1 teaspoon at bedtime for itching). Seen on manufacturers' prepared labels.

Patient Rights

There are many patient rights related to safe medication administration. As you read through a summary of seven major rights, think about the implications should one or more of these rights be violated.

Right Patient

The patient for whom the medication is ordered must be the patient who receives the medication. Because of the number of wrong patient errors, this issue is addressed in the first goal of The Joint Commission (TJC) Patient Safety Council (http://www.jointcommission.org/assets/1/6/2015_NPSG_CAH.pdf). A minimum of two separate written patient identifiers must be used. Identifiers may include the patient's name, an assigned identification number (which may be on the patient's wristband), telephone number, or other person-specific identifiers. Room number and bed number may not be used.

Right Drug

The nurse must be able to interpret drug orders and drug labels and to match the supplied drug exactly to the order. It must be the right drug for the right patient. Any portion of the process that is unclear or unfamiliar needs to be clarified promptly with a current drug reference, the prescriber, or the pharmacist before administering the medication (http://www.ismp.org/tools/confuseddrugnames.pdf).

Right Dose

The nurse needs to know that it is the ordered dose and the dose will be safe for the intended patient. Knowledge of measurement systems, abbreviations, dose calculation, and preparation technique is essential. A reliable current drug reference and/or pharmacist or prescriber must be consulted if there are questions. Attention to detail, decimals, and zeros is also vital to prevent errors.

Right Time

If administration of a medication is delayed, omitted, or given too early, there can be serious consequences. Some drugs must be given at specific, timed intervals to maintain stable blood levels for effectiveness. The Joint Commission and clinical agencies have policies and guidelines pertaining to prioritization of medication administration when several are to be given at about the same time. Certain medications and certain patient conditions take priority (http://www.ismp.org/tools/guidelines/acutecare/tasm.pdf).

> **CLINICAL ALERT!**
> It is very important to ask for help if the workload is too heavy to safely prepare or administer medications on time.

Right Route

The nurse must prepare the medication for the prescribed and safe drug route for the individual patient. Abbreviations are often used to designate the route. Many medications are available in solid and liquid forms for oral, intramuscular, and/or intravenous administration. The label must match the ordered route. If the patient refuses or is unable to tolerate the route ordered, the nurse must document the reason and include an assessment of the mental status of the patient. The prescriber must be reached promptly for a change in the order.

Right Documentation

Accurate and timely reporting and documentation in the patient medication record, as well as other records, is essential for patient safety. Documentation varies among agencies and is best learned during on-site orientation. Most agencies use some form of electronic documentation. "If it wasn't documented, it wasn't done" is an old adage that still holds true. Lack of prompt recording of medications given or omitted can lead to serious errors.

> **CLINICAL ALERT!**
> Documents are confidential. They cannot be photocopied and cannot be altered. Agencies have guidelines for entering amended information.

Right to Refuse a Medication

The patient is entitled to refuse a medication or treatment. The reason should be ascertained, reported promptly, and documented in a timely fashion so that corrective action can be taken if necessary. Include a comment on patient mental status when reporting and recording refusals. This affects subsequent actions to be taken.

> **CLINICAL ALERT!**
> It is illegal for the nurse to change a medication order. The prescriber must be contacted for a new order if any part of an order—the drug, the dose, the route, or the frequency—needs to be changed.

Medication Errors

Estimated rates of medication errors range from 2% to well over 10% when underreporting and wrong time of administration are considered. Many national organizations are working with manufacturers and health care agencies to reduce the error rate. Medication errors by the prescriber, the pharmacist, and the nurse may and do occur at any stage in the process:

- Prescription errors: drug type, dose, route, frequency, use of unapproved abbreviations, directions for use; if handwritten—legibility.
- Pharmacy errors: drug order misinterpretation or contraindication, transcribing and transferal, computer data entry, drug selection, preparation, labeling (including directions for use).
- Nurse errors: wrong patient, drug order misinterpretation or contraindication, drug selection, time, dose calculation and preparation, route, administration technique, and inappropriate follow-up evaluation.

CLINICAL ALERT!
The nurse who prepares and administers the medication offers the last step in administration safeguards to the patient.

CLINICAL ALERT!
Agency policies and needed corrective actions must be carried out promptly by the person who encounters an error *even* if the patient shows no sign of ill effects.

The following are a few of the many web sites that provide updates and articles about medication errors: their causes and prevention.

http://www.fda.gov/drugs/drugsafety/medicationerrors
http://www.ncbi.nlm.nih.gov/books/NBK133373
http://www.ismp.org
http://www.medscape.com
http://www.pharmacist.com

Abbreviations

The trend has been to reduce the number of approved abbreviations used in medical records and to decrease handwritten orders and records because of medication errors due to misinterpretation. Nevertheless, there are still many approved abbreviations to be learned to interpret patient medical records, including prescriber orders, medication administration records, drug literature, and drug labels. The nurse must also avoid writing abbreviations that are on TJC's "Do Not Use" list (Table 3-1) and ISMP's List of Error-Prone Abbreviations, Symbols, and Dose Designations" (Figure 3-1). You will have to double check and review the approved abbreviations frequently. Use the worksheets provided to reinforce your memory.

Table 3-1 The Joint Commission's Official "Do Not Use" List*

Do Not Use	Potential Problem	Use Instead
U, u (unit)	Mistaken for "0" (zero), the number "4" (four), or "cc"	Write "unit"
IU (International Unit)	Mistaken for "IV" (intravenous) or the number "10" (ten)	Write "International Unit"
Q.D., QD, q.d., qd (daily)	Mistaken for each other	Write "daily"
Q.O.D., QOD, q.o.d., qod (every other day)	Period after the Q mistaken for "I" and the "O" mistaken for "I"	Write "every other day"
Trailing zero (X.0 mg)†	Decimal point is missed	Write X mg
Lack of leading zero (.X mg)		Write 0.X mg
MS	Can mean morphine sulfate or magnesium sulfate	Write "morphine sulfate"
MSO_4 and $MgSO_4$	Confused for one another	Write "magnesium sulfate"

From The Joint Commission: Official "Do Not Use" List, 2015. Retrieved from http://www.jointcommission.org/assets/1/18/dnu_list.pdf.
*Applies to all orders and all medication-related documentation that is handwritten (including free-text computer entry) or on preprinted forms.
†Exception: A "trailing zero" may be used only where required to demonstrate the level of precision of the value being reported, such as for laboratory results, imaging studies that report size of lesions, or catheter/tube sizes. It may not be used in medication orders or other medication-related documentation.

Institute for Safe Medication Practices

ISMP's List of *Error-Prone Abbreviations, Symbols,* and *Dose Designations*

The abbreviations, symbols, and dose designations found in this table have been reported to ISMP through the ISMP National Medication Errors Reporting Program (ISMP MERP) as being frequently misinterpreted and involved in harmful medication errors. They should **NEVER** be used when communicating medical information. This includes internal communications, telephone/verbal prescriptions, computer-generated labels, labels for drug storage bins, medication administration records, as well as pharmacy and prescriber computer order entry screens.

Abbreviations	Intended Meaning	Misinterpretation	Correction
μg	Microgram	Mistaken as "mg"	Use "mcg"
AD, AS, AU	Right ear, left ear, each ear	Mistaken as OD, OS, OU (right eye, left eye, each eye)	Use "right ear," "left ear," or "each ear"
OD, OS, OU	Right eye, left eye, each eye	Mistaken as AD, AS, AU (right ear, left ear, each ear)	Use "right eye," "left eye," or "each eye"
BT	Bedtime	Mistaken as "BID" (twice daily)	Use "bedtime"
cc	Cubic centimeters	Mistaken as "u" (units)	Use "mL"
D/C	Discharge or discontinue	Premature discontinuation of medications if D/C (intended to mean "discharge") has been misinterpreted as "discontinued" when followed by a list of discharge medications	Use "discharge" and "discontinue"
IJ	Injection	Mistaken as "IV" or "intrajugular"	Use "injection"
IN	Intranasal	Mistaken as "IM" or "IV"	Use "intranasal" or "NAS"
HS	Half-strength	Mistaken as bedtime	Use "half-strength" or "bedtime"
hs	At bedtime, hours of sleep	Mistaken as half-strength	
IU**	International unit	Mistaken as IV (intravenous) or 10 (ten)	Use "units"
o.d. or OD	Once daily	Mistaken as "right eye" (OD-oculus dexter), leading to oral liquid medications administered in the eye	Use "daily"
OJ	Orange juice	Mistaken as OD or OS (right or left eye); drugs meant to be diluted in orange juice may be given in the eye	Use "orange juice"
Per os	By mouth, orally	The "os" can be mistaken as "left eye" (OS-oculus sinister)	Use "PO," "by mouth," or "orally"
q.d. or QD**	Every day	Mistaken as q.i.d., especially if the period after the "q" or the tail of the "q" is misunderstood as an "i"	Use "daily"
qhs	Nightly at bedtime	Mistaken as "qhr" or every hour	Use "nightly"
qn	Nightly or at bedtime	Mistaken as "qh" (every hour)	Use "nightly" or "at bedtime"
q.o.d. or QOD**	Every other day	Mistaken as "q.d." (daily) or "q.i.d. (four times daily) if the "o" is poorly written	Use "every other day"
q1d	Daily	Mistaken as q.i.d. (four times daily)	Use "daily"
q6PM, etc.	Every evening at 6 PM	Mistaken as every 6 hours	Use "daily at 6 PM" or "6 PM daily"
SC, SQ, sub q	Subcutaneous	SC mistaken as SL (sublingual); SQ mistaken as "5 every;" the "q" in "sub q" has been mistaken as "every" (e.g., a heparin dose ordered "sub q 2 hours before surgery" misunderstood as every 2 hours before surgery)	Use "subcut" or "subcutaneously"
ss	Sliding scale (insulin) or ½ (apothecary)	Mistaken as "55"	Spell out "sliding scale;" use "one-half" or "½"
SSRI	Sliding scale regular insulin	Mistaken as selective-serotonin reuptake inhibitor	Spell out "sliding scale (insulin)"
SSI	Sliding scale insulin	Mistaken as Strong Solution of Iodine (Lugol's)	
i/d	One daily	Mistaken as "tid"	Use "1 daily"
TIW or tiw	3 times a week	Mistaken as "3 times a day" or "twice in a week"	Use "3 times weekly"
U or u**	Unit	Mistaken as the number 0 or 4, causing a 10-fold overdose or greater (e.g., 4U seen as "40" or 4u seen as "44"); mistaken as "cc" so dose given in volume instead of units (e.g., 4u seen as 4cc)	Use "unit"
UD	As directed ("ut dictum")	Mistaken as unit dose (e.g., diltiazem 125 mg IV infusion "UD" misinterpreted as meaning to give the entire infusion as a unit [bolus] dose)	Use "as directed"
Dose Designations and Other Information	**Intended Meaning**	**Misinterpretation**	**Correction**
Trailing zero after decimal point (e.g., 1.0 mg)**	1 mg	Mistaken as 10 mg if the decimal point is not seen	Do not use trailing zeros for doses expressed in whole numbers
"Naked" decimal point (e.g., .5 mg)**	0.5 mg	Mistaken as 5 mg if the decimal point is not seen	Use zero before a decimal point when the dose is less than a whole unit
Abbreviations such as mg. or mL. with a period following the abbreviation	mg mL	The period is unnecessary and could be mistaken as the number 1 if written poorly	Use mg, mL, etc. without a terminal period

FIGURE 3-1 ISMP's List of Error-Prone Abbreviations, Symbols, and Dose Designations. (© ISMP, 2015. Reprinted with permission.)

Continued

Institute for Safe Medication Practices

ISMP's List of Error-Prone Abbreviations, Symbols, and Dose Designations (continued)

Dose Designations and Other Information	Intended Meaning	Misinterpretation	Correction
Drug name and dose run together (especially problematic for drug names that end in "l" such as Inderal40 mg; Tegretol300 mg)	Inderal 40 mg Tegretol 300 mg	Mistaken as Inderal 140 mg Mistaken as Tegretol 1300 mg	Place adequate space between the drug name, dose, and unit of measure
Numerical dose and unit of measure run together (e.g., 10mg, 100mL)	10 mg 100 mL	The "m" is sometimes mistaken as a zero or two zeros, risking a 10- to 100-fold overdose	Place adequate space between the dose and unit of measure
Large doses without properly placed commas (e.g., 100000 units; 1000000 units)	100,000 units 1,000,000 units	100000 has been mistaken as 10,000 or 1,000,000; 1000000 has been mistaken as 100,000	Use commas for dosing units at or above 1,000, or use words such as 100 "thousand" or 1 "million" to improve readability

Drug Name Abbreviations	Intended Meaning	Misinterpretation	Correction
To avoid confusion, do not abbreviate drug names when communicating medical information. Examples of drug name abbreviations involved in medication errors include:			
APAP	acetaminophen	Not recognized as acetaminophen	Use complete drug name
ARA A	vidarabine	Mistaken as cytarabine (ARA C)	Use complete drug name
AZT	zidovudine (Retrovir)	Mistaken as azathioprine or aztreonam	Use complete drug name
CPZ	Compazine (prochlorperazine)	Mistaken as chlorpromazine	Use complete drug name
DPT	Demerol-Phenergan-Thorazine	Mistaken as diphtheria-pertussis-tetanus (vaccine)	Use complete drug name
DTO	Diluted tincture of opium, or deodorized tincture of opium (Paregoric)	Mistaken as tincture of opium	Use complete drug name
HCl	hydrochloric acid or hydrochloride	Mistaken as potassium chloride (The "H" is misinterpreted as "K")	Use complete drug name unless expressed as a salt of a drug
HCT	hydrocortisone	Mistaken as hydrochlorothiazide	Use complete drug name
HCTZ	hydrochlorothiazide	Mistaken as hydrocortisone (seen as HCT250 mg)	Use complete drug name
MgSO4**	magnesium sulfate	Mistaken as morphine sulfate	Use complete drug name
MS, MSO4**	morphine sulfate	Mistaken as magnesium sulfate	Use complete drug name
MTX	methotrexate	Mistaken as mitoxantrone	Use complete drug name
PCA	procainamide	Mistaken as patient controlled analgesia	Use complete drug name
PTU	propylthiouracil	Mistaken as mercaptopurine	Use complete drug name
T3	Tylenol with codeine No. 3	Mistaken as liothyronine	Use complete drug name
TAC	triamcinolone	Mistaken as tetracaine, Adrenalin, cocaine	Use complete drug name
TNK	TNKase	Mistaken as "TPA"	Use complete drug name
ZnSO4	zinc sulfate	Mistaken as morphine sulfate	Use complete drug name

Stemmed Drug Names	Intended Meaning	Misinterpretation	Correction
"Nitro" drip	nitroglycerin infusion	Mistaken as sodium nitroprusside infusion	Use complete drug name
"Norflox"	norfloxacin	Mistaken as Norflex	Use complete drug name
"IV Vanc"	intravenous vancomycin	Mistaken as Invanz	Use complete drug name

Symbols	Intended Meaning	Misinterpretation	Correction
ℨ	Dram	Symbol for dram mistaken as "3"	Use the metric system
ℳ	Minim	Symbol for minim mistaken as "mL"	
x3d	For three days	Mistaken as "3 doses"	Use "for three days"
> and <	Greater than and less than	Mistaken as opposite of intended; mistakenly use incorrect symbol; "< 10" mistaken as "40"	Use "greater than" or "less than"
/ (slash mark)	Separates two doses or indicates "per"	Mistaken as the number 1 (e.g., "25 units/10 units" misread as "25 units and 110" units)	Use "per" rather than a slash mark to separate doses
@	At	Mistaken as "2"	Use "at"
&	And	Mistaken as "2"	Use "and"
+	Plus or and	Mistaken as "4"	Use "and"
°	Hour	Mistaken as a zero (e.g., q2° seen as q 20)	Use "hr," "h," or "hour"
Ø or ∅	zero, null sign	Mistaken as numerals 4, 6, 8, and 9	Use 0 or zero, or describe intent using whole words

**These abbreviations are included on The Joint Commission's "minimum list" of dangerous abbreviations, acronyms, and symbols that must be included on an organization's "Do Not Use" list, effective January 1, 2004. Visit www.jointcommission.org for more information about this Joint Commission requirement.

© ISMP 2013. Permission is granted to reproduce material with proper attribution for internal use within healthcare organizations. Other reproduction is prohibited without written permission from ISMP. Report actual and potential medication errors to the ISMP National Medication Errors Reporting Program (ISMP MERP) via the Web at www.ismp.org or by calling 1-800-FAIL-SAF(E).

FIGURE 3-1, cont'd ISMP's List of Error-Prone Abbreviations, Symbols, and Dose Designations. (© ISMP, 2015. Reprinted with permission.)

The Joint Commission's Official 2015 "Do Not Use" List

The Joint Commission developed its first "do not use" list of abbreviations in 2004. The list was incorporated into the Information Management Standards in 2010. This list currently does not apply to electronic medical records or computerized physician order entry (CPOE) systems, although these systems may be brought into compliance in the future. It is advised that these dangerous abbreviations, acronyms, symbols, and dose designations should be eliminated from future development and upgrades to software used by health care providers.

Answers on page 93

WORKSHEET 3A | Abbreviations, Symbols, and Acronyms

Directions: For medication safety, it is important to be very familiar with The Joint Commission "Do Not Use" list (see Table 3-1) and the Institute for Safe Medication Practices (ISMP) Error-Prone Abbreviations list (see Figure 3-1). Answer the following questions:

TJC: "Do Not Use" List (p. 60)

1. What are three mistakes that can be made if the abbreviation "U" for units is misread?

2. How can periods and "O" be misread?

3. How can trailing zeros and lack of leading zeros result in a dose error?

4. Which documents must be in compliance with the TJC official "Do Not Use" list?

5. Which is the preferred abbreviation for milliliters? cc, ml, or mL? Why?

ISMP: Dose Designation and Symbols Sections (p. 62):

6. How can medication names ending in the letter "l" cause a major dose error?

7. Why should large doses in the thousands have commas?

8. How should a numerical dose and unit of measure such as "ten milligrams" be spaced to avoid 10- to 100-fold overdoses?

9. How can a slash mark be misread, and what word should be used instead of a slash?

10. How can 3xd be misinterpreted, and how can it be avoided?

Medication Forms: Solids and Liquids

Medications can be provided in a variety of forms: solids, liquids, inhalants, skin patches, suppositories, and others. It is very important to distinguish the forms and to ascertain the precise form ordered by the prescriber and supplied for administration. The form affects the rate of absorption and distribution in the body. It also affects the route of administration.

Solid Oral Medications

- Plain tablets (Figure 3-2, *A*): compressed powdered drugs
- Scored tablets (Figure 3-2, *B*): tablets with a dividing line; the *only kind* of tablet that can be cut, if an ordered dose amount is for half a tablet
- Caplets: tablets small or large, oval-shaped like a capsule

- Enteric-coated tablets (Figure 3-2, *C*): tablets with coating to permit them to dissolve in the small intestine instead of the stomach, where it might cause gastric irritation
- Capsules (Figure 3-2, *D*): soluble case—usually gelatin—that holds liquid or dry particles of the drug; can be hard or soft (softgels), in one piece or two pieces
- Delayed release (DR) (Figure 3-2, *E*): extended release (ER), slow release (SR), controlled release (CR), long acting (LA), extra long acting (EL), controlled dose (CD)
- Double strength (DS, ES): extra-strength medications
- Powders and granules (Figure 3-2, *F*): loose or molded drug substance usually to be dissolved in liquid or nonessential food

FIGURE 3-2 Various solid oral drug forms. **A,** Plain tablets. **B,** Scored tablets. **C,** Enteric-coated tablets. **D,** Capsules. **E,** Extended-release tablets. **F,** Granules. (Courtesy Amanda Politte, St. Louis, MO.)

CLINICAL ALERT!
Be aware that the names, abbreviations, and length of release time for these medications vary among tablets and capsules. They are not standardized among manufacturers.

CLINICAL ALERT!
Never crush or cut delayed-release gel or enteric-coated medications. Doing so will accelerate their release into the body's circulation and is a reportable medication error. Only cut scored tablets if needed (Figures 3-3 to 3-5).

CLINICAL ALERT!
Never crush or cut capsules. Occasionally a two-piece capsule may be opened and the contents placed in a nonessential food or liquid for a patient who cannot swallow capsules, but only if the prescriber permits.

Liquid Oral Medications

- Aqueous suspensions: solid particles suspended in liquid that must be mixed well before administration
- Elixirs: sweetened alcohol and water solutions
- Emulsions: fats or oils suspended in liquid by an emulsifier
- Extracts: syrups or derived forms of active drugs
- Fluid extracts: concentrated alcoholic liquid extracts of plants or vegetables
- Solutions: mixtures in which solids are fully dissolved (vs. aqueous suspensions)

FIGURE 3-3 Pill splitter. Pill splitter only splits pills that are scored with an indented line.

FIGURE 3-4 Silent Knight® Tablet Crushing System. A pill crusher that contains disposable pouches for each tablet to prevent cross-contamination with prior crushed medications. (Used with permission by Links Medical Products, Inc., Irvine, California.)

FIGURE 3-5 Scored tablet. A scored tablet may be cut in half if a half dose is ordered. Non-scored tablets may not be cut.

FIGURE 3-6 Prefilled oral syringe.

FIGURE 3-7 **A,** Medicine dropper. **B,** Measuring teaspoon. **C,** Liquid medication in *(1)* a single-unit-dose package, *(2)* liquid measured in medicine cup, and *(3)* oral liquid medicine in syringe. (**A** and **B** from Clayton BD, Willihnganz M: *Basic pharmacology for nurses,* ed. 16, St. Louis, 2013, Mosby. **C** from Perry AG, Potter PA, Ostendorf WR: *Clinical nursing skills and techniques,* ed. 8, St. Louis, 2014, Mosby.)

The trend is to supply liquid oral medications in individual, calibrated unit-dose cups and calibrated plastic droppers and spoons to reduce calculation and measurement errors* (Figures 3-6 and 3-7).

---

*Liquids are also supplied in injectable (also known as parenteral) forms, such as ampules, vials, and prefilled injectable syringes and other devices. These are discussed in Chapter 5 and later chapters.

CHAPTER 3 Safe Medication Administration

Household/metric
Tbs/mL

Household/metric
oz/mL

2 TBSP — 30 ML
— 25 ML
Read here ↓
— 20 ML
1 TBSP — 15 ML
2 TSP — 10 ML
1 TSP — 5 ML
½ TSP —

1 oz — 30 ML
— 25 ML
— 20 ML
½ oz — 15 ML
— 10 ML
— 5 ML

The "Read Here" arrow points to the meniscus, the center of the slightly concave liquid surface where liquid medications should be measured. The meniscus is best seen on a flat surface at eye level.

Occasionally a liquid medication must be poured from a multidose bottle into a metric-calibrated cup. The dose must be measured on a level surface and at eye level.

CLINICAL ALERT!

Teach patients not to substitute household utensils such as spoons and cups when measuring medications at home. The sizes vary considerably and, if used, will result in an underdose or overdose of the medication. The metric-calibrated equipment that is supplied with the medication must be used to obtain the exact dose ordered. Also teach patients to discard unused or excess medication rather than to save it or pour it back into the original container.

Answers on page 93

WORKSHEET 3B | Abbreviations for Drug Forms

Study the abbreviations on the first page of the text. Then provide the abbreviations in the spaces provided.

Term	Recommended Abbreviation
capsule*	
tablet	
fluid	
solution	
suspension	
elixir	
teaspoon	
tablespoon	
liquid	
ounce	
double-strength	
extended release*	
long acting*	
sustained release*	
controlled release*	

*Do not crush these medications.

> **CLINICAL ALERT!**
> Study examples of abbreviations that have caused errors and are best written out (see Table 3-1 and Figure 3-1).

Routes of Medication Administration

There are two major divisions of routes:

1. **Parenteral** (injectables)
   - *Intradermal (ID):* between epidermis and dermis
   - *Intravenous (IV):* into vein
   - *Intramuscular (IM):* into muscle
   - *Subcutaneous (Subcut):* "under the skin" (literal definition); in practice, injected into fatty layer below the dermis
   - *Epidural:* into space between vertebral wall and dura mater (dural membrane that holds spinal fluid and nerve roots)
   - *Intrathecal:* into spinal fluid

2. **Nonparenteral** (all routes administered as a noninjectable)
   - *Oral (PO, po):* swallowed by mouth
   - *Sublingual (SL):* dissolved under the tongue directly into circulation, bypassing the gastrointestinal tract for faster absorption (e.g., nitroglycerin for cardiac-related pain)
   - *Buccal (bucc):* dissolved inside the cheek, absorbed directly into circulation, bypassing the gastrointestinal tract for faster absorption
   - *Topical (top):* applied to skin surface for local effects
   - *Transdermal (skin):* for systemic effects (e.g., transdermal patches deliver pain-relief medication, hormones)
   - *Other:* eyes, ears, lungs (respiratory) (inhalants), nose, nasogastric (NG) (nose to stomach), gastric (g) (stomach), intestine (enteral), rectum, vagina (vag)

CLINICAL RELEVANCE
Most medications are ordered for the oral (po), intravenous (IV), intramuscular (IM), or subcutaneous (Subcut) routes.

> **CLINICAL ALERT!**
> An error with medication routes may result in a serious adverse drug event (ADE). The patient and family must be taught the correct use and/or application of the drug and give return demonstrations during hospitalization and at the time of discharge. One session of teaching is often insufficient. Provide the patient with written follow-up instructions. Patients have been known to apply narcotic transdermal patches over old ones or on the wrong part of the body; to chew or swallow sublingual or buccal medications, or to use bare hands for topically applying a medication when hands should be gloved or an implement used for application to avoid an overdose or injury to the patient (or person applying the medication) and/or contamination of the product.

To reduce the chance of errors, have a family member present and use effective communication, including assessment of mental status and comprehension via feedback.

> **CLINICAL ALERT!**
> The nurse may not legally change the route of medication administration. The provider must be contacted.

WORKSHEET 3C: Abbreviations for Time and Route

Answers on page 94

Study the approved and recommended abbreviations on the first page of the text and their patterns of similarities and differences as well as The Joint Commission's "Do Not Use" list in Table 3-1 and the Institute for Safe Medication Practices List of Error-Prone Abbreviations, Symbols, and Dose Designations (see Figure 3-1). Then enter the approved or recommended abbreviation in the space provided.

Worksheet 3C: Abbreviations for Time and Route Table

Time	Abbreviation (if Applicable)	Time	Abbreviation (if Applicable)
before		after	
before meals		after meals	
daily	Write out daily	three times a day	
twice a day		every other day	Write out every other day
every day	Write out every day	every 6 hours	
every 4 hours		every 12 hours	
whenever necessary		as desired, freely	
immediately, at once		bedtime	Write out bedtime
with		without	
Route	**Abbreviation (if Applicable)**	**Route**	**Abbreviation (if Applicable)**
by mouth		nothing by mouth	
intravenous		intramuscular	
sublingual		subcutaneous	
intradermal		suppository*	
left eye	Write out left eye	right ear	Write out right ear
nasogastric		per gastrostomy tube	

*Orders for suppositories require further route identification per vagina, per rectum, or per urethra.

Measurement Abbreviations

Metric abbreviations for weight and volume are the most frequently seen abbreviations in medication orders. They will be used for calculations in future chapters. Metric abbreviations are the same for single and plural measurements. They are not pluralized. Two milligrams would be written *2 mg* not *2 mgs*.

Answers on page 94

WORKSHEET 3D | Abbreviations for Drug Measurements

Study the abbreviations on the first page of the text. Pay attention to uppercase and lowercase letters when learning the abbreviations. There are only a few instances when uppercase is employed. Then provide the approved abbreviations for the measurements.

Metric Measurement Term*	Abbreviation (if Applicable)
microgram(s)	
milligram(s)	
gram(s)	
kilogram(s)	
milliliter(s)	
milliequivalent(s)	
unit	Write out unit
international unit	Write out international unit
liter	
square meter	
Other Measurement Term	**Abbreviation (if Applicable)**
one half	Write out one half
teaspoon	
tablespoon	
pound	

*The metric abbreviations are the same for singular and plural measurements.

Medication Labels

Medication labels contain required critical information for patient safety. The label must be read carefully to ensure that the medication is precisely what the prescriber ordered.

Drug Names

Drugs may have three names:
1. The **brand name,** which begins with a capital letter, that distinguishes a manufacturer's product from similar products from other manufacturers
2. The **generic name** is the official name by which a drug is commonly available, unprotected by trademark; all drugs, including over-the-counter medications, must have the generic name on the label
3. A long **chemical name,** such as acetylsalicylic acid (the chemical name for aspirin); this name is rarely seen on labels.

CHAPTER 3 Safe Medication Administration

Brand/Trade Name and Registration of Name

Companies that spend millions of dollars and years to be the first to develop an FDA-approved new drug can receive two important official protections from U.S. governmental agencies. The first is registration of the **brand name** (proprietary name) the company selects with the U.S. Food and Drug Administration; it is designated on the label with the **registration symbol** ® after the proprietary name. As long as the registration is maintained, *no other company can use that name.* The second protection is the **patent**, which gives exclusive manufacturing rights to the company for a specific amount of time.

Generic Drugs

Generic drugs are copies of the original drug product that are produced by companies after the original manufacturer's patent expires. The *only* differences permitted by the FDA between the original and the generic product are (1) inactive ingredients, (2) size, (3) color, and (4) shape. There are thousands of generic drugs with and without their own brand names on the market because many patents have expired in recent years. Generic drugs are considerably *less expensive* than the original product because the drug formula has already been invented, tested, and approved and is available.

Examine the following labels. They contain a surprisingly large amount of information in a small space. They *may* contain a trade/brand name, registered or unregistered. They *must* contain a generic (official name); national drug code (NDC) number; manufacturer name; drug concentration (unit dose) and form (tablet, capsule, liquid, suppository, etc.); bar code; total amount in container; route to be administered; expiration date; lot (batch) number; any special storage needs; warnings, if needed; and directions for use.

Additional information, such as the usual dose, may be included. The abbreviations for United States Pharmacopeia (USP) and National Formulary (NF) may appear next to the name, indicating that the product adheres to the national legal standards of identity, purity, quality, strength, labeling, and other specific requirements.

Note that the generic name is in lowercase. The main information on the label is contained in the bar code as well. This lot (batch) expired in 2008. The nurse cannot give an expired medication. "Rx only" means this is a prescription-only medication. The lot (batch) number and expiration date are added when the container is filled and are placed close to each other.

The FDA web site http://www.accessdata.fda.gov/scripts/cder/ndc/dsp_searchresult.cfm maintains all the information on drug labels and more. You can search the site for information on a drug by entering any one of five types of data from the label: proprietary name, application number, active ingredient, NDC number, and labeler. The web site will then show the current status of the drug. It will either state "no match" if the drug is not currently approved or has been withdrawn, or it will list the current manufacturers and all the forms and dosages available by each manufacturer. Additional important information about the medication will be shown.

- **NDC code**
- **Trade name**
- **Generic name**
- **Drug concentration (per tablet)**
- **Total amount in container**
- **Form**
- **Storage**
- **Lot number**
- **Expiration date**
- **Manufacturer**

Registered trademark brand name: Tenormin, the exclusive brand name for this antihypertensive medication.

Generic official name: atenolol; all manufacturers must include the generic official name on all labels of the drug.

Drug dose: 50 mg.

Drug form (tablet, capsule, granules, suppository, inhaler, liquid, etc.): tablet.

Drug concentration (dose per weight or quantity): 50 mg per tablet.

Bar code: placed near the drug dose; contains the NDC code.

NDC code: national drug code contains label information.

Total amount in container: 100 tablets in this multidose container.

Lot (specific batch) and *expiration date:* lot and expiration date appear adjacent to each other on the label when the container was filled.

Storage directions: storage temperatures and conditions (some storage directions pertain to keeping a drug in a dark or light area).

Special warnings: "Keep out of reach of children."

Other information: usual dose.

Note: the implied oral route is not on this label. All new labels must specify the route.

There are about 128 generic copies of Tenormin. Many of the manufacturers have their own brand names, which can be very similar, such as Alol, Adelol, Atol, Atenol, to name a few.

To calculate a dose, enter the drug concentration on the left side of the equation:

WHAT YOU HAVE

$$50 \text{ mg} : 1 \text{ tablet} = \text{ or } \left(\frac{50 \text{ mg}}{1 \text{ tablet}} = \right)$$

Note that the route for this drug is *injectable:* intramuscular (IM) or intravenous (IV). Also note the two types of print on the registered brand name—MethylPREDNISolone—an antiinflammatory drug used for allergies, arthritis, psoriasis, and other indications. The tall letters are called "tall man letters" to draw attention to a drug name that is similar to one or more other drugs by emphasizing the main differences in the spelling. Other examples include medroxyPROGESTERone, a hormone used for female contraception, among other uses; and methylTESTOSTERone, a hormone used to treat testosterone deficiency, among other uses. Many drugs are "look alike, sound alike," which has led to serious medication errors (https://www.ismp.org/tools/confuseddrugnames.pdf). Obviously, confusion about these three names could lead to serious medical issues. Because of medication errors attributed to labels, the FDA, ISMP, and other organizations have been working with manufacturers to reduce errors by improving and standardizing label packaging, design, and content.

This form of Zofran (ondansetron) is a *liquid oral solution* in a multidose container. The usual order for medications is 1 or 2 servings of the supplied concentration, in this case 4 mg per 5 mL or 8 mg per 10 mL. The trend for patient safety is to increase the supply of unit-dose packaging. If this multidose container was mistaken for the unit-dose ordered, such an error would amount to a dose of 40 mg, 10 times the usual dose.

CLINICAL ALERT!
Distinguish unit-dose containers from multidose containers.

Do not use a slash for "per." It can be mistaken for the number 1; for example, 4 mg/5 mL might be misinterpreted as 15 mL.

This oral-route liquid suspension is packaged in a unit-dose (usual single serving) container. Unit-dose containers are not reusable. Acetaminophen is a generic form of the original drug Tylenol. The patent for Tylenol expired in 2011, and over 600 generics containing acetaminophen—many with their own brand names—have been manufactured. This solution concentration is 160 mg per 5 mL and is indicated for pediatric use. The trend is to package more medications specifically in doses that are usually prescribed for children. This reduces the need for calculating a child's fractional portion of an adult dose, thereby reducing the chance of error.

To calculate a dose, place the given concentration per unit on the left side of the equation:

$$160 \text{ mg} : 5 \text{ mL} = \text{ or } \left(\frac{160 \text{ mg}}{5 \text{ mL}} = \right)$$

> **CLINICAL ALERT!**
> Do not confuse aspirin with acetaminophen products. The two often are prescribed for similar conditions. Injury or death can result. They are contained in many hundreds of products. Many have their own brand names.

Answers on page 95

WORKSHEET 3E | Interpreting Medication Labels

Examine the following labels and fill in the requested information.

What you have, the supplied drug concentration (e.g., 100 mg per tablet or 50 mg per 2 mL), is determined from the label and inserted on the left side of your ratio and proportion in colon or fraction form.

1.

   a. National Drug Code number
   b. Proprietary (registered) brand name
   c. Generic (official) name
   d. Drug concentration
   e. Ratio for "what you have" (dose concentration supplied per tablet, capsule, milliliter)

2.

   a. Generic name
   b. Dose in micrograms (mcg) and equivalent dose in milligrams (mg)
   c. Ratio for "what you have"

CHAPTER 3 Safe Medication Administration

3.

AMOXICILLIN for Oral Suspension USP
NDC 0093-4150-80
equivalent to 125 mg per 5 mL amoxicillin when reconstituted according to directions.

Usual Dosage: **Adults** — 250 mg - 500 mg every eight hours, depending on type and severity of infection.
Children — 20 mg - 40 mg/kg/day in divided doses every eight hours, depending on type and severity of infection.

℞ only
See accompanying literature.
WARNING: NOT FOR INJECTION

150 mL (when mixed)

TEVA

Amoxicillin trihydrate equivalent to 3.75 g amoxicillin.
Store dry powder at 20° to 25°C (68° to 77°F) (See USP Controlled Room Temperature).
TO THE PHARMACIST: Prepare suspension at time of dispensing. Add to the bottle a total of 113 mL of water. For ease in preparation, tap bottle to loosen powder, add the water in two portions, shaking well after each addition. The resulting suspension will contain amoxicillin trihydrate equivalent to 125 mg amoxicillin in each 5 mL (teaspoonful).
Oversized bottle permits shaking space.
IMPORTANT
When stored at room temperature or in refrigerator discard unused portion of reconstituted suspension after 14 days.
Date of reconstitution:
Shake well before using. Keep tightly closed.
KEEP THIS AND ALL MEDICATIONS OUT OF THE REACH OF CHILDREN.
Manufactured in Canada By:
NOVOPHARM LIMITED
Toronto, Canada M1B 2K9
Manufactured For:
TEVA PHARMACEUTICALS USA
Sellersville, PA 18960
Rev. E 7/2005

a. Drug form
b. Drug concentration
c. Usual dose for adults
d. Is this a single-dose or multidose container?
e. If multidose, how many times more is total dose in mL after reconstitution than the single dose in mL?
f. Ratio for "what you have"

4.
a. Proprietary name for this compound drug
b. Generic names and dose for each drug
c. Form
d. Meaning of "DS"
e. Ratio for "what you have," if applicable

100 Tablets NDC 0173-0853-55
SEPTRA® DS
Double Strength
(trimethoprim and sulfamethoxazole)
Each scored tablet contains 160 mg trimethoprim and 800 mg sulfamethoxazole.
CAUTION: Federal law prohibits dispensing without prescription.
U.S. Patent No. 4,209,513 (Tablet)
Glaxo Wellcome Inc.
Research Triangle Park, NC 27709
595493
LOT
EXP

Store at 15° to 25°C (59° to 77°F) in a dry place. Dispense in tight, light-resistant container as defined in the U.S.P.
For indications, dosage, precautions, etc., see accompanying package insert.
6505-01-016-1470
Rev. 5/96
Made in U.S.A.

🛑 CLINICAL ALERT!

Compound drugs, such as Septra DS, are usually ordered by name and number of servings of the dose provided. The labels *always* provide the concentration of each drug. The medication *orders* for a compound drug seldom mention the drug concentrations for a compound drug *unless it is a scored tablet* that allows a half dose of the drug on hand.

Three Reasons to Double Check a DS Medication

1. The abbreviation DS reveals that there is also a weaker concentration, "regular strength," available. It alerts the nurse to double check the dose and whether the order is actually for DS or regular strength.
2. The most common order for an oral compound drug is one tablet or capsule. Recheck an order that exceeds a single dose of a compound drug.
3. When medication is provided in a scored tablet, the dose needs to be rechecked. Just because the tablet is scored does not necessarily mean that the order will call for half the dose on hand.

5.

[Nitroglycerin Tablets, USP 0.6 mg (1/100 gr), 100 Sublingual Tablets, Glenmark, NDC 68462-147-01]

    a. Generic name
    b. Route on label and definition
    c. Reason you would assess patient's mental status and experience with this medication before administering
    d. Ratio for "what you have"

Medication Orders

Medication orders must be legible and complete. They may be handwritten, faxed, or entered into a computer (computerized physician order entry [CPOE]) by the provider or pharmacist (Figure 3-8). Handwritten orders are becoming less common because of misinterpretations resulting in medication errors.

GENERAL HOSPITAL

Patient: Greiga, Anna R.   Female ID# C239479 DOB 01/03/60 Age: 56
Allergies: Morphine, Sulfa, Tree nuts
Primary Attending: Jenson, Olaf R. 14589-134
Date: 01/11/16

Medication Orders

Order ID	Order	
122766	Lanoxin (digoxin) tablet 0.25 mg PO AM daily Hold if pulse under 50.	
122767	Calcium 600 + D tablet PO bedtime	
122769	Lantus (insulin glargine) inj 10 units, Subcut, AM daily at same time	
122770	Crestor 10 mg tablet at bedtime (generic allowed)	
122771	Furosemide 20 mg IV push 2 mg per minute in AM after breakfast one time only	
	PRN ORDERS	
122772	Oxycodone tab 30 mg q6h PRN severe pain *	

Electronic Signature: Olaf R Jensen, MD   Date/Time: 01/11/16

A separate signed prescription for controlled substance must accompany this form.

Electronic signature: Olaf R Jensen, MD   Date/Time: 01/11/16 0930 Phone: (602 315 3930)

> This is an example of electronically entered Prescriber Medication Order.
> These orders will be transferred to a Medication Administration Record by Pharmacy with more details if necessary, such as the number of tablets based on what they will supply or a warning about a known side effect to watch for or a flag for controlled substance. The nurse should check for new orders periodically during the shift to see if any orders have been discontinued.

FIGURE 3-8 Sample medication orders.

All medication orders must contain the complete date and time, the name of the patient, the name of the medication, the dosage, the form (if supplied in more than one form), the route, the frequency (dosing) schedule, and the prescriber's signature. Additional directions may be needed for specific medications. Questions about an order need to be clarified with an instructor, pharmacist, and/or the prescriber.

CLINICAL RELEVANCE

Example of a call to a provider: "This is Mark Keene, RN, calling from General Hospital, 5 West, to clarify a medication order for morphine for your patient, Michael Carrana, in Room 600. The patient says that he has an allergy to morphine and gets low blood pressure and feels faint and nauseated."

In most agencies, the pharmacy provides the unit with a printed daily medication administration record (MAR or EMAR) based on the provider's orders. It often includes additional brief but important information for the nurse who administers the medication.

CLINICAL ALERT!

Consult TJC and your clinical agency's policies pertaining to verbal and telephone orders. There are specific requirements limiting verbal and telephone orders to reduce chances of error. This becomes more important each year as more sound-alike drugs appear on the market.

Answers on page 96

WORKSHEET 3F: Identifying Incomplete Medication Orders

Read the physician orders that follow and in a few words state why the order would have to be clarified. Hint: Think of the patient rights list.

1. Cozaar 25 mg daily in AM

2. Aspirin 2 tablets q4h po prn headache

3. Ampicillin 500 mg q6h × 3 days

4. Morphine sulfate 5 mg IV for pain

5. Tylenol 2 teaspoons q6h for fever over 100° F

The 24-Hour Clock

The 24-hour clock is used in most hospitals and governmental and military agencies. It is computer compatible. It runs sequentially from 0001 h (1 minute after midnight) to 2400 h (midnight). Each hour is written in increments of 100: 1200, 1300, 1400, etc. No number is repeated. Use of the 12-hour clock can cause errors because the same number is used twice: once for AM once for PM hours. With an order such as "Give the medicine at 9 o'clock," it is unclear whether 9 AM or 9 PM is intended. Also 12 AM and 12 PM are often misinterpreted.

- Four digits indicate the hours and minutes of the 24-hour clock: 1530 h, 0200 h, etc.
- The 24-hour clock is reset at midnight (2400 h) to 0000 h.
- The AM hours begin at 0001 h (1 minute after midnight) and end at 1159 h (11:59 AM).
- The PM hours begin at 1200 h and end at 2359 h (11:59 PM).
- When saying 24-hour time, say "twelve hundred (hours)" for 1200 h. Do not say "one thousand, two hundred."

Focus on the PM hours to distinguish the major differences between the two clocks (Figure 3-9).

AM HOURS

12-hour clock AM hours	24-hour clock AM hours
12 AM / 12 Midnight	2400 hours Midnight Reset to 0000 hours
1 AM	0100
2 AM	0200
3 AM	0300
4 AM	0400
5 AM	0500
6 AM	0600
7 AM	0700
8 AM	0800
9 AM	0900
10 AM	1000
11 AM	1100
11:59 AM	1159h

PM HOURS

12-hour clock PM hours	24-hour clock PM hours
12 PM Noon	1200 hours Noon
1 PM	1300 hours
2 PM	1400
3 PM	1500
4 PM	1600
5 PM	1700
6 PM	1800
7 PM	1900
8 PM	2000
9 PM	2100
10 PM	2200
11 PM	2300
11:59 PM	2359h

FIGURE 3-9 Comparison of 12- and 24-hour clock.

For faster learning, memorize these 24-hour clock times: noon (1200 h), midnight (2400 h reset to 0000 h), 1 minute after midnight (0001 h) and 1 PM (1300 h).

Examples
1159 = 1 minute before noon
1201 = 1 minute after noon
2359 = 1 minute before midnight
0001 = 1 minute after midnight

It is very helpful to study some key times in your daily schedule. Fill in the space provided in 24-hour clock time.

Your usual breakfast hour: _0700_

The time your shift begins: _____

The time your shift ends: _____

Your usual dinner hour: _1800_

Your usual bedtime hour: _2200_

Noon (12 PM) _1200_

Midnight (12 AM) _0000_

CHAPTER 3 Safe Medication Administration

Worksheet 3G: Converting AM/PM and 24-Hour Clock Time

Answers on page 96

Fill in the requested time in the space provided.

AM/PM Clock	24-Hour Clock (h)	24-Hour Clock (h)	AM/PM Clock
10:30 AM	1030	1200 h	12:00 pm
10:30 PM	2230	2400 h (0000)	12:00 am
1:15 AM	0115	1745 h	5:45 pm
1:15 PM	1315	2345 h	11:45 pm
12:05 AM	0005	0630 h	6:30 am
12:05 PM	1205	1830 h	6:30 pm
4:20 AM	0420	0006 h	12:06 am
7:55 AM	0755	0910 h	9:10 am
1:20 PM	1320	0325 h	3:25 am
8:40 PM	2040	1905 h	7:05 pm

Understanding Medication Administration Records (MARs)

Every nursing institution has its own MAR or electronic (EMAR) forms. Similar in content but different in style, all contain the date, patient name, sex, date of birth, admission date, ID number, room number, allergies, and the name and/or signature of the primary physician. The nurse needs to be oriented to the forms of each clinical agency (Figures 3-10 and 3-11).

All MAR headings include the time span the page covers, such as one shift, three shifts, and/or 1 week or month for long-term facilities. The orders include the date of each order, dosage, route, frequency, time for administration, and the prescriber's name. MARs have codes for data entry. The nurse's entry includes the date and time each medication was administered, in addition to the accompanying code or full signature of the nurse administering the medication.

EMARs provide some additional instructions from the order or from the pharmacy, such as "Hold and report if pulse under 50," "Do not give with grapefruit juice," or "Give with at least 120 mL of water."

During orientation, a nurse who is a new employee must identify hospital policies that are not stated on the form. These policies include, for example, how to record withholding of a medication, how to handle a medication error, and how to correct an incorrect entry.

Problems noted and medication-related assessments need to be recorded on the patient record.

CLINICAL RELEVANCE
Medications are to be recorded as soon as possible after administration to avoid the event of another nurse also giving the medication.

CLINICAL ALERT!
The MAR is a confidential, legal document. It is illegal to erase, backdate, obscure, or make false entries in an MAR, or to photocopy any medical record without authorization.

Brown, John
ID# 45764304
DOB: 01-10-50 Sex: M Rm: 406A
Dr. Marin, Cruz

ALLERGIES: DRUGS: _IV iodine, Aspirin_
FOODS: _Denies_

RN Verification: _Florence Dane, RN_

MAR Date: 05-07-16 0700 - 05-08-16 0659

MEDICATION: Dose Route Freq   Time of Administration, Site, and Initials

	START	STOP	0700 TO 1459	1500 TO 2259	2300 TO 0659
SCH	05-05-16 Digoxin 0.125 mg po Q AM	05-12-16	(0900) JM R		
SCH	05-05-16 Tylenol (acetaminophen) 500 mg po BID	05-12-16	0800 JM	2000	
SCH	05-05-16 Clotrimazole 1% CR TOP bid to affected area	05-12-16	0900 JM L	2100	

> This is a pharmacy-generated MAR for a 24-hr period stated in 24-hour time beginning with the day shift, 5-7-16. The RN who signs the verification is verifying that the medication orders accurately match the provider orders and that the allergies have been noted. SCH means a regularly scheduled medication versus a PRN order. You must use the agency *code* for administration sites. A circled time denotes med NOT given. Additional documentation may need to be added elsewhere in the nurse's record. PRN meds and one-time-only meds have *separate* placeholders. You may add new orders by writing them in (refer to promethazine). This pharmacy prints instructions for diluting intravenous medications. The narcotic (morphine sulfate) has an automatic 48-hr limit and then must have a written renewal order. This hospital policy calls for a yellow highlight to denote discontinued/expired orders. All discontinued orders, automatic or other, must be renewed if it is necessary to continue them. On the SITE CODES, note that if a medication is withheld other than for NPO or surgery, the reason must be documented on the patient record, e.g.: "Alert and oriented; refused acetominophen and states it 'doesn't do anything for him.' Dr. Marin notified."

ONE TIME ONLY AND PRN MEDS

	Start	Stop	Time	Initials	Full Name/Title
PRN	05-07-16 Morphine sulfate 25 mg IV q6h PRN Dilute in 5 mL NS and give over 5 min	05-09-16 0700	2300 C	FD	Florence Dane, RN
	05-07-16 promethazine 25 mg IM STAT	5/7/16	1900 J	TR	Tom Robbins, RN

Sign: _Joe Mack_   Initials: _JM_   Sign: _Tom Robbins_   Initials: _TR_   Sign: _Florence Dane_   Initials: _FD_

SITE CODES   **GENERAL HOSPITAL**

A	Abdomen (L)	J	Gluteus (LUQ)
B	Abdomen (R)	K	Gluteus (RUQ)
C	Arm (L)	L	Thigh (L)
D	Arm (R)	M	Thigh (R)
E	Eyes (both)	N	Ventrogluteal (L)
F	Eyes (left)	O	Ventrogluteal (R)
G	Eyes (right)	P	NPO: Lab
H	Deltoid (mid L)	Q	NPO: Surgery
I	Deltoid (mid R)	R	Withheld/See nurse's notes

FIGURE 3-10 Sample medication administration record.

⚠ CLINICAL ALERT!

Verify pharmacy data on this sheet, including dilution instructions. Remember this form is not a *copy* of the original orders. These data have been recopied into the computer.

Acct: Admitted: 10/05/16 1630 Att Phys: Diagnosis: Gastric ulcer Allergies: Morphine/Beta-Adrenergic blocking agts			MR#: DOB: 05-10-60 Sex: F HT: 5'7.0" / 170.2 cm WT: 224 lbs / 101.606 kg			M A R	MEDICATION AMINISTRATION RECORD

Start Date/Time	Stop Date/Time	RN/ LPN	Medication	0731-1530	1531-2330	2331-0730
			** ****************** **PRN** ****************** **			
10/05/16 2143	10/12/16 2142		Promethazine HCL (Phenergan Equiv) 25 mg = 0.5 mL IV #020 Q6H PRN PRN N/V			
			When administering IV: Must be diluted to a final concentration of 25 mg/mL. IV administration to be at a rate not to exceed 25 mg/minute.			
10/05/16 2100	10/08/16 2059		Zolpidem Tartrate (Ambien) 10 mg = 2 tablet Oral #016 At bedtime PRN for sleep **Narcotic sign-out**			Discontinue
10/05/16 2200	10/11/16 2159		Alum-Mag Hydroxide-Simethicone (Maalox Plus/Mylanta Equiv) 30 mL = 30 mL Oral #022 Q4H PRN nausea, flatulence, upset stomach Stagger one hr from other meds			

This is an example of a computer-generated MAR (cMAR) for PRN orders only. There are many similarities to the MAR in Figure 3-6 and also some differences noted: this MAR states the medication unit dose supplied; the medication nurse must enter the exact time the medication was given. In addition to dilution instructions, scheduling instructions are given with the last medication. The site code is different and the dose omission code is amplified. Even if no medication is given to a patient, the MAR must be signed by the nurse responsible for the patient each shift. Medications which are refused, withheld, or mischarted must be timed and initialed—a standard procedure that may require additional entries on the patient record if the code is not self-explanatory.

Order Date	RN INIT.	Date/Time To Be Given	One Time Orders and Pre-Operatives Medication-Dose-Route	Actual Time Given	Site Codes			Dose Omission Code	
					Arm	LA	RA	A = pt absent	
					Deltoid	LD	RD	H = hold	
					Ventrogluteal	LVG	RVG	M = med absent	
					Gluteal	LG	RG	N = NPO	
					Abdomen	LUQ	RUQ	O = other	
					Abdomen	LLQ	RLQ	R = refused	
								U = unable to tolerate	
					INIT	Signature		INIT	Signature

60321 (8/98)A   CHART

FIGURE 3-11 A, Example of electronic (EMAR) for PRN orders only. **B,** cMAR. (B, From Kee JL, Marshall SM: *Clinical calculations: with applications to general and specialty areas,* ed 7, St Louis, 2013, Saunders.) *N/V = Nausea/Vomiting.

FRIDAY 10/12/16 - 0700 thru SATURDAY 10/13/16 - 0659		ST ANNE HOSPITAL MEDICATION ADMINISTRATION RECORD
Meyer, Lois M. WESOF W303-2 Age: 72 Sex: F Primary Dx: CP	Unit#: Admitted: 10/12/16 Ht: 152.40 cm Wt: kg	Acct#: Page: 1 Attending Dr: Thomas Smith, MD Run Date/Time: 10/12/16 - 2237 DOB: 06/23/1944

ALLERGIES:	Drug: PCN. ERYTHROMYCIN. IV DYE Other: NO ALLERGIES RECORDED Pharmacy: IODINE (INCLUDES RADIOPAQUE AGENTS W/IODINE). MACROLIDE ANTIBIOTICS, PENICILLINS

Init	IV Flushes: Routine	0700-1459	1500-2259	2300-0659
	Sodium Chloride 0.9% **IV** Flush peripheral IV lines with 5 mls 0.9 NS q 8 hours and central lines per protocol.	Time _____ Init _____ # Flushed _____	Time _____ Init _____ # Flushed _____	Time _____ Init _____ # Flushed _____

Init	SCHED MEDS	DOSE		0700-1459	1500-2259	2300-0659
	DOCUSATE SODIUM (DOCUSATE SODIUM) START: 10/12 D/C: 11/11/16 AT 2244	100 MG	PO Q12 RX 002306792			
	PRAVACHOL (PRAVASTATIN SODIUM) Give at: BEDTIME START: 10/12 D/C: 11/11/16 AT 2244	80 MG	PO RX 002306793			
	METOPROLOL TARTRATE (METOPROLOL TARTRATE) HOLD FOR SBP<110 OR HR<55 Check apical rate and BP before drug admin. START: 10/12 D/C: 11/11/16 AT 2244	50 MG	PO Q12 RX 002306794			
	ACCUPRIL (QUINAPRIL HCL) HOLD FOR SBP<120 START: 10/12 D/C: 11/11/16 AT 2244	40 MG	PO Q12 RX 002306795			
	NITROGLYCERIN 2% (NITROGLYCERIN 2%) HOLD FOR SBP<100 START: 10/12 D/C: 11/11/16 AT 2244	1 INCH	TP Q6 RX 002306796			0000 0600
	ALPRAZOLAM (ALPRAZOLAM) START: 10/12 D/C: 10/14/16 AT 1601	0.25 MG	PO Q8 RX 002306791			0000

Init	PRN MEDS	DOSE		0700-1459	1500-2259	2300-0659
	NITROSTAT 25 TABS/BOTTLE (NITROGLYCERIN) Chest discomfort. May repeat q 5 min x 3. If no relief after 3 doses. Stat ECG & call Physician. START: 10/12 D/C: 11/11/16 at 1833	0.4 MG	SL STAT RX 002306718 PRN			

FIGURE 3-11, cont'd B, cMAR. (B, From Kee JL, Marshall SM: *Clinical calculations: with applications to general and specialty areas,* ed 7, St Louis, 2013, Saunders.) *N/V = Nausea/Vomiting.

Answers on page 96

WORKSHEET 3H Interpreting the MAR

Using the MAR in Figure 3-10, briefly answer the following questions.

1. Does the patient have a commonly seen surname? If so, why should the medication nurse take special note of this?

2. Does the patient have any medication allergies? If so, which?

3. This MAR indicates how many days of medication administration?

4. Which drug ordered was withheld or not given as scheduled?

5. By what route is Clotrimazole 1% to be administered?

6. Which order has expired?

7. Which drug was given at 11 PM and in which location?

8. At what date and time must the morphine order be discontinued or reordered to continue administration?

9. When is the next time Tylenol may be given according to the 24-hour clock? According to traditional time? _____

10. Why do you think this form requires both the initials and the full signature of the person giving the medications? _____

Medication Delivery

Hospital pharmacies stock and resupply computerized medication carts as needed. Computerized carts with bar code scanners are thought to reduce medication errors related to patient identification and wrong medication by matching the codes on the patient wristband and the medication with the electronic medical record. Provision of unit-dose (single-serving) medications reduces errors of medication selection and calculation errors. Although certain types of errors have been reduced, no system is foolproof. There are many steps in the process, starting with the medication order and ending with the administration of the medication (Figures 3-12 to 3-15).

FIGURE 3-12 Computer-controlled medication ordering and dispensing system cart stocked with unit-dose (single-serving) packages supplied by the pharmacy daily, based on prescriber orders. The nurse accesses the cart using a code, a password, and/or a fingerprint, then selects the patient's name, the medication profile, and the drugs that are due to be administered. (Used with permission from Cardinal Health, San Diego, Calif.)

FIGURE 3-13 **A,** The nurse removes the selected medications for the specific time period. **B,** The nurse scans the bar code on each one for drug name and dose to match with the order on the computer. If there is a mismatch, the computer will issue an alert. (Used with permission from Cardinal Health, San Diego, Calif.)

82 Drug Calculations: *Ratio and Proportion Problems for Clinical Practice*

FIGURE 3-14 A nurse using the Omnicell Savvy Mobile Medication System at the patient's bedside. (From Omnicell, Inc., Mountain View, Calif.)

FIGURE 3-15 At the bedside, the nurse will use two permitted patient identifiers, one of which will be to scan the medication and the patient's wristband for right drug, right patient via the computer for agencies that provide this equipment. The nurse will also check the label against the complete order three times before administering the drug. (From Kee JL, Marshall SM: *Clinical calculations: With applications to general and specialty areas,* ed. 7, St. Louis, 2013, Saunders.)

Prioritizing Administration of Several Medications

Clinical experience and familiarity with guidelines are necessary when a nurse has several medications that are ordered to be given during the same time frame (e.g., pain medications, insulin, vitamins, and antibiotics). All of the drugs cannot be given at the same time to more than one patient.

Many priorities are obvious, such as medications for acute pain or medications that need to be given a certain time before or after a meal, stat medications, or preoperative medications. Others are not so obvious.

Note: It is important to take a few minutes to review the ISMP website guidelines that follow before moving on to the next chapter, and to review the guidelines periodically thereafter (http://www.ismp.org/tools/guidelines/acutecare/tasm.pdf).

⊖ CLINICAL ALERT!
Always ask for assistance if the priorities are unclear or the workload is too heavy for timely safe medication administration.

Medication incident reports are a confidential report of a medication-related incident (Figure 3-16). They are used to analyze errors, to determine error patterns and methods of error prevention, and to assess liability. They are considered to be administrative records and are not part of the patient medical record. After taking care of any immediate needs of the patient, the supervisor should be notified as well as the patient's physician. Agencies have guidelines about specific and prompt documentation for the patient medical record. Following that, the incident report is to be filled out on the same shift by the nurse *who encounters* the incident and given to the supervisor for signatures. The reports are factual

SAMPLE MEDICATION INCIDENT REPORT

Patient name: _____ Date of incident: _____
                                                Time of incident: _____

Where incident occurred: Hospital: _____ Unit: _____

Admitting diagnosis: _____

Type of incident: _____   Wrong drug
                                     _____   Wrong time
                                     _____   Wrong dose
Check all that apply: _____   Wrong patient
                                     _____   Wrong route
                                     _____   Other

Medication order: _____

Account of incident and intervention(s) taken: _____
_____
_____
_____

Was the physician notified? _____ Time: _____

All persons familiar with incident or involved: _____
_____

_____   _____
Provider signature   Date   Supervisor signature   Date

> Incident reports are used to analyze errors and determine error patterns and methods of error prevention. They also assist agency insurers in assessing risk for liability for incidents. Each agency has its own forms and protocols for incidents.

FIGURE 3-16 Example of a medication incident report.

and are not supposed to be self-incriminating nor to contain causes, excuses, blame, or conjecture about prevention. *All* follow-up assessments and related actions must be recorded on the patient medication record.

> ### CLINICAL ALERT!
> During orientation to a clinical facility, be sure to check agency written policies and procedures, including what may or may not be entered into the patient medical record. Also follow the policy regarding who notifies the patient's family, if necessary.

Medication Reconciliation (National Patient Safety Goal #3)

Measures to reduce the high rate of medication errors upon transfers, admission, and discharges are known as "Medication Reconciliation." The Joint Commission requires that all agencies that administer medications, including long-term care and home health care, provide evidence of Medication Reconciliation. The procedure includes checking allergies and all the medications the patient is taking from all providers, as well as over-the-counter (OTC) medications the patient takes at home. The nurse plays a major role in this review, as do the patient, family, pharmacy, and prescribers. Check your agency's policies, forms, and computerized medical data bank, if available. Frequent updates are required if a patient leaves and returns to the unit for treatment, surgery, or other procedures.

> ### CLINICAL ALERT!
> Failure to perform Medication Reconciliation on admission, transfer, and discharge can result in serious ADE, such as double dosing and other types of wrong doses, missed drugs, incompatible medication reactions with prescription and OTC medications, as well as drugs that have been discontinued but are still being given, to name a few. Agencies have developed their own Medication Reconciliation forms and procedures to meet this challenge. Look for this procedure when you are oriented to each clinical agency. Refer to Appendix D for an example of a thorough hand-off report.

Summary of Safe Medication Practices

Interpretation

- Know the approved and prohibited abbreviations.
- Call the prescriber to clarify unclear orders. Do not guess.
- Be aware of the patient's allergies when reading medication orders.
- Phone orders are only for emergency medication orders and critical laboratory tests. Write the phone order on the record and read it back to the prescriber. Repeat numbers and doses by numeral; for example, for 30 mg say, "Three, zero, milligrams."

> ### CLINICAL ALERT!
> Beware of confusing similar-sounding drugs, such as Xanax (for anxiety) and Zantac (for gastric reflux and ulcers), Klonopin (for seizures) and Clonidine (for hypertension), and so on. There are many such examples.

Preparation

1. Clean and clear the area. Focus on the task. Avoid distractions. Do not leave a current medication preparation unfinished.
2. Recheck the patient's allergies cited on the record. Reconfirm when the medication was last given.
3. If the patient has transferred from another area or is a postoperative patient, check receiving information such as operating room, emergency department, recovery room, and nursing home transfer records to compare medication orders with those that were given, and which medications

were given and the time they were given so that the patient does not receive a double dose, skip a needed medication, or experience an interaction with new orders. (Look for a "Medication Reconciliation" form.)
4. Assess recent laboratory results for abnormal findings that may need attention.
5. Read label and package inserts, and match the label very carefully to the order. If a medication is liquid, check for dilution instructions.
6. Discard improperly labeled medication according to hospital policy.

If the dose will exceed 1 or 2 capsules or tablets, or 1 to 2 mL injectable, or more than two doses of the drug concentration supplied on the label, recheck the original order and a current pharmacology reference. Give the medication if the dose is appropriate. If there is doubt, contact your instructor, the pharmacy, or the prescriber.

Note: Oral liquid dose concentrations on the label often may exceed 1 to 2 mL, but again, the label concentration (e.g., 250 mg per 5 mL) is a guide to the "usual adult dose" ordered and is used for the calculations for "have on hand."

Check for sediment and the presence of discoloration in liquids and for intact seals on controlled substances. Discard according to agency procedures.

With single-dose medications, retain the container at least until the medication has been administered.

CLINICAL ALERT!
The drug order, dose, and label must be checked *three times* before administering the drug to the patient.

CLINICAL ALERT!
Fatal errors have occurred when a nurse miscalculated a dose and gave multiple ampules or multiple pills of a medication instead of looking up safe dose ranges (SDR) and questioning doses that exceed the single-dose amount supplied. Remember also that usual doses for adults are very different from usual doses for children, those who are very ill, or for adults who are above and below average weight.

CLINICAL ALERT!
If hospital policy calls for a second independent nurse check for certain drugs, it is done *before* administering the drug to the patient. An independent check by a second nurse means "look for mistakes" (patient, drug, dose, route, time), and this is achieved by going through all the steps (except preparation) separately from the first nurse. In many cases, the preparation—for example, dilutions and mixes of high-alert drugs—may need to be observed after the order and calculations are verified.

Calculations

Learn to do your dose calculations accurately. Estimate an answer before calculating the dose; this helps to avoid major math errors. Have a reliable current pharmacology drug reference on hand to verify safe dose ranges; usual doses for the age, weight, and condition of your patients; required dilutions; recommended frequency of administration; and administration timing techniques. Call the pharmacy if there are questions.

Administration

The Joint Commission requires that two patient identifiers, such as name, hospital identification number, or birth date, always be used to check with medication records. Room or bed numbers are not valid patient identifiers. Wristbands, if used, must be on the patient, not on a table or taped to a bed. Special precautions for children, such as verification with a parent or other nurse, must be used.

CLINICAL ALERT!
Avoid asking, "Are you Mister or Ms. X?" A patient who is confused or hard of hearing or a child may mistakenly answer "Yes." Instead, ask the patient to state his or her name.

WORKSHEET 31 | Multiple-Choice Practice

Answers on page 97

1. When administering a medication at the bedside, which should be the *first* priority?
   a. Make appropriate assessments.
   b. Identify the patient.
   c. Document the administration of the medication.
   d. Recheck the medication label.

2. If a medication-related problem is identified, which should be the *first* measure the nurse takes?
   a. Assess the patient for side effects.
   b. Notify the supervisor.
   c. Call the physician.
   d. Document the problem in detail on an incident report.

3. Which is the *drug concentration* for the medication shown below?
   a. 50 mg per 5 mL
   b. 1 pint
   c. 473 mL
   d. 200 mg

4. If a handwritten medication order is illegible or unclear, which would be the best nursing decision?
   a. Check with pharmacy.
   b. Rewrite the order to make it more legible.
   c. Give the usual unit dose and clarify.
   d. Clarify with the physician who wrote it.

CHAPTER 3 Safe Medication Administration

5. The nurse gives a medication at 1 PM. The correct equivalent international or military time on the 24-hour clock would be:
   a. 1000
   b. 1300
   c. 1500
   d. 0100

6. Which of the following statements regarding medications is *true*?
   a. Each nurse must be able to perform accurate simple and complex medication calculations.
   b. The unit dose and the total dose in a vial are one and the same.
   c. It is wise to rely on experienced colleagues to calculate drug doses.
   d. Medication errors rarely occur in the hospital setting.

7. The Joint Commission's "Do Not Use" list (p. 60) of abbreviations specifically applies to which documents?
   a. Patient-provided history and medication records brought from home
   b. Laboratory results including x-rays and blood work
   c. All forms in a patient's record that are handwritten
   d. All orders and medication-related documentation that are handwritten or on preprinted forms or free-text computer entry

8. A tablet is ordered for a patient with a nasogastric feeding tube who is NPO. Which is the most appropriate action for the nurse to take?
   a. Crush the tablet, dilute with water, and administer via the tube.
   b. Consult with the charge nurse about the medication routine for NPO patients.
   c. Ask the patient if there have been any problems with swallowing the pill, and then give it by mouth.
   d. Clarify the route with the physician who wrote the order.

9. A physician ordered ceftazidime 1g qh IM at 0800, 1400, and 2400 hours for a patient with an infection. The nurse administered 1 gram of cefepime IM at 0800 hours. Which patient right was violated?
   a. Right drug
   b. Right dose
   c. Right route
   d. Right time

10. An order for morphine sulfate 10 mg IM q4h prn for pain expired after 48 hours, during the previous shift. The patient continues to complain of postoperative pain and requests another pain injection. Which action is an *inappropriate* nursing action?
    a. Attempt alternative measures for pain relief such as repositioning and other comfort measures.
    b. Administer the medication because the patient has had no untoward side effects as the result of any of the prior doses.
    c. Assess the patient for unexplained sources of continued pain.
    d. Explain that the medication order has expired but that you will call for a renewed order.

Critical Thinking Exercises

Critical Thinking Exercises provide math and medication-related patient safety issues for student discussion. Answers are not provided.

Analyze the following examples of medication errors with your peers and/or instructor and discuss the issues suggested in the left-side guidelines, using this chapter and pharmacology references. As you study the error, consider which patient rights on pages 58 and 59 have been violated. What suggestions might you have for procedural changes at the hospital to prevent this from happening again? Include those that might involve pharmacy staff, providers, nurses, and patients.

Example

1. | | |
   |---|---|
   | **Ordered:** | Tylenol #2, stat |
   | **Supplied:** | Tylenol in patient medication drawer and Tylenol #2 (in locked cabinet) |
   | **Given:** | Two Tylenol tablets |
   | **Error(s):** | The wrong medication was given. Two tablets of plain Tylenol were given instead of one tablet of Tylenol #2, which contains a narcotic. (If an incident report must be filed, this is the way the incident should be described in the space provided for a description of the incident.) |
   | **Potential injuries:** | Lack of comfort and its physiologic and emotional effects; lack of security; need for an alternative medication. |
   | **Nursing actions:** | Report to supervisor and provider. |
   | | Obtain orders to give additional pain medication. |
   | | Document on medical record and file incident report per hospital policy. |
   | | Assess patient periodically for side effects, and document the results. |
   | **Preventive measures:** | Familiarize oneself with the medications ordered and commonly used in the unit, as well as with all controlled medications supplied, including those used in emergencies. |

   If this common medication was known to the giver, and a lack of attention or focus was a contributing cause, techniques to avoid distractions must be addressed. If this medication was not known to the giver, a pharmacology review of commonly used medications is in order. Nurses should always look up unfamiliar medications in current pharmacology references or check with the pharmacy before administering them. Nursing students should check with an instructor or supervisor after the reference check if they are unfamiliar with a medication. It is also wise to inform the patient at the bedside exactly which medications are to be given, because the patient may question the order. An informed patient presents the last line of defense in error prevention.

2. | | |
   |---|---|
   | **Ordered:** | Aspirin 650 mg PO, two tablets at bedtime |
   | **Supplied:** | Aspirin 325 mg per tablet |
   | **Given:** | Aspirin 1300 mg by a nurse the first night; Aspirin 650 mg by another nurse the second night. |
   | **Error(s):** | |
   | **Potential injuries:** | |
   | **Nursing actions:** | |
   | **Preventive measures:** | |

3. **Ordered:** Narcotic for pain q3h prn, last noted on record as given by recovery room nurse at 1445 hours

   Given: Narcotic for pain at 1545 hours by nurse who had just started evening shift and admitted patient to unit

   Error(s):

   Potential injuries:

   Nursing actions:

   Preventive measures:

4. **Ordered:** Prednisone 60 mg daily

   Given: Prednisolone 60 mg daily

   Error(s):

   Potential injuries:

   Nursing actions:

   Preventive measures:

5. **Ordered:** Percocet

   Given: 8/11 Percodan. Recorded on the medical record; patient allergic to aspirin

   Error(s):

   Potential injuries:

   Nursing actions:

   Preventive measures:

CHAPTER 3 Final

1. List the seven patient rights stated in the text.
   a. right patient
   b. right drug
   c. right dose
   d. right time
   e. right route
   f. right documentation
   g. right to refuse

2. Fill in the recommended term or abbreviation in the space provided.

Term/Abbreviation	Meaning	Term/Abbreviation	Meaning
c	with	s	without
po	by mouth	npo	nothing by mouth
IV	intravenously	IM	intramuscular
supp	suppository	bid	twice a day
tid	three times/day	q6h	every 6 hours
prn	as needed	ad lib	as desired
ac	before meals	pc	after meals
subcut	subcutaneously	ID	intradermally
SL	sublingually	NG	nasogastric tube
stat	immediately	top	topically

3. Write the approved abbreviation in the space provided.

Term	Abbreviation
milligram	mg
microgram	mcg
gram	g
kilogram	kg
liter	L
milliliter	mL

CHAPTER 3 Safe Medication Administration

4. State the comparable times in the space provided.

Traditional Time	24-Hour Clock	24-Hour Clock	Traditional Time
12 Noon (12 PM)	1200	2100 hours	9:00 pm
Midnight (12 AM)	0000	1400 hours	2:00 pm
1 PM	1300	0145 hours	1:45 am
9 AM	0900	0030 hours	12:30 am
5 PM	1700	1645 hours	4:45 pm

5. Study the label and supply the requested information.

   a. Generic name _acyclovir_
   b. Drug form _capsule_
   c. Dose per capsule _200 mg_
   d. Single-dose or (multidose) container (circle one)

6. How can decimal points lead to errors in medication orders?
   Zeros following decimal points may be mistaken for whole numbers

7. How would you write out this order: Aspirin tab 325 mg po q4h prn headache?
   Give Aspirin tablets 325 mg by mouth every 4 hours as needed for headache

8. What is the purpose of The Joint Commission's "Do Not Use" list?
   prevent errors related to miscommunication

9. What should the nurse do if an order is unclear?
   ask for clarification

10. State nine pieces of information that the medication label may contain:
    a. _trade name_
    b. _generic name_
    c. _dosage_
    d. _expiration date_
    e. _Lot #_
    f. _NDC #_
    g. _cautions_
    h. _recommended route_
    i. _storage information_

Answer Key

3 Safe Medication Administration

WORKSHEET 3A (page 63)

1. Mistaken for "0," "4," or "cc"
2. Periods and O's can be mistaken for "I" (the letter I or the number 1). Do not write Q.D. or Q.I.D. Write out the abbreviations.
3. A decimal point can be missed, which may result in overdoses.
4. All medication-related documents that are handwritten, entered on a computer, and filled in on preprinted forms must abide by The Joint Commission's "Do Not Use" list.
5. The preferred abbreviation is mL. The capital L for milliliter will not be confused with the number 1 as with ml, and cc can be confused with U (units) and aa (of each) if written poorly.
6. The letter "l" can be mistaken for a number 1 if the dose name and dose amount are run together.
7. Large numbers without commas can be easily misread, resulting in very large dose errors.
8. 10 mg, with a space between the numbers and the abbreviation.
9. Slashes have been mistaken as the number 1 in front of the dose.
10. x3d meant to mean times 3 days has been misinterpreted as "times 3 doses." Write out "for 3 days."

WORKSHEET 3B (page 66)

Term	Recommended Abbreviation
capsule	cap
tablet	tab
fluid	fld
solution	sol
suspension	susp
elixir	elix
teaspoon	tsp
tablespoon	tbs, Tbsp
liquid	liq
ounce	oz
double-strength	DS
extended release	XR
long acting	LA
sustained release	SR
controlled release	CR

WORKSHEET 3C (page 68)

Time	Abbreviation (if Applicable)	Time	Abbreviation (if Applicable)
before	a	after	p
before meals	ac	after meals	pc
daily	Write out daily	three times a day	tid
twice a day	bid	every other day	Write out every other day
every day	Write out every day	every 6 hours	q6h
every 4 hours	every 4 hours	every 12 hours	q12h
whenever necessary	prn	as desired, freely	ad lib (fluids and activities only)
immediately, at once	stat	bedtime	Write out bedtime
with	$\bar{c}$	without	$\bar{s}$
Route	**Abbreviation (if Applicable)**	**Route**	**Abbreviation (if Applicable)**
by mouth	po	nothing by mouth	NPO
intravenous	IV	intramuscular	IM
sublingual	SL	subcutaneous	subcut
intradermal	ID	suppository	supp
left eye	Write out left eye	right ear	Write out right ear
nasogastric	NG	per gastrostomy tube	GT

WORKSHEET 3D (page 69)

Metric Measurement Term	Metric Measurement Abbreviation
microgram(s)	mcg
milligram(s)	mg
gram(s)	g
kilogram(s)	kg
milliliter(s)	mL
milliequivalent(s)	mEq
unit	Write out unit
international unit	Write out international unit
liter	L
square meter	m^2
Other Measurement Term	**Abbreviation**
one half	Write out one half
teaspoon	tsp.
tablespoon	tbs, Tbsp
pound	lb

WORKSHEET 3E (page 73)

1. a. NDC: 0071-0155-30
   b. Lipitor®
   c. atorvastatin calcium
   d. 10 milligrams (mg) per tablet
   e. 10 mg : 1 tablet or $\dfrac{10\ mg}{1\ tablet}$

2. a. levothyroxine sodium tablets, USP
   b. 50 mcg (0.050 mg) equivalent
   c. 50 mcg : 1 tablet or $\dfrac{50\ mcg}{1\ tablet}$

⊖ CLINICAL ALERT!
If you have a choice between an equivalent that is stated in whole numbers (e.g., 50 mcg) or one in decimals (e.g., 0.050 mg), use the whole number equivalent. It will simplify the math.

3. a. Liquid oral suspension
   b. 125 milligrams (mg) per 5 milliliters (mL)
   c. Usual dose: 250 mg to 500 mg every 8 hours, depending on type and severity of infection
   d. Multidose container. Contains 150 mL* in small print
   e. 150 mL is 30 times more than 5 mL
   f. 125 mg : 5 mL or $\dfrac{125\ mg}{5\ mL}$

⊖ CLINICAL ALERT!
Multidose containers allow different doses to be drawn as needed for the particular patient and condition. The usual dose is noted on the label. Note that the usual doses for adults and children vary. Serious injuries and death have been caused by failure to read the label and distinguish the single dose from the total contents, especially in a liquid form, thus administering the total contents of a multidose container instead of the ordered single dose. This is one of the reasons that more medicines are being supplied in individual unit-dose containers.

4. a. Septra® DS
   b. Trimethoprim, 160 mg, and sulfamethoxazole, 800 mg.†
   c. Scored tablet, meaning it can be cut in half (only with a pillcutter) if half dose is ordered)
      Note: A half dose would have to be a half dose of each of the drugs in this compound.
   d. DS = "double strength"
   e. No calculation needed

5. a. Nitroglycerin
   b. Sublingual: administer under the tongue
   c. The nurse needs to know that the patient understands and is able to hold the tablet under the tongue until it dissolves. That enables it to be absorbed more rapidly than if it were swallowed because it bypasses the gastrointestinal tract. This medication is given promptly for chest pain to dilate coronary vessels and increase the blood flow to the heart.
   d. 0.5 mg per tablet 1/100 grain (gr) is an outdated measurement but is retained on the label to accommodate patients who have been taking this medicine for many years.

---

*Note: Check storage directions for multidose containers. Check agency policies regarding labeling before storing.
Metric measurements are not italicized. The liter abbreviation is always a capital "L." Most of the metric abbreviations are not capitalized.
†Note the prefix "sulfa" in the name denotes that drug is in the compound. It is a commonly known allergen. Check your patient for allergy to sulfa drugs before administering.

WORKSHEET 3F (page 76)

1. The route is not specified.

2. The dose is not specified. Aspirin is supplied in more than one dose (e.g., 325 mg per tablet, 650 mg per tablet). The number of tablets should *not* be mentioned in the order.

3. The route is not specified. Ampicillin can be administered by more than one route (PO, IM, IV).

4. The time or frequency is not specified—for example, stat, one time only, or more than one time.

5. The dose and form are not specified. Tylenol is supplied in tablet, liquid suspension, intravenous, and suppository forms and in a variety of doses targeted to infants, children, and adults. Teaspoons should not be mentioned in the order.

WORKSHEET 3G (page 78)

AM/PM Clock	24-Hour Clock (h)	24-Hour Clock (h)	AM/PM Clock
10:30 AM	1030h	1200 h	12 PM (Noon)
10:30 PM	2230h	2400 h	12 AM (Midnight)
1:15 AM	0115h	1145 h	11:45 AM
1:15 PM	1315h	2345 h	11:45 PM
12:05 AM	0005h	0630 h	6:30 AM
12:05 PM	1205h	1830 h	6:30 PM
4:20 AM	0420h	0006 h	12:06 AM
7:55 AM	0755h	0910 h	9:10 AM
1:20 PM	1320h	0325 h	3:25 AM
8:40 PM	2040h	1905 h	7:05 PM

CLINICAL ALERT!

"Once" means "eleven" in Spanish. The word for one is "uno" in Spanish or "una vez," one time.

WORKSHEET 3H (page 81)

1. Yes. Care must be taken in distinguishing this patient from other patients with the same or a similar name to avoid giving a medication to the wrong patient.

2. Yes. The patient is allergic to the intravenous iodine used in some contrast media tests and to products that contain aspirin. There are many.

3. One 24-hour day

4. Digoxin was withheld as denoted by a circle and the code "R."

5. Topical

6. Promethazine, a stat order

7. Morphine sulfate; left arm denoted by "C."

8. 05/09/16 at 0700

9. 05/07/16 at 2000; 8 pm

10. Having both the initials and the nurse's signature identifies the nurse who administered the medication more clearly. More than one staff member may have the same initials, or some initials may be illegible.

WORKSHEET 3I (page 87)

1. **b.** Correct identification of patient is always the first priority. Answers a, c, and d would all be appropriate after the patient is identified.

2. **a.** Answers b, c, and d would all be appropriate after the patient was assessed.

3. **a.** Answer b is the total amount of drug in the container. Answer c is the total volume in mL. Answer d is the usual ordered adult dosage on the first day.

4. **d.** Answers a, b, and c are inappropriate actions.

5. **b.** Refer to the international/24-hour clock on page 77.

6. **a.** Answers b, c, and d are false statements.

7. **d.** Refer to the legend below the TJC "Do Not Use" list on page 60.

8. **d.** The right route is usually the one that is ordered but not in this case. There is a conflict, and common sense dictates that the nurse must clarify. The patient is NPO, and there must be a written order to be able to give a medication by mouth. Some medications are totally unsuitable for nasogastric tube administration, and some just obstruct the tube. Some orders may specify to crush the tablet, dilute with water, and give via the tube.

9. **a.** Be very aware that there are many drugs with similar names but different uses.

10. **b.** Giving a medication after the expiration date, whether automatically established by the agency or written by the physician, is illegal. All other actions are appropriate.

CHAPTER 3 FINAL: SAFE MEDICATION ADMINISTRATION (page 91)

1. **a.** Right patient
   b. Right drug
   c. Right dose
   d. Right time
   e. Right route
   f. Right documentation
   g. Right to refuse

2.

Term/Abbreviation	Meaning	Term/Abbreviation	Meaning
c̄	with	s̄	without
po, PO	by mouth	NPO	nothing by mouth
IV	intravenous	IM	intramuscular
supp	suppository	bid	twice a day
tid	three times daily	q6h	every 6 hours
prn	whenever necessary	ad lib*	freely, as desired
ac	before meals	pc	after meals
subcut	subcutaneous	ID	intradermal
SL	sublingual	NG	nasogastric
stat	immediately	top	topical

*ad lib is used for fluids and activity but not for medications.

3.

Term	Abbreviation
milligram	mg
microgram	mcg
gram	g
kilogram	kg
liter	L
milliliter	mL

4.

Traditional Time	24-Hour Clock	24-Hour Clock	Traditional Time
12 Noon (12 PM)	1200 hours	2100 hours	9 PM
Midnight (12 AM)	2400 hours	1400 hours	2 PM
1 PM	1300 hours	0145 hours	1:45 AM
9 AM	0900 hours	0030 hours	12:30 AM
5 PM	1700 hours	1645 hours	4:45 PM

5. **a.** Generic name: acyclovir
   b. Drug form: capsule
   c. Dose per capsule: 200 mg
   d. Single-dose or multidose container: multidose

6. Decimals can be missed altogether or mistaken for the number 1.

7. Aspirin tablet 325 milligrams by mouth every 4 hours as needed for headache.

8. The Joint Commission's "Do Not Use" list contains the prohibited abbreviations that have been misinterpreted and led to medication errors.

9. If an order is unclear, it should be clarified with the prescriber.

10. Generic name; proprietary, trade, or brand name; unit dose; form; total amount in container; recommended routes; preparation directions; storage directions; lot number; NDC code; and expiration date.

Medication Measurements and Oral Dose Calculations

Objectives
- Combine metric base units and prefixes.
- Use approved metric measurement abbreviations.
- Convert metric and household equivalents.
- Estimate and verify dose calculations.
- Solve dose calculation problems with ratio and proportion equations.
- Identify patient safety measures related to oral medication calculations and administration.
- Identify controlled (scheduled) drugs.
- Use critical thinking to analyze medication errors.

Introduction This chapter builds on prior knowledge to solve oral medication dose calculation problems using the metric system and its equivalents. The metric system has replaced the English apothecary system and is now required for medication orders and packaging in the United States. An emphasis is placed on estimation, verification, and knowledge of the measurement-related factors needed for safe clinical practice. The focus is on understanding the calculation process and avoiding behaviors that can lead to medication errors. Mastery of this chapter will provide the reader with a thorough foundation for more complex drug dose calculations.

Vocabulary **Base Units of Metric Measurement:** Three of the base *units* commonly used for metric measurements of medications are **gram** (g) for weight (mass), liter (L) for volume, and **meter** (m) for length.

Household Measurement Systems: Measuring utensils used in the home, such as teaspoons, are a safety risk for measuring medication doses because of various sizes and capacities.

Metric System: A simplified decimal system of measurement based on combinations of base units and prefixes that are related by multiples of the number 10. Modified and adopted by most countries, the metric system is supported in the United States by TJC and ISMP, as well as national nursing, pharmacy, and other health-related organizations to reduce the risk of medication dose errors. It is required for entry into the European Union.

Metric Equivalent Chart

Weight (Mass)

1000 mcg (micrograms) = 1 mg (milligram)

1000 mg = 1 g (gram)

1000 g = 1 kg (kilogram)

lb to kg conversion

2.2 lb (pound) = 1 kg

inch to cm conversion

1 inch = 2.5 cm (approximate)

Volume

1000 mL (milliliter) = 1 L (liter)

Other

1000 milliunits = 1 unit

Length

10 mm (millimeters) = 1 cm (centimeter)

100 cm = 1 m (meter)

1000 mm = 1 m (meter)

Metric Measurements: Base Units

Three base units are commonly used in the medical field. Two are used mainly for medication doses (gram and liter) and one (meter) is used occasionally for topical medications.

Memorize these three base units.

Base Units

Dimension	Metric Base Unit	Approximate English System Equivalent
Weight (or mass)	gram (g)	About 1/3 ounce dry weight
Volume	liter (L)	About 4 measuring cups, a little more than 1 quart
Length	meter (m)	About 39 inches, a little more than 1 yard

The abbreviation for the base unit liter is capitalized (L) to avoid misreading as the number 1. The base unit abbreviations for gram (g) and meter (m) are written in lowercase letters. No other abbreviations are authorized.

Metric Units Number Line

The following Metric Units Number Line illustrates the relationship of the values for selected metric prefixes.

Prefix	Abbreviation		Value
kilo-	k		1000
hecto-*	h		100
deka-*	da		10
			0 (zero)
deci-†	d		0.1
centi-	c		0.01
milli-	m		0.001
micro-	mc		0.000001

*Not seen in medication records.
†Seen in laboratory reports.

Metric Prefixes and Values

Four prefixes are commonly used for medication dose calculations:
- centi- (meaning hundredth)
- milli- (meaning thousandth)
- micro- (meaning millionth)
- kilo- (meaning a thousand times)

Table 4-1 clarifies the relationships of values among the metric measurements most frequently encountered by the nurse on medication labels and orders, laboratory test results, and medication-related literature. It is essential to understand and distinguish them from each other.

Table 4-1 Metric Measurements, Prefixes, Values, and Meanings

Prefix	Multiplier	Exponential Power of 10	Meaning	Examples	Meaning
deci- (d)	.1	10^{-1}	tenth part of	deciliter (dL)	one tenth of a liter
centi- (c)	.01	10^{-2}	hundredth part of	centimeter (cm)	one hundredth of a meter
milli- (m)	.001	10^{-3}	thousandth part of	milliliter (mL)	one thousandth of a liter
				milligram (mg)	one thousandth of a gram
micro- (mc)*	.000001	10^{-6}	millionth part of	microgram (mcg)	one millionth of a gram
kilo- (k)	1000	10^{3}	1000 times	kilogram (kg)	one thousand grams

Note: The prefix value never changes when combined with a base unit (e.g., the prefix *milli* [m] = 0.001).
1 mm = 0.001 (one thousandth of a meter).
1 mL = 0.001 (one thousandth of a liter).
1 mg = 0.001 (one thousandth of a gram).
*Note that "mc" is the only prefix abbreviation with two letters. This distinguishes it from "m" for milli.

CLINICAL ALERT!

The abbreviation "mc" for the prefix "micro" is preferred over the Greek letter μ (mu). A handwritten μg can be mistaken for mg (milligrams).

Answers on page 135

WORKSHEET 4A: Writing Metric Units and Abbreviations

Write the metric name and abbreviation in the space provided.

		Metric Name	Abbreviation
1.	Base unit for weight/mass	_____	_____
2.	Base unit for volume	_____	_____
3.	Base unit for length	_____	_____
4.	Prefix that means 1/1000	_____	_____
5.	Prefix than means 1/100	_____	_____
6.	Prefix that means 1,000,000	_____	_____
7.	Prefix that means 1/10	_____	_____
8.	Prefix that means 1000 times	_____	_____
9.	Name for the base unit "m"	_____	
10.	Name for the prefix "m"	_____	

Finding Equivalent Measurements Using Ratio and Proportion

There are two types of problems that are encountered in basic medication calculations. A dose can be calculated when the measurement units and values are equivalent.
1. Find an equivalent value when two measurement terms are different.
2. Calculate a dose when the terms are the same.

Metric equivalents: 1000 mcg = 1 mg   **1000 mg = 1 g**   **1000 g = 1 kg**

Metric Equivalent Calculation Setup

Examples **Ordered:** 1.5 g of an antibiotic. **Supplied:** 500 mg capsules. How many capsules will you give? The measurement terms are *different*. *They need to be the same in order to calculate the dose.*

Change the ordered 1.5 g to an equivalent amount of (unknown) (*x*) milligrams on hand.

Equivalent formula selected for the conversion: **1000 mg = 1 g**

102   Drug Calculations: *Ratio and Proportion Problems for Clinical Practice*

Step 1: Place the known formula on the left side of the equation, and what you want to know (*x* mg) on the right side of the equation.

USING COLONS	USING FRACTION CROSS PRODUCT
KNOW WANT TO KNOW	KNOW WANT TO KNOW
1000 mg : 1 g = *x* mg : 1.5 g	$\dfrac{1000 \text{ mg}}{1 \text{ g}} = \dfrac{x \text{ mg}}{1.5 \text{ g}}$

Maintain the ratio sequence: (mg : g = mg : g)

Estimate: The answer will be 1500 because the extremes (1000 × 1.5) are being multiplied by 1.

Step 2: Remove the terms, then solve for *x* by multiplying.

KNOW   WANT TO KNOW   KNOW   WANT TO KNOW

1000 : 1 = *x* : 1.5 $\dfrac{1000}{1} \times \dfrac{x}{1.5}$

x = 1000 × 1.5
x = 1500 mg

PROOF
1000 × 1.5 = 1500
1 × 1500 = 1500

Step 3: Check your estimate. Label and prove the answer. Refer to Chapter 2, Ratio and Proportion, if review is needed.

Example 40 mg = ? g (metric equivalent problem)

KNOW   WANT TO KNOW   KNOW   WANT TO KNOW

1000 mg : 1 g = 40 mg : *x* g $\dfrac{1000 \text{ mg}}{1 \text{ g}} = \dfrac{40 \text{ mg}}{x \text{ g}}$
 (mg : g = mg : g)

$\dfrac{\cancel{1000}}{\cancel{1000}} x = \dfrac{\cancel{40}}{\cancel{1000}}$

x = 0.04 g

PROOF
1000 × 0.04 = 40
1 × 40 = 40

ANSWER
40 mg = 0.04 g

Answers on page 135

WORKSHEET 4B | Metric Equivalents

Use ratio and proportion to find the following metric equivalent terms. Prove and label all answers.

remember
1000 mcg = 1 mg
1000 mg = 1 g
1000 g = 1 kg (2.2 lb)
1000 mL = 1 L (liter)

Change milligrams to grams.

1. 200 mg   2. 250 mg   3. 25 mg *0.025 g*

Change grams to milligrams.

4. 2.5 g *2500 mg*   5. 0.5 g *500 mg*   6. 0.01 g

CHAPTER 4 Medication Measurements and Oral Dose Calculations   103

Change micrograms to milligrams.

7. 150 mcg **8.** 500 mcg **9.** 2500 mcg

Change milligrams to micrograms.

10. 5 mg **11.** 0.1 mg **12.** 0.04 mg

Change kilograms to grams.

13. 5.5 kg **14.** 12 kg **15.** 0.5 kg

Change liters to milliliters.

16. 0.5 L **17.** 1.3 L **18.** 2.8 L

Change milliters to liters.

19. 1200 mL **20.** 800 mL

Metric Notation Review

1. Use only the approved abbreviations.*
2. Always abbreviate metric terms when they are accompanied by a number (e.g., the patient drank *2 L* of water).
3. The number comes first; the abbreviation follows.
4. Write out *metric* terms when they are *not* accompanied by a number (e.g., the patient drank a *liter* of water).
5. Leave a space between a number and metric unit (e.g., write *21 mg*, not 21mg; *21 lb*, not 21lb).
6. Capitalize *L* for liter so that it will not be misread as the numeral "1" (e.g., write *4 L*, not 4l or 4 l).
7. Metric terms are not pluralized (e.g., write *50 mL*, not 50 mLs; *5 mg*, not 5 mgs; *2 g*, not 2 gs).
8. There is no period after a metric abbreviation unless it is at the end of a sentence. Periods can be mistaken for the numeral "1."
9. Write out the word "per"; do not use a slash (e.g., write *4 g per kg*, not 4 g/kg).
10. The number 1 is implied, not written when the amount is the number 1 (e.g., write *5 mg per kg*, not *5 mg per 1 kg*).
11. Be aware that *m, w, u, n, v*, and *w* can look like each other, depending on how they are written.
12. The letter *c* can look like a zero or the letter *a* if the *c* is closed up (e.g., *cm* can look like *am*).

*Refer to TJC "Do-Not-Use" List and ISMP Error-Prone Abbreviations in Chapter 3.

⬅ CLINICAL ALERT!

For the sake of patient safety, the nurse must be familiar with all the metric terms, the reason for the medication order, and the safe dosage ranges for the patient's condition and the target population.

⬅ CLINICAL ALERT!

Know the 1000 times numerical difference between *mg* and *g* and between *mcg* and *mg*. Also, know why a patient's condition should or should not receive a smaller or larger dose.

CLINICAL RELEVANCE

Several years ago, a patient was sent for a lab test for hypothyroidism. Thyroid function is tested using a small dose (micrograms [mcg]) of radioactive iodine. Radioactive iodine is also administered in large doses milligrams (mg) to patients with overactive thyroid disease or thyroid cancer. Large doses destroy thyroid cells. The patient to be tested was given a milligram dose in error; family members at home were exposed to the radioactivity after the test, and the patient later died.

Think metric but be prepared to occasionally see unfamiliar terms. Verify questions with the pharmacist or the provider. Never guess. Document the consultation on the medical record.

Finding Metric Equivalents by Moving Decimals

The metric system is a decimal system. When the metric terms in the order and on hand are *different*, another way to verify equivalent measures for *metric* terms is to move decimals. The majority of medications are supplied in grams and milligrams; some are supplied in micrograms.

Moving Decimals for Metric Equivalents

RULE To convert grams to milligrams, multiply by 1000.

Examples
5 g = 5.000. mg = 5000 mg   (1 g : 1000 mg = 5 g : x mg) $\frac{1}{1000} = \frac{5}{x}$

0.2 g = 0.200. mg = 200 mg

0.04 g = 0.040. mg = 40 mg

RULE To convert milligrams to grams, divide by 1000.

Examples
250 mg = 0.250. g = 0.25 g   (1000 mg : 1 g = 250 mg : x g) $\frac{1000}{1} = \frac{250}{x}$

20 mg = 0.020. g = 0.02 g

5 mg = 0.005. g = 0.005 g

RULE To convert milligrams to micrograms, multiply by 1000.

Examples
5 mg = 5.000. mcg = 5000 mcg   (1 mg : 1000 mcg = 5 mg : x mcg) $\frac{1}{1000} = \frac{5}{x}$

0.8 mg = 0.800. mcg = 800 mcg

0.05 mg = 0.050. mcg = 50 mcg

RULE To convert micrograms to milligrams, divide by 1000. Figure 4-1 illustrates the decimal movement.

Examples
2500 mcg = 2.500. mg = 2.5 mg

400 mcg = 0.400. mg = 0.4 mg

10 mcg = 0.010. mg = 0.01 mg

FIGURE 4-1 Metric units number line.

CHAPTER 4 Medication Measurements and Oral Dose Calculations

Answers on page 137

WORKSHEET 4C: Metric Equivalents Practice: Micrograms, Milligrams, and Grams

Fill in the metric equivalents in the space provided.

Grams to Milligrams		Milligrams to Grams	
g	? mg	mg	? g
2		5000	
2.5		3500	
1.5		1200	
0.1		800	
0.5		400	
0.25		350	
0.15		200	
0.03		125	
0.015		80	
0.075		50	

Micrograms to Milligrams		Milligrams to Micrograms	
mcg	? mg	mg	? mcg
7500		1.5	
1200		0.8	
750		0.3	
500		0.25	
100		0.125	

- Division and multiplication by 1000 moves the decimal point three places to the left or the right.
- Always place zero in front of a decimal that is unaccompanied by a whole number.
- Do not let a decimal look like the number "1."
- Do not add "trailing" zeros to the end of decimals. They can be misread as a whole number if the decimal point is not seen.

Memorize

Metric Weight Equivalents	Metric-Household Weight Equivalents (Approximate)
1000 mcg = 1 mg	1 kg = 2.2 pounds (lb)
1000 mg = 1 g	
1000 g = 1 kg	

Medications in micrograms are less frequently encountered than those in milligrams and grams. That makes it all the more important to recognize and distinguish the labels for *mg* and *mcg*. There is a

106 Drug Calculations: *Ratio and Proportion Problems for Clinical Practice*

1000 times difference between a microgram and a milligram. The medications ordered in such small amounts are often very powerful medications.

In clinical agencies, the kilogram is used for weight reporting and dose calculations. At birth, the average baby weighs 3200 g or 3.2 kg (approximately 7 lb). Low-birth-weight babies are those who weigh (less than or equal to) 2500 g (2.5 kg or 5.5 lb) at birth. Weight-based dosages for children and adults are required to be in kilograms. Oral medications contain large ranges of dosages in micrograms and millgrams, from 0.175 mg (175 mcg) to 0.5 mg, 100 mg, 250 mg, 500 mg, or 1 g or more. Calculate your own weight in pounds and kilograms.

Memorize

Metric Volume Equivalents	Metric-Household Equivalents (Approximate)
1000 mL = 1 L	5 mL = 1 teaspoon (tsp)
	15 mL = 1 tablespoon (Tbsp) or 3 teaspoons (tsp)
	30 mL = 1 ounce (oz)
	240 mL = 8 ounces (oz) = 1 cup

CLINICAL RELEVANCE

In clinical agencies, liquids are usually ordered and supplied in milliliters and liters. A calibrated metric medication teaspoon holds 5 mL of fluid. Plastic liquid medication cups are usually supplied with a capacity of 30 mL and occasionally 15 mL. Think metric: 30 mL for an ounce.

The volume of a liter is slightly greater than that of a quart (1 L = 1.06 qt; 1 qt is 0.9 L). Many intravenous solutions are delivered in 1-liter or half-liter containers. Examine water and beverage bottles. Drink 240 mL of water per day instead of 8 ounces or 1 "glass" or 1 "cup."

In many parts of the world, gasoline is purchsed by the liter. There are approximately 4 liters to a gallon. If you normally buy 10 gallons, you would purchase about 40 liters. Although this conversion is not exact, using it when buying gasoline abroad will assist you in deciding how much to buy and give you an idea of what you will owe. Making a quick conversion is safer than saying, "Fill the tank."

> **CLINICAL ALERT!**
> Write the abbreviation *mL* for milliliter. Do not use the abbreviation for cubic centimeter (cc), which is sometimes used to indicate milliliters. The abbreviation "cc" has been misread as two zeros (00), resulting in medication errors.

2 Tbsp — 30 mL
— 25 mL
— 20 mL
1 Tbsp — 15 mL
2 tsp — 10 mL
1 tsp — 5 mL
½ tsp

Answers on page 137

WORKSHEET 4D | Equivalent Measures of Weight

1. How many micrograms are in 5 mg? _____

2. How many milligrams are in 0.5 g? _____

3. How many grams are in 5.5 kg? _____

4. How many milligrams are in 2500 mcg? _____

5. How many kilograms are in 2000 g? _____

Answers on page 138

WORKSHEET 4E | Equivalent Measures of Volume

1. How many mL are in one-half liter of intravenous solution? _____

2. How many mL are in 1 tablespoon (Tbsp)? _____

3. How many mL are in 8 ounces (oz)? _____

4. How many mL are in 0.25 L of an intravenous medicated solution? _____

5. It is recommended that we drink about 1.5 L of fluid per day. How many mL is the equivalent? _____

Memorize

Metric Length Equivalents (Approximate)	Metric-Household Length Equivalents
10 mm = 1 centimeter (cm)	2.5 cm = 1 inch
100 cm = 1 meter (m)	
1000 mm = 1 meter (m)	

108 Drug Calculations: *Ratio and Proportion Problems for Clinical Practice*

CLINICAL RELEVANCE

In the clinical area, measurements of length are used to measure the size of wounds and sometimes to apply a specific amount of topical medication by length to wounds. Pupil size is measured for eye examinations, certain neurological examinations, and health conditions.

CLINICAL RELEVANCE

- When you are assisting with cardiopulmonary resuscitation (CPR), it is helpful to know that fully dilated pupils (10 mm, or 1 cm) can indicate that the patient has been without oxygen for more than 4 or 5 minutes. Assessment of the pupils of the eye provides a clue as to a patient's response to CPR.
- The pinpoint pupil (1 to 2 mm) may be a reaction to strong light or to certain opioids or other medications (Figure 4-2).
- Familiarity with millimeters and centimeters is also helpful when gauging the length of specified areas, such as wounds or scars, or when documenting the application of ointments in the clinical setting.

FIGURE 4-2 Pupil gauge (mm).

If you have any arm scars, freckles, or skin lesions, you can measure them in millimeters and/or centimeters. What is the length in mm or cm?

CLINICAL RELEVANCE

- Once you have established some personal landmarks in millimeters and centimeters, you can estimate the size of skin lesions at the bedside by comparing them with your own landmarks without searching for a ruler.
- Topical prescription ointments usually supply paper tape rulers when exact measurements are needed (Figure 4-3).
- Note that some ointments may be prescribed and measured in inches.

FIGURE 4-3 The nurse is wearing gloves to prevent personal absorption of the medication as well as to avoid skin contact with the patient's wound. (From Clayton BD, Willihnganz M: *Basic pharmacology for nurses*, ed. 16, St. Louis, 2013, Mosby.)

After you learn the major equivalent values, you can infer the equivalent values for quarters, halves, and one and a half units.

Sample Equivalent Metric Values

Row	Length	Volume	Volume	Weight	Weight	Weight	Weight	Weight	Weight
A	10 mm	500 mL	1000 mL	1000 mcg	250 mg	500 mg	1000 mg	1500 mg	1000 g
B	1 cm	0.5 L	1 L	1 mg	0.25 g	0.5 g	1 g	1.5 g	1 kg

Do not confuse micrograms with milligrams. Note the difference in value between 1 mcg and 1 mg. The metric system uses only decimals for numbers less than 1. Note the leading zeros in front of decimals and the elimination trailing zeros after numbers.

Metric Dose Calculation

When the equivalent measurement terms for the medication order and supplied medication *label* are the *same*, the dose can be calculated in one step to find the *amount* of medication to give: x tablets, x capsules, or x mL.

1. Examine the examples of the two ways to set up the ratio and proportion equation using a colon or the fraction cross-multiplication method.
2. Remove the terms and multiply. The proportion is solved in the same way as in all previous examples.

Problem Ordered: 200 mg. On hand: 100 mg per capsule.

Example USING COLONS   USING FRACTION CROSS PRODUCT

HAVE ON HAND   WANT TO HAVE

100 mg : 1 capsule = 200 mg : x capsules $\dfrac{100 \text{ mg}}{1 \text{ capsule}} = \dfrac{200 \text{ mg}}{x \text{ capsules}}$

Note: Maintain the same order in the two ratios—mg : capsule = mg : capsule

Estimate: When the terms are the same and in an equation, make a rough estimate of the answer before completing the problem. Will you give more or less than the single serving on hand? About how much more or less?

Remove the terms and multiply.

USING COLONS   USING FRACTION CROSS PRODUCT

100 : 1 = 200 : x

$100x = 200$

$x = 2$ capsules

PROOF
$100 \times 2 = 200$
$1 \times 200 = 200$

Example Ordered: 50 mg. Unit dose label: 25 mg per tablet.

RULE Place what you have on hand or what you know (the label unit dose) on the left and what is ordered (want to have or know) on the right. Follow through with your math to verify your estimate as shown in the ratio and proportion examples in Chapter 2.

KNOW   WANT TO KNOW

25 mg : 1 tablet = 50 mg : x tablets

$\dfrac{25}{25} \times \dfrac{50}{25} = 2$

$x = 2$ tablets

PROOF
$25 \times 2 = 50$
$1 \times 50 = 50$

ANSWER
Give 2 tablets

> **CLINICAL ALERT!**
> Some of these problems can be easily solved without being written. More complex problems will be more easily solved after practice with easier problems.

Answers on page 138

WORKSHEET 4F | Oral Solid Medication Dose Practice

Estimate and calculate the dose using a ratio and proportion method.

1. Ordered: Prednisone 15 mg tablets daily po for a patient with asthma.
   On hand: Prednisone 5 mg tablets.

   HAVE ON HAND   WANT TO HAVE

   PROOF

2. Ordered: Fortovase (saquinavir) 400 mg soft gel capsule daily for a patient with an HIV infection.

   FORTOVASE® (saquinavir) Soft Gelatin Capsules 200 mg
   Each capsule contains 200 mg saquinavir (free base).
   REFRIGERATE PRIOR TO DISPENSING.
   180 Capsules

   HAVE ON HAND   WANT TO HAVE

   PROOF

   What are the refrigeration directions?

CHAPTER 4 Medication Measurements and Oral Dose Calculations

3. Ordered: Tegretol 200 mg chewable tablet po at bedtime for a patient who has seizures.

Tegretol® 100 mg
carbamazepine USP
Chewable Tablets
NDC 0078-0492-05   Rx only
100 tablets
NOVARTIS

HAVE ON HAND   WANT TO HAVE

$\frac{100}{1}$ :: $\frac{200}{x:1}$ $\frac{200}{100} = 2$

PROOF: 2

4. Ordered: Lanoxin (digoxin) tablet 0.125 mg po daily in AM for a patient with heart failure.

NDC 0173-0249-56
100 Tablets (10 blisterpacks of 10 tablets each)
UNIT DOSE PACK
LANOXIN® (digoxin) Tablets
Each scored tablet contains
250 mcg (0.25 mg)

HAVE ON HAND   WANT TO HAVE

PROOF

5. Ordered: Septra DS 80 mg trimethoprim and 400 mg sulfamethoxazole tablets po daily for a patient with a urinary tract infection.

[Septra DS label: 100 Tablets, NDC 0173-0853-55. SEPTRA® DS Double Strength (trimethoprim and sulfamethoxazole). Each scored tablet contains 160 mg trimethoprim and 800 mg sulfamethoxazole. Glaxo Wellcome Inc., Research Triangle Park, NC 27709.]

HAVE ON HAND	WANT TO HAVE		PROOF
160 mg tri 800 mg sulf	80 mg tri 400 mg sulf	$\frac{160}{1} \cdot \frac{80}{x}$	1/2

HAVE ON HAND	WANT TO HAVE		PROOF
		$\frac{800}{1} \cdot \frac{400}{x}$	1/2

Note: Septra DS is a compound drug that is supplied in more than one concentration.

⊖ CLINICAL ALERT!

DS (double-strength). Do not confuse DS with extended-release or delayed-release products. Those types of products (E-R, S-R, CD, XR, XL,* etc.) are not double strength, and DS is not an abbreviation for an extended-release product.

*Refer to abbreviations on the inside front cover.

Worksheet 4G: Oral Solid Medication Dose Practice

Answers on page 139

Compare the ordered dose with the available dose concentration supplied. Fill in the requested information in the space provided.

Ordered Type or Condition for Rx	Supplied dose	Estimate*: More, Less, or Same as 1 serving of the drug concentration supplied	Actual dose Solve using a ratio and proportion method
1. Rifampin (rifadin) 600 mg po daily for a patient with tuberculosis	300 mg per capsule	a	b
2. Metoprolol XL† 100 mg po at bedtime for a patient with hypertension	100 mg per XL tablet	a	b
3. Lopressor (metoprolol tartrate) 75 mg po daily at bedtime for a patient with hypertension	50 mg per scored tablet	a	b
4. Synthroid (levothyroxine) 175 mcg (0.175 mg) po daily in AM for a patient with hypothyroidism	175 mcg per tablet	a	b
5. Halcion (aprazolam) 0.125 mg po daily at bedtime for anxiety	0.25 mg tablet, unscored	a	b

Note that most of the orders for these commonly ordered drugs are between $\frac{1}{2}$ to 2 servings of the form supplied. Recheck orders that call for more than 2 servings of the supplied form.

*An estimate can be made when the ordered dose and the dose on hand are in the same measurement terms.
†CLINICAL ALERT With XL (extra-long), E-R (extended release), SR (sustained release); the total daily dose is usually given once every 24 hours. The regular form would be given two or more times a day. Many drugs are supplied in different release forms. Be sure to double-check the form on the order and the label.

CLINICAL RELEVANCE

Examples of errors in the clinical setting include the following:*
- Giving 10 mL of a liquid drug instead of 10 mg
- Converting 1 g to 100 mg instead of 1000 mg, a tenfold error.
- Giving 20 mg instead of 200 mg for a 0.2 g order, a tenfold error
- Reading 100U as 1000 because *units* was not spelled out or a space was not left between the number and the *U,* or the *U* was closed and looked like a zero, resulting in a tenfold overdose.
- Reading 7.5 mg as 75 mg because the decimal was not seen
- Reading 100 mEq as 100 mg, two very different measurements

*For more examples of errors, refer to Appendix C.

Drug Calculations: *Ratio and Proportion Problems for Clinical Practice*

Comparison of Metric and Approximate Household Measurements

	METRIC	HOUSEHOLD
Weight	1 kg	2.2 lb
Length	10 cm	2.5 in
	1 m	39 inches, a little more than a yard
Volume	5 mL	1 teaspoon (tsp)
	10 mL	2 teaspoons
	15 mL	1 tablespoon (T, Tbsp, TBSP, tbs) (½ oz) (3 teaspoons)
	30 mL	2 tablespoons (1 oz)
	240 mL	1 measuring cup (8 oz)
	480 ~~500~~ mL	1 pint (16 oz) (2 cups)
	960 mL	1 quart (slightly less than 1 liter)
	4 L	1 gallon (gal) (4 quarts)

CLINICAL RELEVANCE

Explain the importance of using the equipment that is packaged with liquid medications to the patient and/or family when you are administering medications and during discharge from the agency. Many serious dose errors have been reported from use of household equipment.

Answers on page 139

WORKSHEET 4H | Metric and Approximate Household Equivalents Review

Fill in the *approximate* equivalents for household measurements and *exact* amounts for metric equivalents in the space provided:

1. How many tsp are in a Tbsp? _____

2. How many Tbsp are in an ounce? _____

3. How many mL are in a metric-calibrated teaspoon? _____

4. How many mL are in a metric-calibrated tablespoon? _____

5. How many mL are in a metric-calibrated cup? _____

6. How many mL are in a liter? _____

7. How many quarts are approximately in a liter? _____

8. How many pounds are in a kg? _____

9. How many cm are in an inch? _____

10. How many mm are in a cm? _____

Rounding Oral Medication Doses

Round your answers to the nearest measurable dose based on the order and the selected equipment available.

Solids

Tablets and capsules are not rounded. Only scored tablets may be cut in half to give an ordered dose if the dose is exactly $\frac{1}{2}$ of the supplied amount. For example: Ordered—10 mg. What you have—20 mg scored tablet. Cut the 20-mg tablet in half with a pill cutter, and give the $\frac{1}{2}$ tablet (10 mg).

CLINICAL RELEVANCE

Patients who have scored-medication orders often have frequent orders for changed doses based on lab tests and response to the medication. Anticoagulant therapy is an example of various dose orders based on testing.

▶ CLINICAL ALERT!

Remind the patient to avoid mixing scored, unscored, and half tablets in one container. They need to be kept in their original labeled containers at home and during travel to avoid errors in dose. This has become an important safety issue, especially since the patient may be switched to generics of the same brand, which may come in different colors and sizes.

Liquids

The trend is to provide oral liquids in unit-dose packaged medicine cups or prefilled oral syringes. Liquids in mL are rounded, depending on the medication order and the equipment available. Oral liquids of less than 1 or 2 mL are supplied with calibrated droppers (Figure 4-4).

FIGURE 4-4 Calibrated droppers. (From Macklin D, Chernecky C, Infortuna H: *Math for clinical practice,* ed 2, St Louis, 2011, Mosby.)

Amounts of oral liquids less than 5 mL (1 metric teaspoon) are usually prepared in a pleasant-tasting solution to bring the total dose to 5 mL, 1 metric-calibrated teaspoon.

Oral liquids greater than 1 mL can be rounded to the nearest tenth of a milliliter.

Measuring Oral Liquid Doses

On occasion, oral liquid medications need to be prepared by the nurse from a multidose container (Figures 4-5 and 4-6).

FIGURE 4-5 Pour at eye level, on a level surface, to the desired volume of liquid. Read where the meniscus is level with the line on the scale (10 mL).

FIGURE 4-6 Measuring liquid medication on eye level on a level surface. (In Lilley LL, Collins SR, Snyder JS: *Pharmacology and nursing process,* ed. 7, St. Louis, 2014, Mosby. From Rick Brady.)

Liquids for medicine cups can be measured to the nearest tenth of a mL (Figure 4-7). This medicine cup is calibrated in multiples of 5 mL. When a liquid oral dose is not a multiple of 5 mL, fill the cup to the meniscus of the *nearest measurable* calibrated line on the cup and add the remaining precise dose with a syringe.

FIGURE 4-7 Total dose will be 17.5 mL. **A,** 15 mL is prepared in the medicine cup. **B,** 2.6 mL is prepared with a syringe and added to the cup.

CHAPTER 4 Medication Measurements and Oral Dose Calculations

⊖ CLINICAL ALERT!

If the oral medication is to be given with a syringe, it should be administered with an oral syringe (Figure 4-8). Chapter 5, Injectable Medication Calculations, illustrates syringe measurements.

FIGURE 4-8 Oral syringes. Oral syringes are not sterile and are used only for oral medications. (From Clayton BD, Stock YN, Cooper S: *Basic pharmacology for nurses,* ed 15, St. Louis, 2010, Mosby. Courtesy of Chuck Dresner.)

CLINICAL RELEVANCE

Occasionally a small length of tubing needs to be attached to the oral syringe to deliver the medication to facilitate swallowing. Administer very slowly.

⊖ CLINICAL ALERT!

Always be aware of each patient's ability to swallow *before* administering oral liquids. *If a question arises,* check with the patient, the medical history, and the lead nurse on the unit. If no problem is known, offer a couple of sips of water first. If the patient has difficulty, hold the medication and contact the provider promptly for new orders. Document the problem and the contact with the provider.

Answers on page 139

WORKSHEET 4I — Liquid Oral Dose Practice

Liquid doses are calculated using the same setup as with solid medications. Estimate and solve the following liquid dose problems using ratio and proportion. Label and prove answers. Round to the nearest tenth of a mL if applicable.

1. Ordered: Morphine sulfate 5 mg oral solution po q8h for a patient with pain. How many mL will you give?

   NDC 0054-8585
   DELIVERS 5 ml
   MORPHINE SULFATE C-II
   10 mg per 5 ml
   Oral Solution
   (Warning: May be habit forming)
   (SUGAR AND ALCOHOL FREE)
   Caution: Federal law prohibits dispensing without prescription.
   See Package Insert
   Roxane Laboratories, Inc.
   Columbus, Ohio 43216
   PEEL 065

2. Ordered: Potassium chloride oral solution 10 mEq po bid *2x day* for a patient with an electrolyte imbalance. How many mL will you give?

   Delivers 15 mL
   NDC 0121-1465-15
   POTASSIUM CHLORIDE ORAL SOLUTION USP 10%
   20 mEq per 15 mL
   Sugar Free   Alcohol 5%
   DILUTE BEFORE USING
   (01) 0 03 01211 46515 3
   Rx ONLY
   FOR INSTITUTIONAL USE ONLY
   PHARMACEUTICAL ASSOCIATES, INC.
   GREENVILLE, SC 29605
   SEE INSERT

   $\dfrac{20}{10} = \dfrac{15}{x}$ 7.5 mL

CHAPTER 4 Medication Measurements and Oral Dose Calculations

3. Ordered: Dilantin suspension 250 mg po daily in the AM for a patient with seizures. How many mL are needed?

4. Ordered: Zithromax (azithromycin) syrup oral suspension 300 mg daily for a patient with an infection. How many mL should you give?

$\dfrac{200\,mg}{300\,mg} \times \dfrac{5\,mL}{} = 7.5\,mL$

5. Ordered: Lithium citrate syrup 240 mg po bid for a patient with a bipolar disorder. How many mL will you give?

$\dfrac{300}{240} \quad \dfrac{5\,mL}{} = 4\,mL \times 2$

Answers on page 140

WORKSHEET 4J | Liquid Oral Dose Practice

This exercise is not difficult, but it does require focus to avoid confusing the ordered dose with the dose supplied. This can happen even more easily in a busy work environment. Estimation can help prevent major math errors. Many agencies now require silence in the medication preparation area to help reduce distractions.

Fill in the requested answers. Include an estimate of the dose to be administered.

Ordered Action or Condition for Rx	Supplied Dose	State: *More, Less,* or *Same amt* of mL as 1 serving of the drug concentration supplied	Actual dose in mL, calculated using ratio and proportion
1. Tylenol elixir* (acetaminophen) 200 mg q6h po prn headache	Tylenol elixir 125 mg per 5 mL		
2. Oxycodone HCl oral solution 5 mg po stat for patient with severe pain	Oxycodone oral solution 5 mg per 5 mL		
3. Zofran (ondansetron) oral sol. 8 mg po stat for a patient with nausea and vomiting (N/V) related to chemotherapy	Zofran oral sol. 4 mg per 5 mL		
4. Prozac (fluoxetine) oral sol. 30 mg po AM daily for a patient with depression	Prozac liquid 20 mg per 5 mL		
5. Milk of Magnesia 10 mg po daily hs prn constipation	Milk of Magnesia 30 mg per 15 mL		

*Recheck orders for elixirs if patient has known alcohol dependence. Elixirs have an alcohol base.

⊖ CLINICAL ALERT!

If there is an interruption when you are preparing medications, unless it is an emergency, complete the current preparation (and/or administration if possible) *and* the documentation of administration before attending to the interruption, such as a request for help with lifting, transport, coverage, new orders, others' conversations, etc.

Note: Do not give medications someone else has prepared.

⊖ CLINICAL ALERT!

Recheck orders and probable reason if an order is for more than one or two servings of the unit dose supplied.

Identifying Units and Milliequivalents in Medication Dosages

The following measurements in addition to micrograms, milligrams, and grams may be seen in medication orders. They may also be seen in laboratory values.

Term	Abbreviation	Meaning
unit*	write out	Is a quantity that represents a laboratory standard of measurement. It is often used as a unit of measure for products that have some or all animal or plant contents (e.g., heparin, insulin, antibiotics).
milliunit*	write out	Equals 1/1000 of a unit. Pitocin is an example of a medication ordered this way.
milliequivalent	mEq	Represents the number of grams of solute dissolved in a milliliter of solution. Electrolytes are commonly dissolved in solution and measured in milliequivalents (e.g., sodium, potassium, chlorides).
milliequivalent per liter	mEq per L	Equals one thousandth of 1 g of a specific substance dissolved in a liter of a solution. Electrolytes are frequently supplied in milliequivalents per liter for intravenous infusion (e.g., KCl 40 mEq per L).
milliequivalent per milliliter	mEq per mL	Equals one thousandth of 1 g of a specific substance dissolved in 1 mL. (The 1 is implied when a number is absent in front of mL.) 2 mEq per mL would equal two thousandths of a gram dissolved in 1 mL.

CLINICAL ALERT!
"Unit" must be written out to avoid confusion with the zero (0) or the letter "O."

Answers on page 141

WORKSHEET 4K | Measurements Review

1. The provider ordered 1 milligram of a medication for one patient and 1 gram for another. Which is the larger amount?

2. The provider ordered 250 milligrams of an antibiotic for one patient and 0.5 gram for another. Write the abbreviation for the larger amount. _____

3. A patient drank 120 milliliters of juice and 2 Liters of water in 24 h. Write the abbreviation for the larger amount? _____

4. a. If a patient receives 1 milligram instead of 1 microgram of a medication in an intravenous solution, is that an overdose or an underdose? _overdose_
   b. By how many doses is it incorrect? _1000 x_

5. a. The average American consumes about 3400 mg of salt per day. How many grams is this? _3.4 grams_
   b. A recommended amount of daily salt intake is less than 2300 mg per day. How many grams is this? _2.3 g_
   c. Some sources recommend limiting salt intake to 1.5 g per day. How many milligrams is this? _1500 mg_

*Refer to The Joint Commission's Do Not Use list on p. 60.

6. If a patient is supposed to have a 3-cm measured strip of an ointment applied over a wound and 3 mm were applied instead, would that be an underdose or an overdose? (circle one)

7. A popular recommendation is for an adult to drink the equivalent of about eight (8-oz) glasses of fluid per day (fluid from all sources).* One ounce is *approximately* 30 mL.
    a. How many milliliters would there be in an 8-ounce glass? _____
    b. How many total mL would this be for a 24 hr day? _____
    c. How many liters would this be? _____

8. In a few words, state each of the steps in a two-step dose calculation.

    Step 1:

    Step 2:

9. An adult weighs 200 pounds. *Estimate* how many kg would be the equivalent. _____

10. If an order was written for 15 mL of a medicine, how many metric-calibrated teaspoons would be the equivalent? _____

*Fluid needs vary widely, depending on activity and health conditions.

Two-Step Calculation Review

Example Ordered: 100 **mg**. You have 0.05 **g** tablets on hand. How many tablets will you give?

Select the correct equivalents.
Have grams on hand. Need to change **mg** to the equivalent **g** on hand.

Equivalency tables: 1000 mcg = 1 mg
                      1000 mg = 1 g

Step 1 Set up a ratio and proportion problem to find the equivalent measurement.

USING COLONS

KNOW   WANT TO KNOW
1000 mg : 1 g = 100 mg : x g
       (mg : g = mg : g)

$\dfrac{\cancel{1000}}{1000} x = \dfrac{\cancel{100}}{1000} = 0.1$

$x = 0.1$ g   My estimate is that I will give 2 tablets.

USING FRACTION CROSS PRODUCT

$\left(\dfrac{1000}{1} = \dfrac{100}{x} \right)$

PROOF
1000 × 0.1 = 100
1 × 100 = 100

Step 2 Insert the equivalent measure from Step 1 into your ratio and proportion now that all terms of measurement are the same.

HAVE   WANT TO HAVE
0.05 g : 1 tab = 0.1 g : x tab

$\dfrac{\cancel{0.05}}{\cancel{0.05}} x = \dfrac{0.1}{0.05}$ or $0.05 \overline{)0.1}$

$x = 2$ tabs

$\left(\dfrac{0.05}{1} = \dfrac{0.1}{x} \right)$

PROOF
0.05 × 2 = 0.1
1 × 0.1 = 0.1

> **Tips to Avoid Errors**
>
> 1. Analyze your problem. Is it a one-step or two-step calculation? (Are the terms the same or different?)
> 2. Always place a zero in front of a decimal when the number is less than one. It reminds you that the next figure is a decimal, not a number 1 (0.4).
> 3. Eliminate trailing zeros at the end of a decimal (0.75̶0̶).
> 4. Write neatly; estimate and prove your answer. Ask yourself whether this is a reasonable amount of medication. (Close to unit dose?)
> 5. If you doubt your math, recalculate without looking at your original work. If still in doubt, check reliable sources.

Answers on page 141

WORKSHEET 4L | Additional Practice with Metric Problems

Solve the following problems using a ratio and proportion method. If the problem needs to have an equivalent equation first, fill in the measurement terms (a).

1. Ordered: Levoxyl (levothyroxine) tablets 0.35 mg po daily for a patient with hypothyroidism.

[Drug label: LEVOXYL (Levothyroxine Sodium Tablets, USP) 175 mcg, 100 TABLETS, Rx only, King Pharmaceuticals, NDC 60793-859-01]

    a. Equivalent: Change _____ to _____ (if needed)

    b. KNOW   WANT TO KNOW   PROOF

    c. HAVE   WANT TO HAVE   PROOF

2. Ordered: digoxin (Lanoxin) 250 mcg tablet po daily in the AM for a patient with heart failure.

2 tablets

  a. Equivalent: Change _____ to _____ (if needed)

  b. KNOW   WANT TO KNOW   PROOF

  c. HAVE   WANT TO HAVE   PROOF
     125   250

3. Ordered: Dilantin (phenytoin) 0.2 g capsules po daily for a patient with a seizure disorder.

(2)

  a. Equivalent: Change _mg_ to _mg_ (if needed)

  b. KNOW   WANT TO KNOW   PROOF
     grams   mg

  c. HAVE   WANT TO HAVE   PROOF
     100 mg   0.2 g
                      0.200

4. Ordered: Alprazolam oral solution 750 mcg po bid for a patient with anxiety.*

   a. Equivalent: Change ___750 mcg___ to ___mg___ (if needed)

   b. KNOW   WANT TO KNOW
      1000 mcg   750
      ───────   ───
       1 mg   .75 mg

   c. HAVE   WANT TO HAVE

   d. mL after dilution per directions _____

CLINICAL RELEVANCE

Teach the patient to rinse the calibrated dropper that is packaged with the medication after using it and to continue to use the dropper with the specific medication only.

5. Ordered; Morphine Sulfate oral solution 8 mg po stat for a patient with pain.*

   a. Equivalent: Change _____ to _____ (if needed)

   b. KNOW   WANT TO KNOW

   c. HAVE   WANT TO HAVE

*Note that the labels on Problems 4 and 5 each include a "C" with a Roman numeral, symbols that indicate they are controlled substances that carry potential for abuse. They are kept in a locked area separate from other medications. The schedules range from C I, indicating a high potential for abuse and dependence, to Schedule 5, drugs with a relatively lower potential for abuse and dependence.

This order will have to be measured. An oral syringe is preferred to withdraw the needed amount (Figure 4-9). The total dose may be administered with an oral syringe or a calibrated medicine cup. Refer to Figure 4-7 on page 117 for an illustration of precise measurement of oral doses for a medicine cup.

FIGURE 4-9 Transfer of liquid medications into or out of a medicine cup. (From Clayton BD, Willihnganz MJ: *Basic pharmacology for nurses*, ed. 16, St. Louis, 2013, Mosby.)

The red flag in front of the label is an icon reminder that this is an ISMP–identified high-alert drug with the potential to cause serious harm if given in error.

Controlled Drug Schedules

Alprazolam is a C IV-level and morphine is a C II-level drug. C II and C IV are the two most frequently encountered schedules in medication administration. Prescription abuse is a challenging issue for health care providers.

Schedule 1: Highest potential for abuse. These drugs (e.g., peyote and heroin) are not prescribed because they have no currently accepted medical use.

Schedule 2: High potential for abuse and do have currently accepted medical use with severe restrictions and potential for severe dependence. Examples include morphine sulfate, oxycontin, hydrocodone products, and amphetamines.

Schedule 3: Potential for abuse less than Schedule 1 and 2 and potential for moderate dependence. Examples include several codeine products and testosterone products.

Schedule 4: Lower potential for abuse than Schedules 1, 2, and 3. May lead to limited dependence relative to drugs in Schedule 3. Examples include phenobarbital, alprazolam, Halcion, Valium, and Ambien.

Schedule 5: Lower potential for abuse than Schedule 4. May lead to limited dependence relative to drugs in Schedule 4. This level includes cough/cold medicines with codeine.

> **CLINICAL ALERT!**
> Check agency policies if a portion of a controlled substance dose has to be *discarded/wasted*. Do *not* sign as a witness to any procedure unless you witnessed the *entire* medication procedure.

Answers on page 142

WORKSHEET 4M | Multiple-Choice Practice

1. If a patient drinks 0.5 L in 4 hours, how many mL would that be? _____
   - **a.** 25
   - **b.** 100
   - **c.** 500
   - **d.** 5000

2. The correct abbreviations for metric base units are:
   - **a.** L, m, g
   - **b.** m, c, k, mc
   - **c.** mg, mL, cc
   - **d.** mm, cm, mg, kg

3. How many mL are in 2 metric-calibrated teaspoons?
   - **a.** 2
   - **b.** 10 ◯
   - **c.** 5
   - **d.** 20

4. Select the correct equivalent in mg and mcg for 0.2 g:
   - **a.** 200 mg; 200,000 mcg
   - **b.** 2.0 mg; 2000 mcg
   - **c.** 100 mg; 2000 mcg
   - **d.** 2 mg; 200,000 mcg

5. If a current drug reference stated that an antibiotic medication of 500 mg should be given in 4 divided doses, what would you prepare?
   a. 100 mg
   b. 250 mg
   c. 125 mg ✓
   d. 500 mg

   $\frac{500}{4} = 125$

6. Milligram to gram and microgram to milligram conversions require movement of how many decimal places:
   a. 2 decimal places to the right
   b. 3 decimal places to the right
   c. 2 decimal places to the left
   d. 3 decimal places to the left

7. Select the recommended method for preparing a liquid medication of 9 mL from a multidose bottle.
   a. Pour to 5 mL in the cup and add 4 mL with a 5 mL syringe.
   b. Pour to 10 mL in the metric measuring cup, and remove 1 mL with a sterile syringe to be returned to the bottle.
   c. Pour to approximately 9 mL between the 5-mL and 10-mL calibrations.
   d. Remove 9 mL from the bottle with a 10 mL syringe, and place in the cup.

   probably won't fit into bottle!

8. A patient needs 2.5 cm of a topical medication applied to a wound. How many approximate inches would this be?
   a. 0.5
   b. 1
   c. 2
   d. 2.5

9. Which is the recommendation per TJC and ISMP to write the following medication order:
   a. Penicillin, 1,000,000 u
   b. Penicillin 1000000 units
   c. Penicillin 1,000,000 U
   d. Penicillin 1,000,000 Units

10. A patient weighs 80 pounds. Approximately how many kg would be the equivalent?
    a. 20
    b. 120
    c. 40
    d. 160

Critical Thinking Exercises

Critical Thinking Exercises provide math and medication-related patient safety issues for student discussion. Answers are not provided.

Analyze and discuss the following scenarios with a classmate.

1. Mr. R is an alert, anxious-appearing, frail gentleman, 76 years old, weighing 65 kilograms. He was admitted two days before with complaints of chest pain. His medication orders included Lanoxin 0.125 mg daily every morning. This was the only medication ordered for the morning. On hand was digoxin 0.25 mg/tablet (scored).

   After you provided care for him on the evening shift, he mentioned that his doctor must have changed his orders because for 2 days he had been taking only half of a tablet in the morning; then yesterday and today, his new nurse had given him two tablets each day. His wife agreed. He wanted to know if this meant that his heart problem was getting worse.

   Ordered:

   Supplied:

   Given:

   Error(s):

   Potential injuries:

   Nursing actions:

   Preventive measures: How could this have been avoided? If you were on a hospital committee that studies incidents, what sort of recommendations would you make for this specific incident, the nurse involved, and the pharmacy department, keeping in mind that you would not want to discourage the reporting of medication errors?

2. Mrs. D is a housewife who has been admitted to the hospital for surgery for a throat tumor. She has been taking fluoxetine (Prozac) tablets for the past year for depression. The prescriber changed her prescription to Prozac oral solution 60 mg daily because of postoperative throat discomfort. The nurse administered 60 mL (2 oz) of Prozac.

Ordered:

Supplied:

Given:

Error(s):

Potential injuries:

Nursing actions:

Preventive measures (refer to the questions in exercise No. 1):

3. Mr. Z, a 70-year-old nursing home patient who has seizures, has an order for an antiseizure drug daily. The nurse notices he complains of being very tired, sleeps most of the day, and is unwilling to walk since he has been on the new medication. The doctor reduces the order from 0.5 mg po daily at bedtime to 0.1 mg. The 0.1 mg dose has not yet been delivered. The nurse reads the new order and gives two 0.5 mg tablets to the patient. (Read the adverse effects of any antiseizure medications.)

Errors:

What is the amount of the error compared to the new order? And compared to the original order?

Potential injury to the patient:

Nursing actions:

What would you recommend to the Patient Safety Committee?

CHAPTER 4 Final

1. Write the three metric base units and their abbreviations:

   a. __grams__   __g__

   b. __liters__   __L__

   c. __meters__   __m__

2. Write the abbreviations for the following metric terms:

   a. micrograms __mcg__   b. milligrams __mg__   c. kilograms __kg__   d. liter __L__

   e. centimeter __cm__   f. milli __m__   g. meter __m__   h. millimeter __mL__

3. Round the following amounts:

	Nearest tenth	Nearest hundredth
a. 4.556 mL	4.6 mL	4.56 mL
b. 1.928 mL	1.9 mL	1.93 mL
c. 0.893 mL	0.9 mL	0.89 mL
d. 7.467 mL	7.5 mL	7.47 mL
e. 0.785 mL	0.8 mL	0.79 mL

4. a. What kind of tablet can be cut? __Scored__

   b. With what implement must the tablet be cut? __a pill cutter__

5. Why are increasing numbers of medications being supplied in unit-dose packaging in clinical agencies? __prevent errors, reduce waste__

6. An antibiotic medication is ordered four times a day. Would you prepare a (single dose) or the total amount for the day?

7. Your patient has an order for 150 mL of fluid every hour for 10 hours a day. How many liters is the total amount? (Use whole numbers and decimals.) __1500 mL / 1.5 L__

8. Your patient has had 4 oz of juice, 8 oz of coffee, and 1 oz of liquid medication. How many mL of fluid has the patient consumed? __120 + 240 + 30 = 390 mL__   __13 oz × 30 mL/oz = 390 mL__

9. ▶ Ordered: Phenobarbital elixir 40 mg po daily in AM for seizure control. On hand is phenobarbital elixir oral liquid 16.2 mg per 5 mL. How many mL will you give? __16.2 mg / 5 mL = 40 mg / 12.3 mL__

10. ▶ Ordered: Potassium chloride sol. 25 mEq po daily. On hand is potassium chloride 40 mEq per 15 mL. How many mL will you give? __40 mEq / 15 mL 25 mEq / 9.38 mL → 9.4__

132 Drug Calculations: Ratio and Proportion Problems for Clinical Practice

11. What is the patient-safety issue related to telling patients to use only the calibrated equipment supplied with liquid medications?

12. What is the first step that is needed for a calculation when the measurements for the ordered dose and the supplied dose are in different terms?   *equivalent terms, then calculate*

13. If 2.2 lb = 1 kg, how many kg does a 150-lb patient weigh to the nearest tenth of a lb?   [68.2 lbs]

14. Ordered: Diltiazem tablets (E-R) 120 mg po daily for a patient with hypertension. How many tablets will you give?

→ *Label does not state Extended release*

15. Ordered: Dexamethasone tablets 500 mcg po daily in AM for a patient with an inflammatory disorder. How many tablets will you give?   [1 tablet]

0.5 mg = 500 mcg

500 mcg : 1
500 mcg

16. Ordered: Cimetidine 0.8 g at bedtime daily for a patient with a gastric ulcer. How many tablets would you give?

$$\frac{800 \text{ mg}}{1 \text{ dose}} \cdot \frac{1 \text{ tablet}}{400 \text{ mg}}$$

[2 tablets / 1 dose]

[2 tablets]

0.8 g

$$400 \text{ mg} \cdot \frac{1 \text{ g}}{1000 \text{ mg}} = 0.4 \text{ g}$$

CHAPTER 4 Medication Measurements and Oral Dose Calculations   133

17. Ordered: Elixophylline elixir 0.04 g po for a patient with an infection. How many mL would you give?

Handwritten work:
$$\frac{80 mg}{15 mL} \cdot \frac{1 \text{ dose}}{40 mg} = 7.5 \text{ mL/dose}$$

Label: ELIXOPHYLLIN® ELIXIR (THEOPHYLLINE ANHYDROUS) 80 mg / 15 mL, Rx only, 16 OUNCES (473 mL). Each 15 mL (tablespoonful) contains 80 mg theophylline anhydrous. Alcohol 20%.

18. Ordered: Tramadol HCl 0.05 g po q12h for a patient with chronic back pain. How many tablets would you give?

Handwritten work: 0.05 g = 50 mg → 1 tablet

Label: Ultram® (tramadol HCl tablets) 50 mg SCORED TABLET, 100 tablets, Rx only.

19. Name some instances in which a nurse would hold a medication and recheck the order and/or contact pharmacy or the prescriber.

   a. not E-R, patient refuses

   b. wrong route

   c. patient allergy, new side effects

20. What actions would you take if you made or discovered a medication error?

   a. assess patient — FIRST

   b. document in MAR

   c. call prescriber

   d. incident report

   e. follow up assessments

Answer Key

4 Medication Measurements and Oral Dose Calculations

WORKSHEET 4A (page 102)

	Metric Name	Abbreviation
1. Base unit for weight/mass	gram	g
2. Base unit for volume	liter	L
3. Base unit for length	meter	m
4. Prefix that means 1/1000	milli	m
5. Prefix than means 1/100	centi	c
6. Prefix that means 1,000,000	micro	mc
7. Prefix that means 1/10	deci	d
8. Prefix that means 1000 times	kilo	k
9. Name for the base unit "m"	meter	
10. Name for the prefix "m"	milli	

WORKSHEET 4B (page 103)

1. KNOW — WANT TO KNOW
1000 mg : 1 g = 200 mg : x g $\left(\dfrac{1000}{1} = \dfrac{200}{x}\right)$
$\dfrac{\cancel{1000}}{\cancel{1000}} x = \dfrac{200}{1000}$
$x = 0.2$ g
PROOF
$1000 \times 0.2 = 200$
$1 \times 200 = 200$

2. KNOW — WANT TO KNOW
1000 mg : 1 g = 250 mg : x g $\left(\dfrac{1000}{1} = \dfrac{250}{x}\right)$
$\dfrac{\cancel{1000}}{\cancel{1000}} x = \dfrac{250}{1000}$
$x = 0.25$ g
PROOF
$1000 \times 0.25 = 250$
$1 \times 250 = 250$

3. KNOW — WANT TO KNOW
1000 mg : 1 g = 25 mg : x g $\left(\dfrac{1000}{1} = \dfrac{25}{x}\right)$
$\dfrac{\cancel{1000}}{\cancel{1000}} x = \dfrac{25}{1000}$
$x = 0.025$ g
PROOF
$1000 \times 0.025 = 25$
$1 \times 25 = 25$

4. KNOW — WANT TO KNOW
1 g : 1000 mg = 2.5 g : x mg $\left(\dfrac{1}{1000} = \dfrac{2.5}{x}\right)$
$x = 1000 \times 2.5$
$x = 2500$ mg
PROOF
$1 \times 2500 = 2500$
$1000 \times 2.5 = 2500$

135

5. KNOW   WANT TO KNOW
1 g : 1000 mg = 0.5 g : x mg $\left(\dfrac{1}{1000} = \dfrac{0.5}{x}\right)$
x = 1000 × 0.5
x = 500 mg
PROOF
1 × 500 = 500
1000 × 0.5 = 500

6. KNOW   WANT TO KNOW
1 g : 1000 mg = 0.01 g : x mg $\left(\dfrac{1}{1000} = \dfrac{0.01}{x}\right)$
x = 1000 × 0.01
x = 10 mg
PROOF
1 × 10 = 10
1000 × 0.01 = 10

7. KNOW   WANT TO KNOW
1000 mcg : 1 mg = 150 mcg : x mg
$\dfrac{\cancel{1000}}{1000} x = \dfrac{150}{1000}$ $\left(\dfrac{1000}{1} = \dfrac{150}{x}\right)$
x = 0.15 mg
PROOF
1000 × 0.15 = 150
1 × 150 = 150

8. KNOW   WANT TO KNOW
1000 mcg : 1 mg = 500 mcg : x mg $\left(\dfrac{1000}{1} = \dfrac{500}{x}\right)$
$\dfrac{\cancel{1000}}{1000} x = \dfrac{500}{1000}$
x = 0.5 mg
PROOF
1000 × 0.5 mg = 500
1 × 500 = 500

9. KNOW   WANT TO KNOW
1000 mcg : 1 mg = 2500 mcg : x mg
$\dfrac{\cancel{1000}}{1000} x = \dfrac{2500}{1000}$ $\left(\dfrac{1000}{1} = \dfrac{2500}{x}\right)$
x = 2.5 mg
PROOF
1000 × 2.5 = 2500
1 × 2500 = 2500

10. KNOW   WANT TO KNOW
1 mg : 1000 mcg = 5 mg : x mcg
x = 1000 × 5 $\left(\dfrac{1}{1000} = \dfrac{5}{x}\right)$
x = 5000 mcg
PROOF
1 × 5000 = 5000
1000 × 5 = 5000

11. KNOW   WANT TO KNOW
1 mg : 1000 mcg = 0.1 mg : x mcg
x = 1000 × 0.1 $\left(\dfrac{1}{1000} = \dfrac{0.1}{x}\right)$
x = 100 mcg
PROOF
1 × 100 = 100
1000 × 0.1 = 100

12. KNOW   WANT TO KNOW
1 mg : 1000 mcg = 0.04 mg : x mcg
x = 1000 × 0.04 $\left(\dfrac{1}{1000} = \dfrac{0.04}{x}\right)$
x = 40 mcg
PROOF
1 × 40 = 40
1000 × 0.04 = 40

13. KNOW   WANT TO KNOW
1 kg : 1000 g = 5.5 kg : x g $\left(\dfrac{1}{1000} = \dfrac{5.5}{x}\right)$
x = 1000 × 5.5
x = 5500 g
PROOF
1 × 5500 = 5500
1000 × 5.5 = 5500

14. KNOW   WANT TO KNOW
1 kg : 1000 g = 12 kg : x g $\left(\dfrac{1}{1000} = \dfrac{12}{x}\right)$
x = 1000 × 12
x = 12,000 g
PROOF
1 × 12,000 = 12,000
1000 × 12 = 12,000

15. KNOW   WANT TO KNOW
1 kg : 1000 g = 0.5 kg : x g $\left(\dfrac{1}{1000} = \dfrac{0.5}{x}\right)$
x = 1000 × 0.5
x = 500 g
PROOF
1 × 500 = 500
1000 × 0.5 = 500

16. KNOW   WANT TO KNOW
1 L : 1000 mL = 0.5 L : x mL $\left(\dfrac{1}{1000} = \dfrac{0.5}{x}\right)$
x = 1000 × 0.5
x = 500 mL
PROOF
1 × 500 = 500
1000 × 0.5 = 500

17. KNOW WANT TO KNOW

1 L : 1000 mL = 1.3 L : x mL $\left(\dfrac{1}{1000} = \dfrac{1.3}{x}\right)$

x = 1000 × 1.3
x = 1300 mL
PROOF
1 × 1300 = 1300
1000 × 1.3 = 1300

18. KNOW WANT TO KNOW

1 L : 1000 mL = 2.8 L : x mL $\left(\dfrac{1}{1000} = \dfrac{2.8}{x}\right)$

x = 1000 × 2.8
x = 2800 mL
PROOF
1 × 2800 = 2800
1000 × 2.8 = 2800

19. KNOW WANT TO KNOW

1 L : 1000 mL = x L : 1200 mL $\left(\dfrac{1}{1000} = \dfrac{x}{1200}\right)$

$\dfrac{\cancel{1000}}{\cancel{1000}} x = \dfrac{1200}{1000}$

x = 1.2 L
PROOF
1 × 1200 = 1200
1000 × 1.2 = 1200

20. KNOW WANT TO KNOW

1 L : 1000 mL = x L : 800 mL $\left(\dfrac{1}{1000} = \dfrac{x}{800}\right)$

$\dfrac{\cancel{1000}}{\cancel{1000}} x = \dfrac{800}{1000}$

x = 0.8 L
PROOF
1 × 800 = 800
1000 × 0.8 = 800

WORKSHEET 4C (page 106)

Grams to Milligrams	
g	? mg
2 g	2000
2.5 g	2500
1.5 g	1500
0.1 g	100
0.5 g	500
0.25 g	250
0.15 g	150
0.03 g	30
0.015 g	15
0.075 g	75

Milligrams to Grams	
mg	? g
5000 mg	5
3500 mg	3.5
1200 mg	1.2
800 mg	0.8
400 mg	0.4
350 mg	0.35
200 mg	0.2
125 mg	0.125
80 mg	0.08
50 mg	0.05

Micrograms to Milligrams	
mcg	? mg
7500	7.5
1200	1.2
750	0.75
500	0.5
100	0.1

Milligrams to Micrograms	
mg	? mcg
1.5	1500
0.8	800
0.3	300
0.25	250
0.125	125

WORKSHEET 4D (page 108)

1. 5000 mcg
2. 500 mg
3. 5500 g
4. 2.5 mg
5. 2 kg

WORKSHEET 4E (page 108)

1. 500 mL
2. 15 mL
3. 240 mL
4. 250 mL
5. 1500 mL

WORKSHEET 4F (page 111)

1. HAVE   WANT TO HAVE
   5 mg : 1 tablet = 15 mg : x tablets

   $\dfrac{5}{5}x = \dfrac{15}{5}$

   x = 3 tablets

   $\left(\dfrac{5}{1} = \dfrac{15}{x}\right)$

   PROOF
   5 × 3 = 15
   1 × 15 = 15

2. HAVE   WANT TO HAVE
   200 mg : 1 capsule = 400 mg : x capsules

   $\dfrac{200}{200}x = \dfrac{400}{200}$

   x = 2 capsules

   $\left(\dfrac{200}{1} = \dfrac{400}{x}\right)$

   PROOF
   200 × 2 = 400
   1 × 400 = 400

   Refrigeration directions: Refrigerate prior to dispensing.

3. HAVE   WANT TO HAVE
   100 mg : 1 tablet = 200 mg : x tablets

   $\dfrac{100}{100}x = \dfrac{200}{100}$

   x = 2 tablets

   $\left(\dfrac{100}{1} = \dfrac{200}{x}\right)$

   PROOF
   100 × 2 = 200
   1 × 200 = 200

4. HAVE   WANT TO HAVE
   0.25 mg : 1 tablet = 0.125 mg : x tablets

   $\dfrac{0.25}{0.25}x = \dfrac{0.125}{0.25}$

   $x = \dfrac{1}{2}$ tablet

   $\left(\dfrac{0.25}{1} = \dfrac{0.125}{x}\right)$

   PROOF
   $0.25 \times \dfrac{1}{2} = 0.125$
   1 × 0.125 = 0.125

5. HAVE   WANT TO HAVE
   160 mg : 1 tablet = 80 mg : x tablets

   $\dfrac{160}{160}x = \dfrac{80}{160}$

   x = 0.5 tablet

   $\left(\dfrac{160}{1} = \dfrac{80}{x}\right)$

   PROOF
   1 × 80 = 80
   160 × 0.5 = 80

   HAVE   WANT TO HAVE
   800 mg : 1 tablet = 400 mg : x tablets

   $\dfrac{800}{800}x = \dfrac{800}{400}$

   x = 0.5 tablet

   $\left(\dfrac{800}{1} = \dfrac{400}{x}\right)$

   PROOF
   1 × 400 = 400
   800 × 0.5 = 400

   Note: ½ tablet contains the total dose for the two drugs

WORKSHEET 4G (page 114)

1. a More	b 2 capsules (300 : 1 = 600 : x) $\frac{300}{300}x = \frac{600}{300}$ x = 2	$\left(\frac{300}{1} = \frac{600}{x}\right)$
2. a Recheck tablet supplied, regular or XL; must be XL	b 1 XL tablet (100 : 1 = 100 : x) $\frac{100}{100}x = \frac{100}{100}$ x = 1	$\left(\frac{100}{1} = \frac{100}{x}\right)$
3. a More	b 1.5 tablets (50 : 1 = 75 : x) $\frac{50}{50}x = \frac{75}{50}$ x = 1.5	$\left(\frac{50}{1} = \frac{75}{x}\right)$
4. a Same	b 1 tablet (175 : 1 = 175 : x) $\frac{175}{175}x = \frac{175}{175}$ x = 1	$\left(\frac{175}{1} = \frac{175}{x}\right)$
5. a Contact pharmacy.	b Cannot cut unscored tablets	N/A

WORKSHEET 4H (page 115)

1. 3 tsp = 1 Tbsp
2. 2 Tbsp = 1 ounce
3. 5 mL = 1 tsp
4. 15 mL = 1 Tbsp
5. 240 mL = 1 cup
6. 1000 mL = 1 L
7. 1 quart = 1 liter
8. 2.2 lb = 1 kg
9. 2.5 cm = 1 inch
10. 10 mm = 1 cm

Note: Use metric measurements for medications.

WORKSHEET 4I (page 119)

1. 2.5 mL
10 mg : 5 mL = 5 mg : x mL
$\left(\frac{10}{5} = \frac{5}{x}\right)$
$\frac{10x}{10} = \frac{25}{10}$ x = 2.5 mL
PROOF 10 × 2.5 = 25
5 × 5 = 25

2. 7.5 mL
20 mEq : 15 mL = 10 mEq : x mL
$\left(\frac{20}{15} = \frac{10}{x}\right)$
$\frac{20}{20}x = \frac{150}{20}$ x = 7.5 mL
PROOF 20 × 7.5 = 150
15 × 10 = 150

3. 10 mL
125 mg : 5 mL = 250 mg : x mL
$\left(\frac{125}{5} = \frac{250}{x}\right)$
$\frac{125x}{125} = \frac{1250}{125}$ x = 10 mL
PROOF 125 × 10 = 1250
5 × 250 = 1250

4. 7.5 mL
200 mg : 5 mL = 300 mg : x mL
$\left(\frac{200}{5} = \frac{300}{x}\right)$
$\frac{200}{200}x = \frac{1500}{200}$ x = 7.5 mL
PROOF 200 × 7.5 = 1500
5 × 300 = 1500

Answer Key 139

5. 4 mL

300 mg : 5 mL = 240 mg : x mL

$$\left(\frac{300}{5} = \frac{240}{x}\right)$$

$$\frac{300x}{300} = \frac{1200}{300} \quad x = 4 \text{ mL}$$

PROOF 300 × 4 = 1200
  5 × 240 = 1200

WORKSHEET 4J (page 121)

1. a More	b 15 mL 125 mg : 5 mL = 200 mg : x mL) $\left(\frac{125}{5} = \frac{200}{x}\right)$ $\frac{125}{125}x = \frac{1000}{125} \quad x = 8 \text{ mL}$ **PROOF** 125 × 8 = 1000 5 × 200 = 1000
2. a Same	b 5 mL 5 mg : 5 mL = 5 mg : x (1 mg : 1 mL = 5 mg : x mL) $\left(\frac{1}{1} = \frac{5}{x}\right) \quad x = 5 \text{ mL}$ **PROOF** 5 × 5 = 25 (1 × 5 = 5) 5 × 5 = 25 (1 × 5 = 5)
3. a More	b 10 mL 4 mg : 5 mL = 8 mg : x mL) $\left(\frac{4}{5} = \frac{8}{x}\right)$ $\frac{4}{4}x = \frac{40}{4} \quad x = 10 \text{ mL}$ **PROOF** 4 × 10 = 40 5 × 8 = 40
4. a More	b 7.5 mL 20 mg : 5 mL = 30 mg : x mL) $\left(\frac{20}{5} = \frac{30}{x}\right)$ $\frac{20}{20}x = \frac{150}{20} \quad x = 7.5 \text{ mL}$ **PROOF** 20 × 7.5 = 150 5 × 30 = 150
5. a Less	b 5 mL 30 mg : 15 mL = 10 mg : x mL) $\left(\frac{30}{15} = \frac{10}{x}\right)$ $\frac{30}{30}x = \frac{150}{30} \quad x = 5 \text{ mL}$ **PROOF** 30 × 5 = 150 15 × 10 = 150

WORKSHEET 4K (page 122)

1. 1 g
2. g
3. L
4. a. overdose   b. 1000 times overdose
5. a. 3.4 g   b. 2.3 g   c. 1500 mg
6. underdose
7. a. 240 mL   b. 1 mL   c. 1.92 L
8. Step 1: Find equivalent terms. Step 2: Calculate the dose using the equivalent terms.
9. 100 kg (divide lb by 2)
10. 3 metric teaspoons

WORKSHEET 4L (page 124)

1. a. Change mg to mcg

   b. KNOW   WANT TO KNOW
   1000 mcg : 1 mg = x mcg : 0.35 mg
   $x = 1000 \times 0.35$
   $x = 350$ mcg

   PROOF
   $1000 \times 0.35 = 350$
   $1 \times 350 = 350$

   c. HAVE   WANT TO HAVE
   175 : 1 tablet = 350 : x tablets
   $\dfrac{\cancel{175}}{\cancel{175}} x = \dfrac{350}{175}$
   $x = 2$ tablets

   PROOF
   $2 \times 175 = 350$
   $1 \times 350 = 350$

2. a. Change mcg to mg

   b. KNOW   WANT TO KNOW
   1000 mcg : 1 mg = 250 mcg : x mg
   $\dfrac{\cancel{1000}}{\cancel{1000}} x = \dfrac{250}{1000}$
   $x = 0.25$ mg

   PROOF
   $1000 \times 0.25 = 250$
   $1 \times 250 = 250$

   c. HAVE   WANT TO HAVE
   0.125 mg : 1 scored tablet = 0.25 mg : x tablets
   $\dfrac{\cancel{0.125}\,x}{\cancel{0.125}} = \dfrac{0.125}{0.125}$
   $x = 2$ tablets

   PROOF
   $0.125 \times 2 = 0.25$
   $1 \times 0.25 = 0.25$

3. The order does not specify the extended release form.

   [Dilantin label: Store at 20-25°C (68-77°F) [See USP Controlled Room Temperature]. Preserve in tight, light-resistant containers. Protect from moisture. Dispense in tight, light-resistant container (USP). NOTE TO PHARMACISTS - Do not dispense capsules which are discolored. DOSAGE AND USE: See accompanying prescribing information. Each capsule contains 100 mg phenytoin sodium, USP. Distributed by Parke-Davis, Division of Pfizer Inc, NY, NY 10017. ALWAYS DISPENSE WITH MEDICATION GUIDE. NDC 0071-0369-24. Rx only. Pfizer Dilantin® (extended phenytoin sodium capsules, USP) 100 mg. 100 Capsules. 7630]

   a. Not needed. The order needs to be rechecked with the record and with pharmacy.

   The prescriber may need to be contacted to confirm the order.

   Document the clarification.

4. a. Change mcg to mg

   b. KNOW   WANT TO KNOW
      1000 mcg : 1 mg = 750 mcg : x mg

      $\dfrac{1000}{1000} x = \dfrac{750}{1000}$

      x = 0.75 mg

      PROOF
      1000 × 0.75 = 750
      1 × 750 = 750

   c. HAVE   WANT TO HAVE
      1 mg : 1 mL = 0.75 mg : x mL
      x = 0.75 mL

      PROOF
      1 × 0.75 = 0.75
      1 × 0.75 = 0.75

   d. 30 mL

   CLINICAL RELEVANCE
   Teach the patient to rinse and reuse the equipment that is packaged with this medication.

5. a. Conversion not needed.

   b. KNOW   WANT TO KNOW
      N/A

      PROOF
      N/A

   c. HAVE   WANT TO HAVE
      10 mg : 5 mL = 8 mg : x mL
      10x = 40

      $\left(\dfrac{10}{5} = \dfrac{8}{x} \right)$

      $\dfrac{10}{10} x = \dfrac{40}{10}$

      x = 4 mL

      PROOF
      10 × 4 = 40
      8 × 5 = 40

WORKSHEET 4M (page 128)

1. c. 1000 mL : 1 L = x mL : 0.5 L $\left(\dfrac{1000}{1} = \dfrac{x}{0.5} \right)$
      x = 1000 × 0.5
      x = 500 mL

2. a. 1000 mg = 1 g

142   Answer Key

3. b. (5 mL per teaspoon)

4. a. 1000 mg = 1g   200 mg = 0.2 g   1000 mcg = 1 mg; 200,000 mcg = 200 mg
   Note: it helps to write the metric base equivalents in mg and mcg

5. c. 1000 mg ÷ 6 = 125 mg per dose. Only the current dose is prepared.

6. d. 3 places to the left

7. a. Excess medication needs to be discarded. The other methods risk wasting medication.

8. b. 2.5 cm = 1 inch

9. d. Units needs to be written out with a capital "U" and commas.

10. c. 2.2 lb = 1 kg. Dividing pounds by 2 gives a rough estimate of the equivalent for the kg.

CHAPTER 4 FINAL: MEDICATION MEASUREMENTS AND ORAL DOSE CALCULATIONS (page 132)

1. a. (weight/mass) gram (g)
   b. (volume) liter (L)
   c. (length) meter (m)

2. a. mc + g = mcg
   b. m + g = mg
   c. k + g = kg
   d. L (capitalized) (small l's look like a number 1)
   e. c + m = cm
   f. m
   g. m
   h. m + m = mm

3. **Nearest tenth**   **Nearest hundredth**
   a. 4.6   4.56
   b. 1.9   1.93
   c. 0.9   0.89
   d. 7.5   7.47
   e. 0.8   0.79

4. a. scored tablet   b. a pill cutter

5. Unit-dose packaging reduces underdose and overdose errors and reduces waste that occurs with multidose containers.

6. You would only calculate and/or prepare a single dose, not the daily dose.

7. 1500 mL; 1.5 L

8. 120 + 240 + 30 = 390 mL have been consumed. (1 oz = 30 mL)

9. 6.17 rounded to 6.2 mL (16.2 mg : 5 mL = 20 mg : x mL) $\left(\frac{16.2}{5} = \frac{20}{x}\right)$

10. 6.87 rounded to 6.9 mL (40 mEq : 15 mL = 25 mEq : x mL) $\left(\frac{40}{15} = \frac{25}{x}\right)$

11. Household equipment varies widely in size and capacity. This assures a risk of underdose or overdose.

12. Obtain equivalent terms first. Then calculate the dose.

13. 68.18 rounded to 68.2 kg (2.2 lb : 1 kg = 150 lb : x kg) $\left(\frac{2.2}{1} = \frac{150}{x}\right)$

14. The label does not state extended release (E-R or S-R). Hold the medication. Recheck the order. If the patient has been taking the medication at home, get some information from the patient, if possible, about type and how many times a day the medication has been taken. Recheck the order with pharmacy and/or the prescriber. Note: Color of pills changes if manufacturer of brand or generic company is changed.

15. 1 tablet (1000 mcg : 1 mg = 500 mcg : x mg) (0.5 mg : 1 tablet = 0.5 mg : x tablets)

    Note: What you have on hand is the first entry, on the left, in the dose calculation equation step.

16. 2 tablets (1000 mg : 1 g = x mg : 0.8 g) (400 mg : 1 tablet = 800 mg : x tablets)

17. 7.5 mL (1000 mg : 1 g = x mg : 0.04 g) (80 mg : 15 mL = 40 mg : x mL)

18. 1 tablet (1000 mg : 1 g = x mg : 0.05 g) (50 mg : 1 tablet = 50 mg : 1 tablet)

19. a. order or label unclear

    b. patient states allergic to the medication or similar medications

    c. patient states medication looks different from what was being taken

    d. patient is complaining of new issue (rash, diarrhea, nausea, etc.), which could be result of a side effect of this particular medication

    e. patient refuses the medication

20. a. Assess patient and attend to immediate needs with help if necessary to take corrective action

    b. Notify supervisor promptly and prescriber (many agency policies have the supervisor notify the prescriber if it is necessary).

    c. Follow agency policy about what is to be recorded on the patient MAR.

    d. Document frequent follow-up assessments on the MAR in a timely manner.

    e. Fill out an incident report according to agency policy the same day, and give it to the supervisor or appropriate department.

Injectable Medication Calculations

Objectives
- Read and measure syringe capacities and volumes.
- Identify the lowest measurable dose on various syringes.
- Identify critical information on injectable labels.
- Calculate injectable doses.
- Differentiate tuberculin and insulin syringes.
- State three criteria for needle selection.
- State safety measures to protect the patient from injectable medication errors.
- State safety measures to protect the nurse from needlestick injuries.

Introduction

The trend for pharmacies to supply unit-dose injectable medications reduces contamination, dose errors, and waste. This chapter focuses on intradermal, subcutaneous, and intramuscular routes.* The medications that may be encountered for these routes include vaccines, antidiabetic agents, insulin products, anticoagulants, pain medications, and emergency drugs, as well as a variety of medications that are to be given relatively infrequently or for a short period. Injectable medications that have to be given frequently are often given by the intravenous route to avoid the emotional and/or physical trauma of multiple needlesticks.

Dose calculations for injectable medications are the same as for oral liquid medications.

Vocabulary

Calibration: A set of gradations on a scale to indicate values, such as seen on a ruler or a syringe.

cc: An abbreviation for cubic centimeter (ccm) occasionally used interchangeably with milliliter. May be seen on some syringes. *Write mL.* Do not write cc.† It has been misinterpreted as aa or two zeros, 00, when not written carefully.

---
*Intravenous medications are covered in later chapters.
†See ISMP Error-Prone Abbreviations in Appendix B.

Hypodermic: Meaning literally "under the skin," a "hypodermic" is an injection that delivers medication under the skin to the intradermal, subcutaneous, muscular, and intravenous layers.

Parenteral route: Any route *excluding* the gastrointestinal tract. Parenteral routes include intravenous, subcutaneous, intradermal, and intramuscular routes, among others.

Units: A standardized measurement used to quantify selected products with biological activity such as vitamins, vaccines, blood products, and hormones, including insulin.

Viscosity: Fluid resistance to flow seen in some injectable medications that are thick or sticky and require larger-diameter needles.

Syringe Selection

There are a variety of syringe sizes available—from 1 mL, 3 mL, 5 mL, and 10 mL up to 60 mL. The larger syringes may be used for infusion devices or for administration into the spinal cord (intrathecal) and other special procedures. The nurse most frequently uses the 1-, 3-, 5-, and 10-mL syringe sizes (Figure 5-1).

FIGURE 5-1 Comparison of syringe sizes and calibrations. Note the red arrows are where the 0.8-mL dose is measured. **A,** 5-mL syringe. **B,** 3-mL syringe. **C,** 1-mL tuberculin syringe.

5-mL syringe
0.2 mL increments
A (arrow to 0.8 mL)

3-mL syringe
0.1 mL increments
B (arrow to 0.8 mL)

1-mL syringe
(tuberculin syringe)
0.01 mL increments
C (arrow to 0.8 mL)

The selection of a syringe depends on several practical factors:
- The *volume* of the medication to be administered and the capacity of the syringe so that the nearest measurable dose ordered can be given. For a medication dose of 3 mL, you would not select three (1-mL) syringes or a 10-mL syringe.

CLINICAL ALERT!

If the syringe is at full capacity, be aware there is risk of disconnection of the plunger from the syringe. Figure 5-2 illustrates a half-filled syringe with the plunger in partial extensions.

FIGURE 5-2 Parts of a syringe. (From Kee JL, Marshall SM: Clinical calculations: with applications to general and specialty areas, ed 7, St Louis, 2013, Saunders.)

CLINICAL RELEVANCE

Check agency policies regarding slight, gentle withdrawal of the plunger after the needle is inserted to check for blood return. Blood return may indicate that the needle is in a blood vessel. The procedure is standard for administration of intravenous injections, but the benefits are controversial for subcutaneous and intramuscular injections.

- The *calibrations* on the syringe. If you need to give 2.7 mL, the syringe size has to have 0.1 increments to measure the portion of the dose.
- The *route* to be administered. Larger-barrel syringes deliver with lower pressure than narrow barrels. This is important when delivering viscous medications or delivering directly into veins or narrow tubing.
- The *viscosity* of the medication ordered. Very thick medications need to be administered in a syringe that is large enough to accommodate more pressure without the needle detaching from the syringe. Syringes are usually chosen on the basis of the volume of the medication and the syringe capacity in order to give the nearest measurable dose of the medication for intradermal, intramuscular, and subcutaneous routes. Some syringes are selected based on the route.

To measure doses and read syringe volumes, examine the illustrated syringes in this *suggested order:*

Steps for Reading and Measuring Amounts in a Syringe

1. **Identify the *total liquid capacity* of the syringe and the capacity between two adjacent bold calibrations.** The major calibrations are bolder with longer lines. Different-sized syringes will have different capacities between the calibrations.
2. **Divide the measured capacity by the number of spaces within two adjacent bold lines.** This gives you the **capacity *per calibration*—the lowest measurable dose, which will be in increments of 0.01 mL, 0.1 mL, 0.2 mL, 1 mL, or larger.**
3. **Identify the minimum and maximum range** of doses that may be given with the syringe.

Note the 3-mL syringe illustration (Figure 5-3). The 3-mL syringe is frequently used for subcutaneous and intramuscular injections, depending upon the size of the patient.

FIGURE 5-3 3-mL syringe calibrated in 0.1-mL increments.

Total Capacity:	3 mL
Capacity between 2 adjacent bold calibrations:	1 mL
Lowest measurable dose (capacity each calibration):	0.1 mL (1 mL ÷ 10 spaces)
Minimum/maximum dose range:	0.1 mL to 3 mL in increments of tenths of a mL

CHAPTER 5 Injectable Medication Calculations

Doses in tenths of a milliliter, such as 1.4 mL or 2.8 mL up to 3 mL, may be given. Doses of *less than 0.1 mL* or more than 3 mL *cannot* be measured on this syringe. Doses of hundredths of a milliliter, such as 1.04 mL or 2.07 mL, cannot be measured.

Examples Examine the 5-mL syringe (Figure 5-4). This syringe is used for intramuscular injections.

Total Capacity:	5 mL
Capacity between 2 adjacent bold calibrations:	1 mL
Lowest measurable dose (capacity each calibration):	0.2 mL (1 mL ÷ 5 spaces)
Minimum/maximum dose range:	0.2 mL to 5 mL in 0.2-mL increments

FIGURE 5-4 5-mL syringe calibrated in 0.2-mL increments.

Doses that end with an even number, such as 1.2 mL or 3.6 mL, can be measured. Odd-numbered doses cannot be measured.

The 1 mL tuberculin syringe is used for skin tests and injectable volumes of 1 mL or less.

Total Capacity:	1-mL tuberculin syringe
Capacity between 2 adjacent bold calibrations:	0.2 mL
Lowest measurable dose (capacity each calibration):	0.01 mL (0.2 mL ÷ 20 spaces)
Minimum/maximum dose range:	0.01 mL to 1 mL in increments of 0.01 mL

Doses of less than and up to 1 mL can be given in hundredths and tenths of a milliliter. For example, doses such as 0.05 mL, 0.36 mL, 0.8 mL, and 0.91 mL can be given. Doses that exceed 1 mL cannot be given.

remember To give the nearest measurable dose of a medication, the total capacity and the capacity of each calibration need to be known for syringe selection.

Example Differentiate 1-mL tuberculin syringe calibrated in milliliters from a 1-mL insulin syringe calibrated in units. The insulin syringe is to be used only for insulin (Figure 5-6).

Prefilled syringes are thought to reduce medication dose errors by simplifying home use, delivering precise doses, and minimizing medication waste. Some need to be attached to compatible equipment as shown in Figure 5-7, *A* to *D*. Others are provided as a syringe and may have a needle attached (Figure 5-7, *E* and *F*).

Prefilled Auto-injector syringes contain a hidden fine needle that is released immediately when the barrel contacts the skin. Figure 5-7, *F* is an example of a single-use autoinjector pen.

1 mL syringe (tuberculin syringe) 0.01 mL increments (arrow to 0.8 mL)

FIGURE 5-5 1-mL syringe.

FIGURE 5-6 **A,** 1-mL tuberculin syringe. **B,** 100-unit 1-mL insulin syringe. (From Perry AG, Potter PA, Ostendorf WR: *Clinical nursing skills and techniques,* ed 8, St Louis, 2014, Mosby.)

148 Drug Calculations: *Ratio and Proportion Problems for Clinical Practice*

FIGURE 5-7 **A,** Carpuject syringe holder. **B,** Tubex syringe holder. **C,** Tubex prefilled cartridge syringe in holder. **D,** Tubex prefilled cartridge syringe with calibrations (enlarged). **E,** B-D Hypak prefilled syringe. **F,** Epipen—a prefilled autoinjector containing epinephrine (Adrenalin) for treatment of extreme emergency allergic reactions (anaphylactic shock). (**A** and **B** from McCuistion LE, Kee JL: *Pharmacology: A nursing process approach,* ed. 7, St Louis, 2012, Saunders. **C** and **D** from Macklin D, Chernecky C: *Math for clinical practice,* ed. 2, St. Louis, 2010, Mosby. **E** from Becton, Dickinson and Company, Franklin Lakes, New Jersey. **F** from Mylan Specialty, I.P, Basking Ridge, New Jersey.)

CHAPTER 5 Injectable Medication Calculations

CLINICAL RELEVANCE

The trend is to supply more prefilled autoinjector medications. There is no plunger on an autoinjector. This design permits faster administration and is simpler for use by a caretaker or for self-administration than a standard syringe with a plunger. There are also autoinjector insulin syringe pens that have been designed for multiple use for patients with diabetes.

CLINICAL ALERT!

As with all medication, the nurse needs to carefully examine the label, calibrations, dose, and expiration date on prefilled equipment to ensure a safe match with the medication order.

CLINICAL ALERT!

Distinguish injectable from oral syringes. Oral syringes are not to be connected to injectable equipment (Figure 5-8).

FIGURE 5-8 Various sized oral syringes for liquid medications. (From Potter PA, Perry AG: *Essentials for nursing practice*, ed. 8, St. Louis, 2015, Mosby.)

Needle Selections

Needle sizes refer to length and gauge (diameter). For most injections, they range in length from $\frac{3}{8}$ of an inch to 3 inches. Longer needles are used for special procedures such as spinal taps and biopsies. The finest gauges are 32 G for skin tests and insulin administration up to larger 18 G for the administration of blood and other viscous substances (Figures 5-9 and 5-10).

remember   **Mnemonic: The Lower the gauge, the Larger the diameter of the needle.**

FIGURE 5-9 Parts of a needle. (From Kee JL, Hayes ER, McCuistion LE: *Pharmacology: A nursing process approach*. ed. 7, Philadelphia, 2012, Saunders.)

FIGURE 5-10 Needle length and gauge. (From Clayton BD, Willihnganz M: *Basic pharmacology for nurses*, ed 16, St Louis, 2013, Mosby.)

Gauge	Length
15G	1½"–2"
18G	1½"–2"
20G	1"–1½"
22G	1"–1½"
23G	1"–1½"
25G	⅝"
26G	½"–⅜"
28G	½"–⅜"

Selection of needles varies widely and depends upon the following criteria:

- Patient size
- Location to be administered
- Condition of skin
- Development of muscle
- Type and viscosity of medication
- Equipment available

Intramuscular injections may consist of larger volumes than injections to the subcutaneous or intradermal layers of the skin. Older children and adults can tolerate larger amounts of medication in one site than babies or frail, underweight, malnourished people.

The following chart shows examples of syringe and needle sizes and syringe medication volumes.*

	Intradermal	Subcutaneous	Intramuscular
Length	3/8" to 1/2"	1/2" to 5/8"	1" to 2"
Gauge	25 to 27	26 to 32	20 to 23
Usual syringe size	1 mL	3 mL	3 mL
Volume	0.01 to 1 mL	0.5–1 to 2 mL	0.5 to 3 mL

Needle comfort depends on prior experiences, feelings about needles, length and gauge of the needle, sharp polishing (finishing) of the needle, and skill of the nurse who administers it.

CLINICAL ALERT!

Fear of needles is not uncommon. Try to obtain a history of previous injection experiences. Patients big and small do sometimes faint from "needles." Give injections with the patient lying down or seated to avoid injury.

CLINICAL RELEVANCE

Injections are emotionally and/or physically traumatic for many patients, young and old. Do not give false reassurance, such as "You won't feel a thing." Prepare the patient for a little discomfort. It is better to warn about "A little stick!" seconds before administration to avoid having the patient suddenly move. Do the preparation out of sight of the patient. Good technique takes supervised practice. Provide some distraction if needed and an empathetic physical or verbal pat on the shoulder before leaving to document the medication.

---

*Lengths, sizes, best location, and angles of injection are highly indivualized.

CLINICAL ALERT!

Avoid needlestick injuries and contact with blood. Keep the syringe pointed down, away from you, visitors, and bedside curtains. Dispose of the syringe and needle immediately in the nearest sharps container (Figures 5-11 and 5-12).

FIGURE 5-11 Sharps container. (From Lilley LL, Collins SR, Snyder JS: *Pharmacology and nursing process,* ed 7, St Louis, 2014, Mosby.)

FIGURE 5-12 Sharps disposal one hand. (From Perry AG, Potter PA, Ostendorf WR: *Clinical nursing skills and techniques,* ed 8, St Louis, 2014, Mosby.)

CLINICAL ALERT!

The major cause of needlestick injuries is the recapping of needles (Figure 5-13).

FIGURE 5-13 Recapping needle. From Perry AG, Potter PA, Ostendorf WR: *Clinical nursing skills and techniques,* ed 8, St Louis, 2014, Mosby.

CLINICAL ALERT!

Needlestick injuries and the handling of blood-contaminated syringes or sponges can result in the transmission of blood-borne illnesses such as hepatitis B and C and HIV (human immunodeficiency virus). Do not add or force syringes or needles into a sharps container that is almost full. Do not *reuse* needles. It dulls the point and can cause injuries and breakage.

CLINICAL ALERT!

Be very careful when clearing an area where a procedure using needles, such as a spinal tap, has been carried out. Needlestick injuries have occurred from unseen needles under linens.

The incidence and dangers of needlestick injuries have resulted in production of an increasing variety of safety syringes. The trend to create and provide needleless equipment is growing. There are syringes manufactured with various types of covers that reduce the chance of needlesticks (Figure 5-14).

The Luer-Lok syringe tip locks the needle in the syringe (Figure 5-14, *E*).

FIGURE 5-14 Safety syringes. **A** and **B**, Safety guard before and after. **C**, Needle-less 5-mL syringe. **D**, Safety glide. **E**, 3-mL Luer-Lok syringe. (**A** and **B** from Potter PA, Perry AG: *Essentials for nursing practice,* ed. 8, St Louis, 2014, Mosby. **C** from McCuistion LE, Kee JL: *Pharmacology: A patient-centered nursing process approach,* ed. 8, St Louis, 2015, Saunders. **D** From Becton Dickinson and Company, Franklin Lakes, New Jersey. **E** from Potter PA, Perry AG, Stockert P, Hall A: *Fundamentals of nursing,* ed. 9, St. Louis, 2013, Mosby.)

Answers on page 171

WORKSHEET 5A | Reading Syringe Measurements

Examine the following syringes. Note the total capacity and the 1 mL markings. Indicate the filled-in dose measurements in the space provided.

1. a. Total capacity: _____ mL   b. Smallest measurable dose: _____ mL
   c. Indicated dose: _____

2. a. Total capacity: _____ mL   b. Smallest measurable dose: _____ mL
   c. Indicated dose: _____

3. a. Total capacity: __1__ mL   b. Smallest measurable dose: __0.01__ mL
   c. Indicated dose: __0.25__

4. a. Total capacity: _____ mL   b. Smallest measurable dose: _____ mL
   c. Indicated dose: _____

5. a. Total capacity: __20__ mL   b. Smallest measurable dose: __0.4__ mL
   c. Indicated dose: __13.2__

154   Drug Calculations: *Ratio and Proportion Problems for Clinical Practice*

Answers on page 172

WORKSHEET 5B: Syringe Volume Practice

Examine the following syringes. Note the total capacity and the 1 mL and 0.5 mL markings. Fill in the blanks and the dose on the syringe. If possible, practice with real syringes.

1. Total capacity: _____ mL. Calibrated in 0.1, 0.2, or 0.01 of a milliliter? (Circle one)
   Indicated dose _____

2. Total capacity: _____ mL. Calibrated in 0.1, 0.2, or 0.01 mL increments? (Circle one)
   Indicated dose _____

3. Total capacity: _____ mL. Calibrated in 0.1, 0.2, or 0.01 mL increments? (Circle one)
   Indicated dose _____

4. Total capacity: _____ mL. Calibrated in 0.1, 0.2, or 0.01 mL increments? (Circle one)
   Indicated dose _____

5. Total capacity: _____ mL. Calibrated in 0.1, 0.2, or 0.01 mL increments? (Circle one)
   Indicated dose _____

CHAPTER 5 Injectable Medication Calculations

Answers on page 172

WORKSHEET 5C | Additional Syringe Volume Practice

Examine the following syringes. Note the total capacity and the 1 mL and 0.5 mL markings. Fill in the blanks and shade the syringe to the volume requested. If possible, practice with real syringes.

1. Total capacity: _____ mL. Calibrated in tenths or hundredths of a milliliter? (Circle one)
   Indicate 1.6 mL.

2. Total capacity: _____ mL. Calibrated in 0.1, 0.2, or 0.1 mL increments? (Circle one)
   Indicate 4.6 mL.

3. Total capacity: _____ mL. Calibrated in 0.1, 0.2, or 0.1 mL increments? (Circle one)
   Indicate 3.4 mL.

4. Total capacity: _____ mL. Calibrated in tenths or hundredths of a milliliter? (Circle one)
   Indicate 2.5 mL.

5. Total capacity: _____ mL. Calibrated in tenths or hundredths of a milliliter? (Circle one)
   Indicate 0.75 mL.

156   Drug Calculations: *Ratio and Proportion Problems for Clinical Practice*

Ampules and vials that are amber colored and/or made of glass require special care.

Amber-colored containers such as ampules (Figure 5-15) are provided for medications that are unstable in light.

FIGURE 5-15 A, Injectable liquid supplied in ampules. **B,** Injectable liquid supplied in vials. **C,** Filter needle. (**A & B** From Perry AG, Potter PA, Ostendorf WR: *Clinical nursing skills and techniques,* ed 8, St Louis, 2014, Mosby. **C** From Becton, Dickinson and Company, Franklin Lakes, NJ.)

Filter needles are used to withdraw medications from glass ampules and multidose vials. They filter out particles of glass or rubber that might be withdrawn into the syringe.

CLINICAL ALERT!
Vials with rubber latex stoppers may also contain latex in the medication if it has been in contact with the stopper. Allergic reactions to even very small amounts of an allergen can be very serious. Manufacturers are being asked to include latex on the vial label when it is present. Be sure to check the patient for latex allergy and document it on the chart. Latex allergy may be overlooked because it is not a medicine.

CLINICAL ALERT!
The filter needles *must be removed* and *replaced* with a traditional needle *before* administering the medication. Otherwise, the filtered glass or particles would be injected into the patient.

Parenteral Routes

Injectable medication routes known as parenteral (outside the gastrointestinal [GI] tract) include the routes mentioned below as well as the intravenous route, which is taught in a later chapter. All equipment and sites are based upon patient size and condition, the type of medication, and the route. Refer to clinical skills manuals for injection techniques.

Many injectables are provided in ampules and vials and prefilled syringes.

Intradermal (ID) Injections

These are small-volume injections usually administered as skin tests. The usual dose for a skin test administered with a 1-mL syringe and a 25- to 30-gauge needle is 0.1 mL (Figure 5-16).

Subcutaneous (subcut) Injections

Nonirritating substances up to 1 mL may be injected into subcutaneous fatty tissue sites usually with a 25- to 30-gauge needle. Insulin and anticoagulants are examples of medications that may be delivered by this route. The most common sites for subcutaneous injections are noted in Figure 5-17.

A 2-inch zone around the umbilicus is to be avoided when giving abdominal subcutaneous injections (see Figure 5-17).

Intramuscular (IM) Injections

Intramuscular (IM) injections are selected to deliver medications for faster absorption. They tolerate more concentrated substances than subcutaneous sites. Doses up to 3 mL may be injected into a single site, depending on the patient's skin integrity and muscle size. The most common sites are noted in Figure 5-18. The angle of injection is shown in Figure 5-19.

FIGURE 5-16 During intradermal injection, note formation of small bleb (blister-like raised area) on the skin's surface. (From Perry AG, Potter PA, Ostendorf WR: *Clinical nursing skills and techniques,* ed 8, St Louis, 2014, Mosby.)

FIGURE 5-17 Sites recommended for subcutaneous injections. (From Perry AG, Potter PA, Ostendorf WR: *Clinical nursing skills and techniques,* ed 8, St Louis, 2014, Mosby.)

FIGURE 5-18 **A,** Deltoid site. **B,** Ventrogluteal site. **C,** Vastus lateralis site. (From Kee JL, Hayes, ER, & McCuistion LE: *Pharmacology: A patient-centered nursing process approach,* ed 8, St Louis, 2015, Saunders.)

Handwritten annotations:
- three fingers down from acromion process
- palm on greater trochanter, fingers up — spread fingers and inject between
- hand breadth below trochanter and above knee

FIGURE 5-19 Angles of injection. **A** from Perry AG, Potter PA, Ostendorf WR: *Clinical nursing skills and techniques,* ed 8, St Louis, 2014, Mosby. **B** from Kee JL, Marshall SM: *Clinical calculations,* ed. 7, St. Louis, 2013, Saunders.)

CHAPTER 5 Injectable Medication Calculations

Answers on page 173

WORKSHEET 5D: Injectable Label Interpretation

1. **MethylPREDNISolone Sodium Succinate for Injection, USP**
   FOR IM OR IV USE
   40 mg*
   Rx ONLY
   Recommended Diluent Contains Benzyl Alcohol as a Preservative.
   NDC 55390-209-10 Single Dose Vial
   Reconstitute with 1.2 mL of Bacteriostatic Water for Injection with benzyl alcohol.
   *Each 1 mL (when mixed) contains: Methylprednisolone sodium succinate equiv. to 40 mg methylprednisolone. Lyophilized in container.
   Protect from light.
   Manufactured for: Bedford Laboratories™
   Bedford, OH 44146   MPNL-V01

   a. What is the label concentration of this male hormone (have on hand), to be entered on the left side of an equation for this product?
   b. What precaution does the label lettering indicate to the nurse?
   c. What routes can be ordered for administration?

2. **LOVENOX® (enoxaparin sodium) Injection**
   40 mg/0.4 mL Syringe
   RHÔNE-POULENC RORER PHARMACEUTICALS INC.
   COLLEGEVILLE, PA 19426
   Made in France   L-5560A

   a. What is the label concentration of this anticoagulant?
   b. How is the medication "packaged"?

3. **BICILLIN® C-R 900/300**
   (900,000 units penicillin G benzathine and 300,000 units penicillin G procaine injectable suspension)
   1,200,000 UNITS per 2 mL
   Not for the Treatment of Syphilis
   FOR DEEP IM INJECTION ONLY
   WARNING: NOT FOR INTRAVENOUS USE
   Mfg. by: King Pharmaceuticals, Inc., Bristol, TN
   3000970

   a. What is the label concentration of this antibiotic?
   b. What does the unit of measurement mean: "units"?
   c. What are the three warnings for this product?
   d. What does C-R mean?

4.

   Dilaudid®
   hydromorphone HCl
   Injection
   C II 4 mg/mL
   ℞ only
   Mfd for: Purdue Pharma L.P.
   Stamford, CT 06901-3431

   a. What is the drug concentration?*
   b. What does *C II* mean?
   c. How many mcg are equal to the mg per mL concentration?
   d. Will this product be in a regular medicine drawer or a locked drawer?
   e. State briefly what the meaning of an ISMP-identified high-alert drug is.

5.

   NDC 10019-179-44
   Morphine
   Sulfate Inj., USP
   15 mg/mL   C II
   FOR SC, IM OR SLOW IV USE
   1 mL
   DOSETTE® Vial
   PROTECT FROM LIGHT
   DO NOT USE IF PRECIPITATED
   Mfd. for an affiliate of
   Baxter Healthcare Corporation
   by: Elkins-Sinn
   Cherry Hill, NJ 08003
   400-833-00
   Lot:
   Exp.:

   a. What is the drug concentration?†
   b. How is this narcotic packaged?
   c. How many mg are supplied?

6.

   NDC 0641-1410-31   2 mL Ampul
   Digoxin Injection, USP
   500 mcg/2 mL   ℞ only
   0.5 mg/2 mL (250 mcg/mL)
   FOR SLOW IV OR DEEP IM USE
   Distr. by: WEST-WARD
   Lot:
   Exp:

   a. What is the drug concentration in mcg?
   b. What is the drug concentration in mg?
   c. What are the warnings on the label?

---

*Note: The estimated potency of Dilaudid to morphine is a ratio of 7.5 to 1.
†Note: Concentrations are not comparable among products of same or different types. For example, 4 mg of morphine per mL is not equal to 4 mg of Dilaudid.

7.

KETOROLAC TROMETHAMINE INJECTION USP
30 mg/mL
1 mL Vial
FOR IM OR IV USE ONLY
NDC 55390-481-01
1 mL Single-dose Vial
Protect from light.
Rx ONLY
Manufactured for:
Bedford Laboratories™
Bedford, OH 44146
KC-KRLVA03

a. What is the concentration of this nonsteroidal antiinflammatory drug?
b. Which routes are specified for this medication?
c. What is the warning on the label?

8.

40 mEq Potassium Chloride for Inj. Concentrate, USP (2 mEq/mL)
25 Units/NDC 0074-6653-05
20 mL Single-dose
For I.V. use.
CONCENTRATE — MUST BE DILUTED BEFORE USE.
Rx only
ABBOTT LABORATORIES, NORTH CHICAGO, IL 60064, USA

a. What is the concentration of this high-alert electrolyte medication?
b. What does the word *concentrate* convey to the nurse?
c. What route is specified for this medication?
d. Is this a reusable container?

9.

ACYCLOVIR FOR INJECTION USP
FOR IV INFUSION ONLY
Equivalent to 1000 mg acyclovir
Rx ONLY
NDC 55390-613-20
Usual Dosage - See package insert.
Preparation of Solution: Inject 20 mL Sterile Water for Injection into vial. Shake vial until a clear solution is achieved and use within 12 hours. DO NOT USE BACTERIOSTATIC WATER FOR INJECTION CONTAINING BENZYL ALCOHOL OR PARABENS.
Dilute to 7 mg/mL or lower prior to infusion.
See package insert for additional reconstitution and dilution instructions.
Store between 15° to 25°C (59° to 77°F).
Manufactured by: Ben Venue Labs, Inc. Bedford, OH 44146
Manufactured for: Bedford Laboratories™ Bedford, OH 44146
ACYVA05

Method of Preparation: Each 10 mL vial contains acyclovir sodium equivalent to 500 mg of acyclovir. Each 20 mL vial contains acyclovir sodium equivalent to 1000 mg of acyclovir. The contents of the vial should be dissolved in Sterile Water for Injection as follows:

Contents of Vial	Amount of Diluent
500 mg	10 mL
1000 mg	20 mL

The resulting solution in each case contains 50 mg acyclovir per mL (pH approximately 11). Shake the vial well to assure complete dissolution before measuring and transferring each individual dose. DO NOT USE BACTERIOSTATIC WATER FOR INJECTION CONTAINING BENZYL ALCOHOL OR PARABENS.

a. What is the concentration in mg per mL after dilution?
b. What is the specified route?
c. What is the warning on the label?

10.

AMINOPHYLLINE Inj., USP Rx only
20 mL Single-dose
500 mg (25 mg/mL)
Protect from light.
DO NOT USE IF CRYSTALS HAVE SEPARATED FROM SOLUTION.
HOSPIRA, INC., LAKE FOREST, IL 60045 USA
RL-0561 (9/04)

NDC 0409-5922-01

Each mL contains aminophylline (calculated as the dihydrate) 25 mg (equivalent to 19.7 mg/mL of anhydrous theophylline). May contain an excess of ethylenediamine for pH adjustment. pH 8.8 (8.6 to 9.0). Sterile, nonpyrogenic. Use only if clear and seal is intact and undamaged. Contains no bacteriostat; use promptly; discard unused portion. For intravenous use.
Usual dosage: See insert.

a. What is the concentration of mg per mL?
b. What are the two warnings on the label?

Answers on page 174

WORKSHEET 5E — Injectable Dose Calculation

Estimate an answer. Use a ratio and proportion method to calculate the dose. Label and prove the answer. Indicate the dose on the syringe.

1. Ordered: Diazepam 7.5 mg IM stat for a patient with agitation. How many mL will you administer?

DIAZEPAM Injection, USP
10 mL Multiple-dose Rx only
5 mg/mL
HOSPIRA, INC, LAKE FOREST, IL 60045 USA

NDC 0409-3213-02
Each mL contains 5 mg diazepam; 40% propylene glycol; 10% alcohol; 5% sodium benzoate and benzoic acid added as buffers and 1.5% benzyl alcohol added as a preservative. pH 6.6 (6.2 to 6.9). Store at 20 to 25°C (68 to 77°F). For I.V. or I.M. use. Usual dosage: See insert. NOTE: Solution may appear colorless to light yellow.
RL-0644 (10/04)

2. Ordered: Solu-Cortef (hydrocortisone sodium succinate) 0.2 g IM for a patient with a severe allergic reaction. How many mL will you administer?

Single-Dose Vial For IM or IV use Rx only 2 mL Act-O-Vial NDC 0009-0909-08
Contains Benzyl Alcohol as a Preservative.
DOSAGE AND USE: See accompanying prescribing information.
Lyophilized in container.
*Each 2 mL (when mixed) contains hydrocortisone sodium succinate equivalent to 250 mg of hydrocortisone.
Protect solution from light. Discard after 3 days.
Reconstituted
Distributed by Pharmacia & Upjohn Co
Division of Pfizer Inc, NY, NY 10017
Solu-Cortef® hydrocortisone sodium succinate for injection, USP
250 mg*

$\dfrac{2\,mL}{X} = \dfrac{0.25\,g}{0.2}$

1.6 mL

$\dfrac{2\,mL}{X} = \dfrac{250\,mg}{200\,mg}$

CHAPTER 5 Injectable Medication Calculations 163

3. Ordered: Diphenhydramine HCl Injection 0.1 g IM for a patient with nausea.* How many mL will you administer?

4. Ordered: Naloxone 1 mg IM stat for an adult with a heroin overdose. How many mL will you administer?†

0.4 mg
4 mg 10 ml
─────────
1 mg   2.5 mL

5. Ordered: Aranesp (darbepoetin alfa) 45 mcg per kg subcut for a patient with anemia related to chemotherapy. Pt wt is 80 kg.

40   1
─────── ─
3600 mcg x

90 mL

---

*Note the Tall Man letters on this label. The tall letters help differentiate the product from a look-alike, sound-alike drug—dimenhyDRINATE—to reduce the chance of medication error.

†A multidose vial is supplied because more than one dose may have to be given every few minutes up to a maximum of 10 mg to reverse the overdose.

Worksheet 5F: Multiple-Choice Practice

Answers on page 176

1. What are the increments of the calibrations on a 1-mL syringe?
   a. 1
   b. 0.1
   c. 0.01
   d. 0.001

2. Which of the following statements about needle gauge is true?
   a. The lowest-gauge needles have the largest diameters.
   b. An 18-gauge needle would be used for intradermal skin tests.
   c. The needles for intramuscular injections have the smallest diameters.
   d. The gauge of the needle selected is determined by the length of the needle to be used.

3. Which site is to be avoided for intramuscular injections, particularly for infants and toddlers, because of potential injury to the sciatic nerve and blood vessels in the area?
   a. deltoid
   b. dorsogluteal
   c. vastus lateralis
   d. ventrogluteal

4. Which size syringe would you select for an intramuscular injection of 3.1 mL?
   a. A 3-mL syringe with 0.1 mL calibrations
   b. A 5-mL syringe with 0.1 mL calibrations
   c. A 5-mL syringe with 0.2 mL calibrations
   d. A 10-mL syringe with 0.2 mL calibrations

5. Which is a major cause of needlestick injuries and serious blood-borne diseases?
   a. Recapping the needle
   b. Failure to wear gloves
   c. Lack of cooperation of the patient
   d. Poor injection technique

6. Which of the following situations would necessitate a lower-gauge syringe?
   a. Viscous medications
   b. Large-size patients
   c. Undeveloped muscle
   d. Intradermal medication

7. Which is the first important nursing responsibility before preparing an injection mix of more than one medication?
   a. Check the dilution instructions.
   b. Inspect the patient's previous injection sites.
   c. Clear and clean the area of preparation.
   d. Check the medications' compatibility.

8. If a patient states that there has been some kind of previous problem with a medication the nurse plans to administer, what action should the nurse take next?
   a. Give the medication and monitor the patient for side effects.
   b. Give half the dose and monitor the patient for side effects.
   c. Hold the medication and call the physician for another order.
   d. Hold the medication and find out what kind of problem occurred.

9. Which of the following reactions to a new or recently changed medication indicates a possible allergic reaction and reason to hold the medication?
   a. Skin color changes, swollen joints, and/or chest pain
   b. Blurred vision, ringing in the ears (tinnitus), white patches on the tongue
   c. Rash, respiratory difficulty, diarrhea
   d. Brittle nails, hair loss, flaking skin

10. Which of the following statements is *true* about the use of filter needles?
    a. They should be used with the preparation of all injectable medications.
    b. They need to be placed on the syringe before injecting the medication in the patient.
    c. Filter needles are to be used to withdraw medication from glass ampules and multidose vials with rubber stoppers.
    d. The filter needle can be reused because it doesn't come in contact with the patient.

Critical Thinking Exercises

Critical Thinking Exercises provide math and medication-related patient safety issues for student discussion. Answers are not provided.

1. Ordered: Phenergan 50 mg IM stat for a patient who has nausea.

   On hand: Phenergan Injection (Promethazine HCl Injection, USP) 50 mg/mL, 25 x 1 mL Vials, FOR DEEP INTRAMUSCULAR USE ONLY. NDC 0641-6085-25. Manufactured by West-Ward, Eatontown, NJ 07724 USA.

   Given: Phenergan 50 mg IM using a 1-inch needle in a patient weighing 109.1 kg (240 lb).

   Error:

   Potential problem for patient:

   Recommendations for the Patient Safety Committee for this nurse:

2. Ordered: Glycopyrrolate 0.2 mg IM stat preop for an operative patient to reduce secretions during surgery.

On Hand: [Glycopyrrolate Injection, USP 1 mg/5 mL (0.2 mg/mL), 5 mL Multiple Dose Vial]

Given: Glycopyrrolate 2 mL

Error:

Potential injury to patient:

Recommendations for the Patient Safety Committee for this nurse:

3. Ordered: Cyanocobalamin 0.5 mg IM for a frail patient with vitamin B-12 deficiency. Patient weight 40 kg. The patient developed a sciatic nerve injury.

On Hand: [Cyanocobalamin Injection, USP 1,000 mcg/mL, 1 mL Multiple Dose Vial]

Given: 0.5 mg IM in the dorsogluteal muscle.

Error:

Recommendations for the Patient Safety Committee for this nurse:

CHAPTER 5 Final

Directions: Solve the problems using a ratio and proportion method. Estimate, label, and prove your answer. Indicate the dose on the syringe.

1. Ordered: Lorazepam 2 mg deep IM stat, a sedative and antianxiety agent, for an agitated patient. Note: Ativan is a very irritating substance and should be given undiluted deep IM.

    a. Drug concentration _____
    b. Route _____
    c. How many mL will you prepare? _____

Note that Ativan (lorazepam) is labeled C IV (controlled substance Schedule IV). Drugs in this category have less potential for abuse or addiction than Schedule I, II, or III drugs. Schedule IV drugs include phenobarbital and certain other antianxiety agents.

2. Ordered: Atropine 0.1 mg subcut on call to OR. How many mL will you prepare? Indicate the dose on the syringe.

$$\frac{0.4 \text{ mg mL}}{0.1 \text{ mg}} \times 0.25$$

168 Drug Calculations: Ratio and Proportion Problems for Clinical Practice

3. Ordered: Lanoxin (digoxin), a cardiotonic, 0.25 mg deep IM daily for three days for a patient with heart failure.

Digoxin Injection, USP
NDC 0641-1410-31   2 mL Ampul
500 mcg/2 mL   Rx only
0.5 mg/2 mL (250 mcg/mL)
FOR SLOW IV OR DEEP IM USE
Distr. by: WEST-WARD

How many mL will you prepare? _____

4. Ordered: Meperidine HCL 50 mg IM stat for a patient allergic to other analgesics.
   hydroxyzine 30 mg

$\dfrac{100\,mg}{50\,mg} \times \dfrac{1\,mL}{x} = 0.5\,mL$

0.5 mL

Meperidine HCl Injection, USP 100 mg/mL
NDC 0641-6054-25 Rx only
25 x 1 mL Single Dose Vials
FOR INTRAMUSCULAR, SUBCUTANEOUS OR SLOW INTRAVENOUS USE
WEST-WARD

Vistaril (hydroxyzine hydrochloride)
NDC 0049-5460-74
10 mL
Intramuscular Solution
50 mg/mL
Pfizer Roerig

$\dfrac{50\,mg}{30\,mg} \times \dfrac{1\,mL}{} = 0.6\,mL$

a. How many mL of meperidine will you prepare? __0.5 mL__
b. How many mL of hydroxyzine will you prepare? __0.6 mL__

Indicate the combined dose on the syringe.

1.1

Note: Combined injectables are seldom ordered. If they are, it's best to prepare each dose in a separate syringe and then add them together in one of the two syringes.

🛑 CLINICAL ALERT!
Always check a current reliable reference for incompatibility when a mixture of solutions is to be administered. If a question arises, check with pharmacy.

5. Ordered: Furosemide 34 mg IM stat for a patient with heart failure and edema. Draw an arrow pointing to the nearest measurable dose on the syringe provided.

6. Ordered: Tuberculin skin test ID for an adult patient. The volume for this test is 0.1 mL. Draw an arrow pointing to the nearest measurable dose on the syringe provided.

7. Ordered: Imitrex (sumaTRIPtan) 10 mg subcut bid prn for a patient with acute migraine headaches. Available: Imitrex vial 12 mg per mL.
   a. How many mL will you prepare for the nearest measurable dose?
   b. Indicate the dose with an arrow on the syringe provided.

8. Indicate 4.7 mL on the syringe.

9. State the volume prepared in the syringe.

10. State three practices that can protect the nurse from needlestick injuries.

170   Drug Calculations: Ratio and Proportion Problems for Clinical Practice

Answer Key

5 Injectable Medication Calculations

WORKSHEET 5A (page 154)

1. a. 3 mL
   b. 0.1 mL
   c. 1.2 mL

2. a. 5 mL
   b. 0.2 mL
   c. 4.4 mL

3. a. 1 mL
   b. 0.01 mL
   c. 0.25 mL

4. a. 10 mL
   b. 0.2 mL
   c. 6.8 mL

5. a. 20 mL
   b. 0.4 mL
   c. 13.2 mL

WORKSHEET **5B** (page 155)
 1. 1.8 mL
 2. 8.2 mL
 3. 4.6 mL
 4. 5.2 mL
 5. 0.15 mL

WORKSHEET **5C** (page 156)
 1. a. 3 mL
    b. tenths

 2. a. 10 mL
    b. 0.2

 3. a. 5 mL
    b. 0.2

 4. a. 3 mL
    b. tenths

 5. a. 1 mL
    b. hundredths

172   Answer Key

WORKSHEET 5D (page 160)

Reading labels carefully is a critical patient-safety responsibility, in addition to knowing why the medication was ordered for the patient. The nurse who administers the medication provides the last protection from a medication error for the patient.

1. **a.** 40 mg per mL
   b. There are other medications with similar names that may be confused with this name, so special care must be taken when identifying the order, including matching the patient condition with the drug activity and reason for the order.
   c. IM or IV

2. **a.** 40 mg per 0.4 mL
   b. In a syringe

3. **a.** 1,200,000 Units per mL
   b. Units are standardized measure used to quantify the biological activity of selected products, including vitamins, hormones, vaccines, and blood products (see Vocabulary section).
   c. Not for treatment of syphilis; for deep IM injection only; not for intravenous use
   d. Controlled-release product (see Abbreviations on inside front cover)

4. **a.** 4 mg per mL of this high-alert narcotic
   b. A federally controlled substance. Schedule II drugs have a high potential for abuse and physical and/or psychological dependence.
   c. 4000 mcg per mL
   d. Locked drawer
   e. High-alert drugs have the potential to cause serious harm if given in error.

5. **a.** 15 mg per mL of this high-alert narcotic
   b. Sterile cartridge (prefilled) with Luer-Lok connector (a leak-free connector)

6. **a.** 500 mcg per 2 mL of this high-alert cardiotonic medication
   b. 0.5 mg per 2 mL
   c. For *slow* IV or *deep* IM route

7. **a.** 30 mg per mL
   b. For IM or IV use
   c. Protect from light. Product is unstable when exposed to light.

8. **a.** 40 mEq per mL
   b. *Concentrate* alerts the nurse to be sure to look for dilution instructions on the label or in the accompanying literature or in a current drug reference if the label does not specify dilution.
   c. For IV route
   d. No single dose

9. a. 50 mg per mL
   b. IV route
   c. WARNING re: dilution with Sterile Saline or Sterile Water for Injection. It is very important to note that Sterile Saline and Sterile Water for injection are NOT interchangeable. Sterile Saline and Sterile Water for injection containing *preservatives* are also NOT interchangeable with the non-preservative equivalents. A label with preservatives will usually say BACTERIOSTATIC. It may contain phenol and/or other products.

   ALWAYS check dilution solution labels and literature for preservatives. The label with preservatives will usually say *bacteriostatic*. Injectables with preservatives *cannot* be administered via the intravenous or spinal, epidural, or any central nervous system route. The preservatives are usually harmless via the subcutaneous and intramuscular route. Sterile saline for injection is most commonly used for injection dilutions because it is an isotonic solution. Sterile water for injection is used *only* for specific purposes because it is hypotonic. Recheck with Pharmacy if there are any questions.

10. a. 25 mg per mL
    b. Protect from light. Do not use if crystals have separated from solution.*

WORKSHEET 5E (page 163)

1. 1.5 mL

   HAVE   WANT TO HAVE

   5 mg : 1 mL = 7.5 mg : x mL $\left(\dfrac{5}{1} = \dfrac{7.5}{x}\right)$

   Estimate: Will give more than the unit dose on hand

   $\dfrac{5}{5}x = \dfrac{7.5}{5}$

   x = 1.5 mL

   Answer supports the estimate.

   PROOF
   5 × 1.5 = 7.5
   1 × 7.5 = 7.5

---

*Always check fluids for discoloration and crystals and foreign bodies. Hold them up to a good light. If problems are noted, return fluids to pharmacy and obtain a replacement.

2. 1.6 mL

KNOW   WANT TO KNOW

1000 mg : 1 g = x mg : 0.2 g $\left(\dfrac{1000}{1} = \dfrac{x}{0.2}\right)$

x = 200 mg

HAVE   WANT TO HAVE

250 mg : 2 mL = 200 mg : x mL $\left(\dfrac{250}{2} = \dfrac{200}{x}\right)$

Estimate: Will give less than the unit dose 2 mL on hand.*

$\dfrac{\cancel{250}}{\cancel{250}}x = \dfrac{\cancel{400}}{\cancel{250}}$

PROOF
255 × 1.6 = 400
2 × 200 = 400

x = 1.6 mL

Answer supports the estimate.

3. 2 mL

KNOW   WANT TO KNOW

1000 mg : 1 g = x mg : 0.1 g $\left(\dfrac{1000}{1} = \dfrac{x}{0.1}\right)$

x = 100 mg

Estimate: Will give 2 times the unit dose on hand.

HAVE   WANT TO HAVE

50 mg : 1 mL = 100 mg : x mL $\left(\dfrac{50}{1} = \dfrac{100}{x}\right)$

$\dfrac{\cancel{50}}{\cancel{50}}x = \dfrac{100}{50}$

PROOF
50 × 2 = 100
1 × 100 = 1

x = 2 mL

Answer supports the estimate.

---

*Make your estimate when the terms are equal.

4. KNOW   WANT TO KNOW

1000 mcg = 1 mg = x mcg : 1 mg $\left(\dfrac{1000}{1} = \dfrac{x}{2}\right)$

x = 1000 mcg

HAVE   WANT TO HAVE

400 mcg : 1 mL = 1000 mcg : x mL $\dfrac{400}{1} = \dfrac{2000}{x}$

Estimate: Will give about $2\tfrac{1}{2}$ times more than 1 mL.

400 x = 2000

x = 2.5 mL

Answer supports the estimate.

PROOF
400 × 2.5 = 1000
1 × 1000 = 1000

5. 0.9 mL

KNOW   WANT TO KNOW

0.45 mcg : 1 kg = x mcg : 80 mg $\left(\dfrac{0.45}{1} = \dfrac{x}{80}\right)$

x = 36 mcg

HAVE   WANT TO HAVE

40 mcg : 1 mL = 36 mcg : x mL $\left(\dfrac{40}{1} = \dfrac{36}{x}\right)$

Estimate: Will give slightly less than 1 mL.

$\dfrac{\cancel{40}}{\cancel{40}} x = \dfrac{36}{40}$

x = 0.9 mL

Answer supports the estimate.

PROOF
40 × 0.9 = 36
1 × 36 = 36

WORKSHEET 5F (page 165)

1. c
2. a
3. b
4. b
5. a
6. a
7. d
8. d
9. c*
10. c

---

*All of the choices present a reason to hold the medication and contact the prescriber.

CHAPTER 5 FINAL (page 168)

1. a. 4 mg per mL
   b. Deep IM
   c. 0.5 mL

2. a. 0.25 mL

3. a. 1 mL

4. a. 1 mL meperidine
   b. 0.6 mL Vistaril

5. 3.4 mL

6.

Answer Key 177

7. 0.83 mL

8.

9. 0.75 mL

10. a. Dispose of used needles and syringes immediately in the nearest hazardous waste container.
   b. Use safety syringes and needles if available.
   c. Take care in handling the linens and equipment of bedside procedures that involve injections.
   d. Wear gloves with any procedure involving injections and/or potential contact with blood.

Note: Report any incident of potential contamination immediately according to agency procedure. Do not wait to see if a problem arises.

Reconstitution of Medications From Powders and Crystals: Oral and Intramuscular

Objectives
- Read reconstitution labels to determine specific diluents, diluent amounts, specific doses, conditions for storage, and expiration dates.
- State the importance of initialing and writing the date and time of reconstitution on the medication vial or bottle on multidose medications.
- Determine the best dilution strength to use for multiple-dosage-strength vials.
- Calculate doses in milligrams, grams, and milliliters for oral and parenteral routes.
- Reconstitute and measure liquid medications using a medicine cup and syringe.
- Reconstitute oral and injectable medications from powders and crystals.

Introduction

Preparation of reconstituted medications, mostly antibiotics, from powders and crystals is usually the nurse's responsibility. The medications are reconstituted by adding a diluent (liquid) recommended by the manufacturer as the vehicle for administration. The shelf life of reconstituted medications is usually short; therefore careful consideration must be given to how they are stored, the date and time of reconstitution (initialed by the nurse), the expiration date, and the route of administration. This chapter teaches the steps for safely preparing medications from powders and crystals. The measurement of units will be spelled out in the physician's orders and is used in the problem setups.

Vocabulary

Diluent (Solvent): The liquid that is added to the powder or liquid concentrate. The type and amount of diluent (solvent) used is indicated by the manufacturer and found on the medication label. If this information is not printed on the label or accompanying literature, consult the pharmacist, the Physicians' Desk Reference (PDR), the hospital formulary, or the manufacturer's website.

Dilution: The process of adding the diluent (sterile water, sodium chloride, or other liquid) to the dry powder, crystals, or concentrate to produce a solution. The more diluent added = less concentrated medication. The less diluent added = more concentrated medication.

Displacement: The volume of the powder, crystals, or concentrated liquid that occupies space in the vial (0.6 mL). This volume is added to the amount of the diluent used (2.7 mL). 0.6 + 2.7 = 3.3 mL of medication.

Reconstitution: The process of adding a liquid to the powder or crystals or liquid to return the medication to its original state.

Solute: The powder, crystal, or liquid concentrate to be diluted or dissolved.

Solution: The liquid medication that results after the diluent has been added.

Reconstitution is necessary for medications that are in powdered or crystal form. These medications must be diluted with a liquid (diluent) before they can be administered. Most medications should be reconstituted just before administration. Medications that require reconstitution are stable for only a short time after a diluent is added. In their powdered or crystal form, medications are stable, but when a diluent is added, such as sterile water, normal saline, or an accompanying diluent provided by the manufacturer, the medication begins its "shelf life." That is the time the medication will be stable and able to be used. Labels will indicate whether the reconstituted medication needs to be refrigerated or can be stored at room temperature. The label will also state the number of days the medication will be stable, or able to be used. If multiple doses are prepared, the label must be clearly marked with the diluent used, the strength prepared, the date and time of reconstitution, the preparer's initials, and the date the medication must be discarded to avoid giving an ineffective medication.

CLINICAL RELEVANCE

Reconstituted medications are expensive, as most have a short shelf life. Therefore it is important for the nurse to check that the medication order is current and has not been discontinued before reconstituting. Reconstituted medications are cost effective if all doses are used.

Parenteral reconstituted medication labels will state for intravenous (IV), intramuscular (IM), or subcutaneous (subq) use. Oral medications will be reconstituted with tap water or sterile water. If the directions for reconstitution are unclear, consult the pharmacist, the hospital drug formulary, the Physicians' Desk Reference (PDR), or the manufacturer's website.

Measuring Liquid Medications

When measuring a liquid medication, put the transparent measuring device on a flat surface, then measure at eye level. The curved surface of the liquid is called *the meniscus* (Figure 6-1). The meniscus is caused by the surface tension of the medication against the side of the medication cup. All liquid medication is measured at the meniscus level.

Medications can be measured in a medicine cup and transferred to an oral syringe for ease in administration and accuracy (Figure 6-2).

However, liquid medications can be measured more accurately in a syringe than in a medicine cup (Figure 6-3).

FIGURE 6-1 Measuring cup showing meniscus. Meniscus is the lowest level. Always measure the meniscus on a flat surface.

FIGURE 6-2 Filling a syringe directly from medicine cup. (From Clayton BD, Stock YN, Cooper S: *Basic pharmacology for nurses,* ed 15, St Louis, 2013, Mosby.)

FIGURE 6-3 Oral syringes. Oral syringes are not sterile and are used only for oral medications. (From Clayton BD, Stock YN, Cooper S: *Basic pharmacology for nurses,* ed 15, St Louis, 2013, Mosby. Courtesy of Chuck Dresner.)

CHAPTER 6 Medications From Powders and Crystals: Oral and Intramuscular

Reconstitution: Medication Labels

Labels for medications that require reconstitution contain information about the amount of diluent to use and the resulting concentration. The important information is as follows:

- Strength-reconstitution directions
- Usual dose
- Route
- Name—generic and proprietary
- Expiration date
- Storage conditions/shelf life

CLINICAL ALERT!

If the vial is a multiple-dose vial, the nurse must note on the label the date, time, amount of diluent used, and his or her initials.

Many solutions are unstable after being reconstituted. Read labels carefully for directions on storing the solution in the refrigerator or in a dark place. There is usually a time limit or expiration date on the vial. It is important to date, label, and initial all reconstituted medications.

Answers on page 213

WORKSHEET 6A: Practice in Reconstituting, Administering, and Measuring Liquid Medications

Show your calculations and proofs in the following problems. Shade in the correct dose on the medicine cup. Draw a line on the syringe showing the correct dose.

1. Ordered: Biaxin 300 mg po bid for lung infection.
   Follow mixing directions on the label.
   a. How many total milliliters of water are needed?
   b. How many total milligrams of Biaxin are in the bottle?
   c. How many milliliters will provide 300 mg of Biaxin? Draw the amount you will give on the medicine cup and the syringe.
   d. How many doses are in the bottle?

Label information:
Store granules at 15° to 30°C (59° to 86°F).
CONSTITUTING INSTRUCTIONS:
VOLUME OF WATER: 55 mL
Measure the required volume of water using a graduated cylinder. Add half the volume of water to the bottle and shake vigorously. Add the remainder of water to the bottle and shake.
Contains 5 g clarithromycin.
When mixed as directed, each teaspoonful (5 mL) contains:
Clarithromycin .... 250 mg
in a fruit punch-flavored, aqueous vehicle.
DOSAGE MAY BE ADMINISTERED WITHOUT REGARD TO MEALS.
Usual dose: Children: 15 mg/kg/day divided in 2 equal doses. See enclosure for adult dose and full prescribing information.
Abbott Laboratories
North Chicago, IL 60064, U.S.A.

NDC 0074-3188-13
100 mL (when mixed)
BIAXIN® GRANULES
clarithromycin for oral suspension, USP
250 mg per 5 mL when reconstituted
℞ only

CHAPTER 6 Medications From Powders and Crystals: Oral and Intramuscular

2. Ordered: Cefprozil 300 mg po stat, then 125 mg every 6 hours for a urinary tract infection.
   a. How many milliliters of water will you add?
   b. How many milliliters will you administer for the stat dose?
   c. How many doses are remaining after administering the stat dose?

3. Ordered: 350 mg of clarithromycin suspension bid po for mastoiditis.
   a. How many milligrams are in the bottle?
   b. How many milliliters will you administer? Draw the amount you will give on the medicine cup and syringe.

184 Drug Calculations: *Ratio and Proportion Problems for Clinical Practice*

4. Ordered: cefadroxil suspension 200 mg po q8h for acute sinusitis.
   a. How many milliliters of water will you add?
   b. How many total milliliters are in the bottle?
   c. How many milliliters of cefadroxil will you administer? Draw the amount you will give on the medicine cup and syringe.

5. Ordered: Lorabid 400 mg po q12h times 14 days 1 hour ac for pneumonia. Follow mixing directions on the label.
   a. How many total milliliters of water are needed?
   b. How many total milligrams of Lorabid are in the bottle?
   c. How many milliliters will provide 400 mg? Draw the amount you will give on the medicine cup.
   d. How many doses are in the bottle?

6. Ordered: 40 mg Pepcid po four times a day for a duodenal ulcer.
   a. How many milliliters of diluent will you add?
   b. How many total milliliters of Pepcid are in the bottle?
   c. How many milliliters will you administer?
   d. How many doses are in the bottle?

DIRECTIONS FOR CONSTITUTION: Slowly add 46 mL of Purified Water. Shake vigorously for 5-10 seconds immediately after adding the water.

Inactive ingredients: citric acid, flavors, microcrystalline cellulose and carboxymethylcellulose sodium, sucrose, and xanthan gum, with sodium benzoate 0.1%, sodium methylparaben 0.1%, and sodium propylparaben 0.02% added as preservatives.

NDC 0006-3538-92

PEPCID®
(FAMOTIDINE) FOR ORAL SUSPENSION

400 mg of famotidine

Constituted to 50 mL, each 5 mL contains 40 mg famotidine

SHAKE WELL BEFORE USING
NOT FOR INJECTION

Rx only

MERCK & CO., INC.
Whitehouse Station, NJ 08889, USA

7. Ordered: cefaclor 350 mg po every 8 hours for otitis media. Follow mixing directions on the label.
   a. How many milliliters of distilled water are needed?
   b. How many total milligrams of cefaclor are in the bottle?
   c. How many doses are in the bottle?
   d. How many milliliters of cefaclor will provide 350 mg? Draw the amount you will give on the medicine cup and syringe.

NDC:16571-071-12

CEFACLOR
For Oral Suspension, USP

250 mg per 5 mL

150 mL (when mixed)
SHAKE WELL BEFORE USE

Prior to Mixing, store at 20° to 25°C (68° to 77°F). [See USP Controlled Room Temperature]. Protect from moisture.
Directions for Mixing: Add 106 mL of water in two portions to dry mixture in the bottle. Shake well after each addition.
Each 5 mL (Approx. one teaspoonful) will then contain Cefaclor USP monohydrate equivalent to 250 mg anhydrous cefaclor.
Oversize bottle provides extra space for shaking.
Store in a refrigerator. May be kept for 14 days without significant loss of potency. Keep tightly closed. Discard unused portion after 14 days.
Usual Dose:
Pediatric Patients - 20 mg/kg/day (40 mg/kg per day in otitis media) in three divided doses every 8 hours.
Adults - 250 mg every 8 hours.
See literature for complete dosage information.
Bottle contains a total of Cefaclor Monohydrate equivalent to 7.5 g anhydrous cefaclor in a dry, strawberry flavored mixture.
Rev. 09/12

△PACK™
Pharmaceuticals

Rx only

186 Drug Calculations: *Ratio and Proportion Problems for Clinical Practice*

8. Ordered: Augmentin 450 mg po every 8 hours for 24 hours then 250 mg twice a day for 4 days for endocarditis prophylaxis.
   a. How many milliliters of diluent will you add?
   b. How many milliliters will you administer per dose for 24 hours? Draw the amount you will give on the medicine cup and syringe.
   c. How many milliliters are left after the 24 hr doses?
   d. Will you have enough medication for the next 4 days?

CLINICAL ALERT!

For accuracy, read the medication's level at the meniscus.

9. Ordered: Fluconazole 50 mg po twice a day as a prophylaxis of candidiasis.
   a. How many mL of sterile water will be added to the powder?
   b. How many mL will you administer?
   c. How many 50-mg doses are in the bottle?

CHAPTER 6 Medications From Powders and Crystals: Oral and Intramuscular   187

10. Ordered: 200 mg of Biaxin po two times a day for laryngitis.
   a. How many mL of water should be added?
   b. How many mL will you administer?
   c. How many doses are in the bottle?

Reconstituting Medications for Parenteral Use

Reconstituting medications is much like making a cup of soup out of dried soup mix from a package or using freeze-dried coffee crystals to make a cup of coffee. The concept is the same. When a lot of liquid, or diluent, as it is referred to when mixing medications, is used, the soup or coffee becomes weaker. The less liquid or diluent used, the stronger the soup or coffee. For some medications that must be reconstituted, various amounts of diluent or liquid can be added to produce various strengths of the medicine. As an example, if you add 16 oz, or 1 pint, of water to 1 Tbsp of instant coffee, you will have very weak coffee. If you add 8 oz of water to 1 Tbsp of instant coffee, you will have stronger coffee and less total volume. The main point is that the amount of instant coffee remains constant; only the amount of liquid (diluent) changes to make a stronger or weaker dilution. Reconstituting medications works in the same manner.* There is always a certain amount of powder or crystals in the container before the diluent is added. The drug manufacturer tells you what the displacement factor is. This amount is added to the amount of diluent to give the total number of milliliters (volume). The label on the medication vial states the strength (amount) of medication in the vial. That amount never changes. The only thing that can change is the amount of diluent (liquid) that is added.

*Directions for dissolving medications in vials can be found in the accompanying literature. What will be given is the volume of the powder after it is dissolved in the diluent. For instance, the directions may read: *Add 1.4 mL NS to make 2 mL of reconstituted solution*. These directions tell the user that the powder takes up 0.6 mL of space. The displacement factor is 0.6 mL.

1.4 mL + 0.6 mL = 2 mL of medication

Types of Diluents

🚩 **It is important to use the type of diluent described in the directions for reconstitution.** The diluents used to reconstitute powders vary based on the chemical properties of the powder. For example, erythromycin must be reconstituted with sterile water. If normal saline (NS) is used, the powder clumps and will not go into solution. The bacteriostatic agent used in bacteriostatic water is benzyl alcohol. If sterile water is used instead of bacteriostatic water, it may cause some products to clump instead of going into solution. The choice of diluent is based on the pH and the physical properties of the product (medication).

Dibasic sodium is added to some powders to correct the final pH of the product.

Lidocaine is added to ease pain during IM administration. The amount of lidocaine added to the medication would not affect vasoconstriction.

> **CLINICAL ALERT!**
> *Always* use the diluent recommended for reconstitution.

Two-Vial Reconstitution Method

When parenteral drugs are supplied with two vials, one vial will have the diluent and the other the powdered medication. Both vials are cleaned with alcohol swabs. The amount of diluent needed is stated on the medication label. The required amount of the diluent is withdrawn from its vial (Figure 6-4) and injected into the powdered-drug vial. The mixture is then rotated until it is thoroughly mixed.

Example Read the medication label to find out how many units, grams, milligrams, or micrograms are in each milliliter of the reconstituted drug.

Begin by adding 2.7 mL of air to the sterile water for injection (diluent) vial, and then invert the vial to withdraw the 2.7 mL of diluent. Add the 2.7 mL of diluent to the oxacillin sodium vial to make 500 mg of medication in 3 mL.

FIGURE 6-4 Diluting oxacillin sodium in sterile water for injection.

Sterile water for injection. **Add** 2.7 mL of air to allow for withdrawal.

Sterile water for injection. **Withdraw** 2.7 mL of diluent.

Add 2.7 mL sterile water for injection to oxacillin sodium.

Oxacillin sodium 500 mg per 3 mL.

Ordered: 250 mg oxacillin sodium IM q6h. Use either ratio and proportion or fraction cross product.

KNOW   WANT TO KNOW

3 mL : 500 mg = x mL : 250 mg
500x = 3 × 250 = 750
  x = 1.5 mL

$$\frac{3 \text{ mL}}{500 \text{ mg}} = \frac{x \text{ mL}}{250 \text{ mg}}$$

PROOF
500 × 1.5 = 750
3 × 250 = 750

Give 1.5 mL of reconstituted solution for each 250 mg.

CLINICAL ALERT!
When giving intramuscular injections, always aspirate before injecting. If blood is returned, discard the dose.

Drug Calculations: *Ratio and Proportion Problems for Clinical Practice*

Prefilled Vials and Syringes

When medications to be reconstituted are packaged with the diluent attached, the sterility and accuracy of the reconstituted powder are ensured (Figure 6-5). Some medications are reconstituted by the manufacturer and are delivered in prefilled cartridges or syringes. With this technique there is less chance for contamination.

FIGURE 6-5 Mix-o-vial directions. **A,** Remove lid protector. **B,** Powdered medication is in lower half; diluent is in upper half. **C,** Push firmly on the diaphragm-plunger. Downward pressure dislodges the divider between the two chambers. (From Clayton BD, Stock YN, Cooper S: *Basic pharmacology for nurses,* ed 16, St Louis, 2013, Mosby. Courtesy of Chuck Dresner.)

Most reconstituted medications are antibiotics and have similar-sounding generic and trade names. The following chart is an example of some common sound-alike and look-alike drugs.

Generic Name	Trade Name
Cefaclor	Ceclor
Cefprozil	Cefzil
Cefuroxime	Ceftin
Cephalexin	Keflex
Cephazolin	Kefzol
Ciprofloxacin	Cipro
Gatifloxacin	Tequin
Gemifloxacin	Factive

> Figure 6-6 is a pharmacy-generated MAR for 24 hours stated in military time for 8-hour shifts beginning at 0700. At the top, the orders must be signed by an RN indicating that the original order has been verified and is correct and allergies have been noted. SCH is a regularly scheduled medication. The start and stop dates are printed. PRN orders and One Time Only Meds are written in a separate space. Narcotic orders must be rewritten q48h. Discontinued orders are highlighted according to hospital policy and must be renewed if it is necessary to continue them. Site codes are in alpha order. Withheld meds use the code R circled with a nurse's note on the chart. The nurses giving the meds must initial each dose and sign the bottom of the MAR to identify their initials.

Doe, John
ID# 45764304
Age: 50 Sex: M Rm: 406A
Dr. Marin, Cruz

ALLERGIES: DRUGS: Codeine
FOODS: none

RN Verification: Mary Smith

Date: 11-09-16 (Beg)
11-13-16 (End)

MEDICATION: Dose Route Freq   Time of Administration, Site, and Initials

	START	STOP	0700 TO 1459	1500 TO 2259	2300 TO 0659
SCH	11-09-16 Kefzol 300 mg IM q8h	11-13-16	0700 N MS	1500 O IB	2300 N JB

Each health care agency will have a protocol for charting injection sites. This is one example

ONE TIME ONLY AND PRN MEDS

Start	Stop	Time	Initials	Full name/title
Lasix 11-16-16 40 mg IV STAT		2000	IB	Irene Butler, RN

Sign: Mary Smith   Initials: MS   Sign: Irene Butler   Initials: IB   Sign: Jill Beck   Initials: JB

SITE CODES   GENERAL HOSPITAL

A	Abdomen (L)	J	Gluteus (LUQ)
B	Abdomen (R)	K	Gluteus (RUQ)
C	Arm (L)	L	Thigh (L)
D	Arm (R)	M	Thigh (R)
E	Eyes (both)	N	Ventrogluteal (L)
F	Eyes (left)	O	Ventrogluteal (R)
G	Eyes (right)	P	NPO: Lab
H	Deltoid (mid L)	Q	NPO: Surgery
I	Deltoid (mid R)	R	Withheld/see nurse's notes

FIGURE 6-6 Medication administration record (MAR).

CLINICAL RELEVANCE

Ask patients who are receiving antibiotics if they have ever had an allergic reaction to antibiotics. If the answer is yes, ask which medication and what type of reaction they had. Report any previous reactions to the physician before administering the medication.

CLINICAL RELEVANCE

When all of the medication in a prefilled syringe is not used, the unused portion must be discarded, and this action must be witnessed by another health professional. The syringe is intended only for a one-time injection.

WORKSHEET 6B — Practice in Reconstituting Parenteral Dosages With Multiple-Strength Decisions

Answers on page 218

Show your calculations and proofs in the following problems. Shade in the correct doses on the syringes.

1. Ordered: Pfizerpen (penicillin G potassium) 300,000 units IM bid to prevent bacterial endocarditis. Available: 1 million units.
   Calculate the strength closest to the ordered amount.
   a. How many milliliters of diluent will you add?
   b. How many milliliters will you administer?
   c. How many doses are in the multidose vial?

2. Ordered: Ceftriaxone 0.5 g IM q4h for gonorrhea.
   a. How many milliliters of diluent will you add?
   b. How many milligrams per milliliter will this make?
   c. How many milliliters will you administer?
   d. How many doses are in the vial?

CHAPTER 6 Medications From Powders and Crystals: Oral and Intramuscular

3. Ordered: Ampicillin 1000 mg q6h IM for tonsillitis. Available: Ampicillin 1 g.
   a. How many milliliters will you administer?
   b. How many milliliters will you give in each site?

CLINICAL ALERT!

The maximum single injection for adults is 3 mL. Not all patients can tolerate a 3-mL injection. Assess the patient for adequate muscle mass at the site of injection to determine the ability for absorption, which aids in patient comfort as well as therapeutic value.

4. Ordered: Oxacillin sodium 500 mg for a leg infection. Available: A multidose vial.
   a. How many mL of diluent will you add?
   b. How many mL of oxacillin will you administer?

194 Drug Calculations: *Ratio and Proportion Problems for Clinical Practice*

5. Ordered: Cefobid 1000 mg IM q12h for pelvic inflammatory disease. Available: Cefobid 1 g. Reconstitute IM doses with 2.2 mL of bacteriostatic water for injection (taken from insert). The powder displaces 0.4 mL. How many milliliters will be administered?

6. Ordered: Ceftriaxone 450 mg IM twice a day times 3 days for meningitis. Available: A vial containing 500 mg.
   a. How many mL of 1% Lidocaine will you add?
   b. What amount will you administer?

CHAPTER 6 Medications From Powders and Crystals: Oral and Intramuscular

7. Ordered: Tazicef 250 mg IM q8h for otitis media.
   Available: Tazicef 1 g for IM or IV use.
   Follow insert directions for reconstitution directions.
   a. How many mL of diluent will be added to the powder?
   b. How many mg/mL will this make?
   c. How many mL will you administer IM?

RECONSTITUTION

Single Dose Vials:
For I.M. injection, I.V. direct (bolus) injection, or I.V. infusion, reconstitute with Sterile Water for injection according to the following table. The vacuum may assist entry of the diluent. SHAKE WELL.

Table 5

Vial Size	Diluent to Be Added	Approx. Avail. Volume	Approx. Avg. Concentration
Intramuscular or Intravenous Direct (bolus) Injection			
1 gram	3.0 ml.	3.6 ml.	280 mg./ml.
Intravenous Infusion			
1 gram	10 ml.	10.6 ml.	95 mg./ml.
2 gram	10 ml.	11.2 ml.	180 mg./ml.

Withdraw the total volume of solution into the syringe (the pressure in the vial may aid withdrawal). The withdrawn solution may contain some bubbles of carbon dioxide.

NOTE: As with the administration of all parenteral products, accumulated gases should be expressed from the syringe immediately before injection of 'Tazicef'.

These solutions of 'Tazicef' are stable for 18 hours at room temperature or seven days if refrigerated (5C.). Slight yellowing does not affect potency.

For I.V. infusion, dilute reconstituted solution in 50 to 100 ml. of one of the parenteral fluids listed under COMPATIBILITY AND STABILITY.

(Tazicef label: equivalent to 1 gram ceftazidime, NDC 0007-5082-01, TAZICEF CEFTAZIDIME FOR INJECTION, SmithKline Beecham)

8. Ordered: 100 mg ampicillin IM q12h to treat a skin ulcer.
   a. How many milliliters of diluent will be added?
   b. What is the shelf life after reconstitution?
   c. What is the total amount of medication in the vial?
   d. How many milliliters of ampicillin will you administer?

(Ampicillin for Injection, USP, 1 gram per vial, For I.M. or I.V. use, Claris — This vial contains ampicillin sodium equivalent to 1 gram ampicillin. For I.M. use, add 3.5 mL diluent (read accompanying insert). Resulting solution contains 250 mg ampicillin per mL. Use solution within 1 hour. Usual Dosage: Adults - 250 to 500 mg I.M. q.6.h. READ ACCOMPANYING INSERT for detailed indications, I.M. or I.V. dosage and precautions. Store dry powder at 20° to 25°C (68° to 77°F) [See USP].)*

196   Drug Calculations: *Ratio and Proportion Problems for Clinical Practice*

9. Ordered: Cefadyl 700 mg IM q6h for bronchitis. Available: Cefadyl 1 g. Follow directions on label.
   a. How many milliliters will you administer per injection?
   b. How many milligrams will the patient receive in 24 hours?
   c. How many vials will you need for a 24-hour period?

> **CLINICAL ALERT!**
> Do not confuse units of medication with milligrams.

10. Ordered: Cefobid 2 g IM q12h for a respiratory tract infection. Available: Cefobid 2 g vial. Reconstitution for IM use is found on the package insert. Directions read: Add 3.4 mL of sterile water for injection. The Cefobid powder displaces 0.6 mL. Administer the entire dose.
    a. How many milliliters will you give for the first dose?
    b. How many injections will you administer?
    c. What sites will you select?

WORKSHEET 6C — Additional Practice in Reconstituting Parenteral Dosages With Multiple-Strength Decisions

Answers on page 221

Answer the questions in the following problems. Show your calculations and proofs; then shade in the correct dose on the syringes.

1. Ordered: Streptomycin 0.5 g IM q12h for a patient with *Klebsiella* pneumonia.
   a. If you add 1.8 mL of diluent, what mg per mL concentration will you have?
   b. How many mL will you give?

Streptomycin for Injection USP — 1 gram/vial
For Intramuscular Use

Volume (mL) to be added	Approx. Conc. mg/mL
4.2	200
3.2	250
1.8	400

2. Ordered: Cefadyl (cephapirin) 500 mg IM q6h for infected bone (leg).
   a. How many milliliters of sterile water will you add?
   b. How many mg/per 1.2 mL will you have?
   c. How many milliliters will you administer?

CEFADYL® — Sterile Cephapirin Sodium, USP — 1 gram CEPHAPIRIN
For IM or IV Use
Usual Dosage: Adults—500 mg to 1 g every 4 to 6 hours. For IM use, add 2 mL Sterile or Bacteriostatic Water for Injection, USP. Each 1.2 mL contains 500 mg of cephapirin.

198 Drug Calculations: *Ratio and Proportion Problems for Clinical Practice*

3. Ordered: Ceftriaxone 500 mg IM bid for a urinary tract infection.
   Directions: For IM use, add sterile water for injection according to directions. Withdraw entire contents to yield 500 mg. Give deep in a large muscle. Aspirate before giving. Calculate both dosages to determine which amount is appropriate for your patient.

Vial Dose Size	Amount of Diluent to Be Added
	1.8 mL ——— 250 mg/mL
500 mg	1 mL ——— 350 mg/mL

   Which concentration did you choose? Measure it on the syringe.

CLINICAL ALERT!
Check patient's medication history of drug sensitivity before administration of antiinfectives. Keep epinephrine, an antihistamine, and resuscitation equipment nearby in the event of an anaphylactic shock reaction.

4. Ordered: 400,000 units Pfizerpen IM q6h for pneumococcal pneumonia.
   Available: Pfizerpen 1 million units with mixing options.
   Choose between adding 4 mL and adding 1.5 mL of diluent.
   a. How many units/mL will you administer if you use 4 mL of diluent? Mark the syringe.
   b. How many units/mL will you administer if you use 1.5 mL of diluent? Mark the syringe.

CHAPTER 6 Medications From Powders and Crystals: Oral and Intramuscular 199

5. Ordered: Methylprednisolone 125 mg IM q6h for ulcerative colitis.
   a. How many milliliters of diluent will you add?
   b. How many milligrams per milliliters will this make?
   c. How many milliliters will you give?
   d. How many doses are in the vial?
   e. The medication has to be used within how many hours after reconstituting?
   f. Will all of the doses for this order be given within the recommended time frame?

6. Ordered: Pfizerpen 400,000 units IM every 12 hours for a patient with a streptococcal infection.
   a. Which strength will you prepare for your patient. Show the different calculations.
   b. How many mL's will you give? How will you determine which strength to give?

3 Strengths to Determine Dosage
18.2 mL =   250,000 units/mL
8.2 mL =   500,000 units/mL
3.2 mL = 1,000,000 units/mL

7. Ordered: Ticar 750 mg IM q8h for peritonitis.
   a. How many milliliters of diluent will be added?
   b. 2.6 mL of Ticar contains how many grams?
   c. What is the shelf life of the medication?
   d. What is the total amount of medication in the vial?
   e. How many milliliters will you administer?

8. Ordered: ampicillin 0.5 g IM q6h for a patient with an URI (upper respiratory infection).
   a. How many milliliters of diluent will you add?
   b. What is the resulting concentration?
   c. How many milliliters of medication will you administer?
   d. What is the shelf life?

CHAPTER 6 Medications From Powders and Crystals: Oral and Intramuscular

9. Ordered: Ampicillin 500 mg IM q6h times 3 days for a streptococcal throat infection.
   a. How many milliliters of diluent are needed to reconstitute the medication?
   b. How many mg/mL will it make?
   c. What is the shelf life of the medication?
   d. How many milliliters will you administer?

10. Ordered: Oxacillin sodium 450 mg IM q6h for actinomycosis.
    a. How many milliliters of sterile water will be used for reconstitution?
    b. How many mg/mL will it make?
    c. What is the shelf life of the medication after reconstitution?
    d. What is the total amount of medication in the vial?
    e. How many milliliters will you administer?

> **CLINICAL ALERT!**
> Always make sure that the patient's body mass is adequate for the amount of medication that will be given intramuscularly.

Worksheet 6D: Multiple-Choice Practice

Answers on page 225

1. Ordered: Levothyroxine 60 mcg IM for a thyroid condition.
   How many milliliters will you administer?
   a. 2 mL   b. 1.5 mL   c. 2.2 mL   d. 2.5 mL

   LEVOTHYROXINE SODIUM FOR INJECTION
   NDC 55390-880-10
   Usual Dosage: See insert for complete information.
   Vial contains 200 mcg levothyroxine sodium, 10 mg mannitol, 0.7 mg tribasic sodium phosphate, and sodium hydroxide for pH adjustment.
   FOR IM OR IV USE ONLY
   200 mcg
   LYOPHILIZED
   Rx ONLY
   Use immediately after reconstitution with 5 mL of 0.9% sodium chloride injection, USP only. Reconstituted concentration is 40 mcg/mL. Preservative free. Discard any unused portion.
   Store at controlled room temperature, 15° to 30°C (59° to 86°F).
   Manufactured for:
   Bedford Laboratories™
   Bedford, OH 44146
   LTR-V04

2. Ordered: Ampicillin 250 mg IM q12h to treat an infected surgical site.
   Available: Ampicillin 125 mg.
   How many milliliters of diluent will you add?
   a. 2 mL   b. 1.2 mL   c. 3 mL   d. 1.5 mL

   How many vials will you need in 24 hours?
   a. 1 vial   b. 2 vials   c. 3 vials d. 4 vials

   NDC 0015-7401-20
   EQUIVALENT TO
   125 mg AMPICILLIN
   Ampicillin for Injection, USP
   For IM or IV Use
   Rx only
   APOTHECON®
   A Bristol-Myers Squibb Company
   Princeton, NJ 08540 USA

3. Ordered: Methylprednisolone 35 mg IM every day times 3 days for arthritis.
   Available: Methylprednisolone 40 mg/mL.
   How many milliliters of sterile water will you add?
   a. 2.1 mL   b. 12 mL   c. 3.1 mL   d. 1.2 mL

   How many milliliters will you administer?
   a. 1.5 mL   b. 1 mL   c. 0.8 mL   d. 0.9 mL

   MethylPREDNISolone Sodium Succinate for Injection, USP
   NDC 55390-209-10 Single Dose Vial
   Reconstitute with 1.2 mL of Bacteriostatic Water for Injection with benzyl alcohol.
   FOR IM OR IV USE
   40 mg*
   Rx ONLY
   Recommended Diluent Contains Benzyl Alcohol as a Preservative.
   *Each 1 mL (when mixed) contains: Methylprednisolone sodium succinate equiv. to 40 mg methylprednisolone.
   Lyophilized in container.
   Protect from light.
   Manufactured for:
   Bedford Laboratories™
   Bedford, OH 44146   MPNL-V01

4. Ordered: Cefobid 1.5 g IM q12h for bacterial endocarditis.
   Available: Cefobid 1 g vial.
   Directions read: Add 1.4 mL of sterile water for injection. Each 2 mL yields 1 g.
   How many milliliters will you administer?
   a. 2.5 mL   b. 3 mL   c. 2 mL   d. 1.5 mL

   How many vials will you need for 24 hours?
   a. 2 vials   b. 2.5 vials   c. 3.5 vials   d. 3 vials

5. Ordered: Cefobid 1g IM q12h for a respiratory tract infection.
   Available: Cefobid 2 g vial.
   Directions for IM use read: Add 3.4 mL of sterile water for injection. Each 4 mL yields 2 g.
   How many milliliters will you administer?
   a. 3.5 mL   b. 4 mL   c. 2 mL   d. 2.5 mL

6. Ordered: Ticar 500 mg IM tid for a pseudomonas infection.
   Available: Ticar 1 g.
   Directions read: Add 2 mL of sterile water for injection.
   How many milliliters will you administer?
   a. 2.6 mL   b. 2 mL   c. 1.3 mL   d. 3 mL

7. Refer to question 6.
   How many vials of Ticar will be needed in 24 hours?
   a. 3 vials   b. 4 vials   c. 2 vials   d. 5 vials

8. Ordered: Pfizerpen 400,000 units IM bid to treat diphtheria.
   Available: Pfizerpen (penicillin G potassium) 1 million units.
   How many milliliters of diluent will you add?
   a. 5 mL   b. 10 mL   c. 1.5 mL   d. 20 mL

   How many milliliters will you administer?
   a. 2 mL   b. 2.5 mL   c. 1.6 mL   d. 0.8 mL

9. Ordered: Streptomycin 500 mg IM bid for meningitis.
   Available: Streptomycin sulfate 5 g.
   What is the concentration after dilution?
   a. 500 mg/mL   b. 1 g/mL   c. 400 mg/mL   d. 0.5 g/mL

   How many milliliters will you administer?
   a. 1.3 mL   b. 1 mL   c. 2.2 mL   d. 1.8 mL

10. Ordered: Ancef 250 mg IM q6h for a urinary tract infection.
    Available: Ancef 1 gram for reconstitution.
    How many mL will you administer?
    a. 2 mL   b. 0.5 mL   c. 0.8 mL   d. 4.5 mL

Critical Thinking Exercises

Critical Thinking Exercises provide math and medication-related patient safety issues for student discussion. Answers are not provided.

Analyze the following scenarios.

1. A 1-million-unit multiple-dose vial of penicillin G potassium has these directions for reconstitution:

Add Diluent	Concentration of Solution
9.6 mL	100,000 units/mL
4.6 mL	200,000 units/mL
1.6 mL	500,000 units/mL

   The medication was reconstituted with 9.6 mL of diluent and 200,000 units per mL circled.

   Ordered: Penicillin G potassium 200,000 units IM q6h

   Given: Penicillin G potassium 1 mL IM q6h

   Error(s):

   Potential injuries:

   Discussion
   How many units of penicillin G potassium were given?
   What were the potential injuries?
   Which concentration would have provided the ordered amount in 1 mL?
   How could this error have been prevented?

2. Ordered: Cefadyl 250 mg IM every 12 hours times 4 doses for dermatitis.

   The Cefadyl (cephapirin) vial was reconstituted with 2 mL of sterile water for injection. The vial was labeled with the date, time, amount of diluent (2 mL of sterile water) circled, and the nurse's initials. The nurse gave the first injection (0.6 mL) of Cefadyl IM at 0800 hours. The next nurse gave the 250 mg dose (0.3 mL) at 2000 hours. The next dose of 250 mg (0.3 mL) was given at 0800 hours. The nurse noted that the vial was empty and discarded it.

   How many doses of 250 mg were in the 1 gram vial?

   How many doses were given?

   What should you do if you found that a medication error had been made by another nurse?

   Was the patient's safety jeopardized in any way?

   How could this error have been prevented?

3. Multiple-dose vials have various reconstitution directions for both IM and IV administration along with different shelf life and storage requirements.

   Discuss how each of these steps for reconstitution of drugs could cause potential harm to a patient if not followed properly.

   a. Adding the wrong diluent
   b. Adding the wrong amount of diluent
   c. Administering the wrong amount of reconstituted medication
   d. Administering via the wrong route
   e. Storing the medication in the wrong place after reconstitution
   f. Keeping the medication longer than the recommended shelf life
   g. Not labeling the date and time and initialing the label

CHAPTER 6 Final

1. Ordered: Biaxin 150 mg po twice a day for helicobacter gastritis.
   Shade in medicine cup to the appropriate measurement.
   a. How much diluent will you add?
   b. When reconstituted, how many milligrams per milliliter will be in the bottle?
   c. How many milliliters will you administer?

2. Ordered: Vibramycin 200 mg the first day followed by a maintenance dose of 100 mg for 5 days for a patient with an intestinal infection.
   a. How many mg will the patient receive during the course of treatment?
   b. What is the generic name for Vibramycin?

3. Ordered: Ampicillin 250 mg IM q4h for endocarditis prophylaxis.
   a. How much diluent will you add?
   b. How many milliliters will you administer? Shade in the amount on the syringe.

CHAPTER 6 Medications From Powders and Crystals: Oral and Intramuscular   209

4. Ordered: Ticar 0.5 g IM q6h for salpingitis.
   a. How much diluent will you add?
   b. How many milliliters will you administer? Shade in the amount on the syringe.

5. Ordered: Pfizerpen 300,000 units IM q12h for chronic obstructive pulmonary disease.
   Available: Pfizerpen 5 million units.
   If you add 18.2 mL of diluent to the Pfizerpen:
   a. How many units/mL will this yield?
   b. How many milliliters will you administer?
   c. How many doses are in the multidose vial?

210   Drug Calculations: *Ratio and Proportion Problems for Clinical Practice*

6. Ordered: Carbenicillin 750 mg IM q8h for endocarditis.
   Available: Geopen (carbenicillin) 5 g for reconstitution.
   a. How many mL of diluent will you add?
   b. How many mL will you administer? Shade in the syringe.

7. Ordered: Ceftazidime 0.5 g IM, an antibiotic, for a patient with *Klebsiella* pneumonia.
   a. How much diluent will you add for an IM injection?
   b. What is the concentration per mL after dilution.
   c. How many mL will you give?

8. Ordered: Penicillin G potassium 100,000 units IM q4h for pneumonia. The directions read: *Sterile solution may be kept in refrigerator for 7 days without significant loss of potency. Add diluent 9.6 mL for 100,000 units/mL concentration of solution; add diluent 4.6 mL for 200,000 units/mL; add diluent 1.6 mL for 500,000 units/mL.*
   a. Which dilution will you use? Why?
   b. How many milliliters will you administer? Shade in the amount on the syringe.

9. Ordered: Oxacillin sodium 250 mg IM q4h for a urinary tract infection (UTI).
   a. How many milliliters of diluent will you add?
   b. How many milliliters of oxacillin sodium will you administer? Shade in the amount on the syringe.

10. Ordered: Keflin 400,000 units IM q12h for a kidney infection.
    Available: a vial with 600,000 units/mL. How many milliliters will you administer? Shade in the amount on the syringe.

evolve   Refer to the Basic Calculations section on Drug Calculations Companion, version 5 on Evolve for additional information.

Answer Key

6 Reconstitution of Medications From Powders and Crystals: Oral and Intramuscular

WORKSHEET 6A (page 183)

1. **a.** Add 55 mL of water, half at a time.
   b. 6 mL

KNOW	WANT TO KNOW
250 mg : 5 mL = 300 mg : x mL	
250x = 5 × 300 = 1500	
x = 6 mL	

   PROOF

   5 × 300 = 1500

   6 × 250 = 1500

   CROSS FRACTION

   $$\frac{25 \text{ mg}}{5} = \frac{30}{x \text{ mL}}$$

   25x = 5 × 30 = 150

   x = 6 mL

   c. 6.6 doses per bottle

   KNOW — WANT TO KNOW
   6 mL : 1 dose = 100 mL : x dose

   6x = 100
   x = 16.6

   PROOF

   1 × 100 = 100

   16.6 × 6 = 99.6 = 100

   $$\frac{6 \text{ mL}}{1} = \frac{100 \text{ mL}}{x}$$

   6x = 100
   x = 16.6

213

2. a. Add 35 mL of water, half at a time.
   b. 12 mL stat dose

KNOW	WANT TO KNOW	PROOF	CROSS FRACTION
125 mg : 5 mL = 300 mg : x mL		5 × 300 = 1500	$\dfrac{125 \text{ mL}}{5} = \dfrac{300 \text{ mg}}{x}$
125x = 5 × 300 = 1500		12 × 125 = 1500	125x = 1500
x = 12 mL			x = 12 mL

   c. 7.6

KNOW	WANT TO KNOW	PROOF	CROSS FRACTION
5 mL : 1 dose = 38 mL : x doses		1 × 38 = 38	$\dfrac{5 \text{ mL}}{1} = \dfrac{38 \text{ mL}}{x}$
5x = 38		5 × 7.6 = 38	5x = 38
x = 7.6 doses			x = 7.6 doses

3. a. 1250 mg

KNOW	WANT TO KNOW	PROOF	CROSS FRACTION
5 mL : 125 mg = 50 mL : x mg		1250 × 5 = 6250	$\dfrac{5 \text{ mL}}{125} = \dfrac{50 \text{ mL}}{x \text{ mg}}$
5x = 125 × 50 = 6250		125 × 50 = 6250	5x = 125 × 50 = 6250
x = 1250 mg			5x = 6250
			x = 1250 mg

   b. 14 mL. Use a larger syringe.

KNOW	WANT TO KNOW	PROOF	CROSS FRACTION
5 mL : 125 mg = x mL : 350 mg		14 × 125 = 1750	$\dfrac{5 \text{ mL}}{125 \text{ mg}} = \dfrac{x \text{ mL}}{350 \text{ mg}}$
125x = 5 × 350 = 1750		5 × 350 = 1750	125x = 5 × 350 = 1750
x = 14 mL			x = 14 mL

4. a. Add 67 mL in two portions.
  b. 100 mL
  c. 4 mL

KNOW	WANT TO KNOW	PROOF	CROSS FRACTION
250 mg : 5 mL = 200 mg : x mL		$4 \times 250 = 1000$	$\dfrac{25 \text{ mg}}{5 \text{ mL}} = \dfrac{20 \text{ mg}}{x}$
$25x = 5 \times 20 = 100$		$5 \times 200 = 1000$	$25x = 5 \times 20 = 100$
$x = 4$ mL			$x = 4$ mL

5. a. Add 60 mL of water in two portions.
  b. 200 mg : 5 mL = x mg : 100 mL
  $5x = 200 \times 100 = 20{,}000$
  $5x = 20{,}000$
  $x = 4000$ mg in bottle

PROOF
$200 \times 100 = 20{,}000$
$5 \times 4000 = 20{,}000$

CROSS FRACTION
$\dfrac{200 \text{ mg}}{5 \text{ mL}} = \dfrac{x \text{ mg}}{100 \text{ mL}}$
$5x = 200 \times 100 = 20{,}000$
$5x = 20{,}000$
$x = 4000$ mg

  c. 10 mL

KNOW	WANT TO KNOW	PROOF	CROSS FRACTION
200 mg : 5 mL = 400 mg : x mL		$5 \times 400 = 2000$	$\dfrac{200 \text{ mg}}{5 \text{ mL}} = \dfrac{400 \text{ mg}}{x \text{ mL}}$
$200x = 5 \times 400 = 2000$		$200 \times 10 = 2000$	$200x = 2000$
$x = 10$ mL			$x = 10$ mL

  d. 10 doses in the bottle.

KNOW	WANT TO KNOW	PROOF	CROSS FRACTION
10 mL : 1 dose = 100 mL : x dose		$1 \times 100 = 100$	$\dfrac{10 \text{ mL}}{1 \text{ dose}} = \dfrac{100 \text{ mL}}{x \text{ doses}}$
$10x = 1 \times 100 = 100$		$10 \times 10 = 100$	$10x = 100$
$x = 10$			$x = 10$ doses

6. a. Add 46 mL of purified water
   b. 50 mL total
   c. KNOW WANT TO KNOW

   400 mg : 50 mL = 40 mg : x mL

   $400x = 50 \times 40 = 2000$
   $x = 5$ mL/dose

   PROOF

   $400 \times 5 = 2000$
   $50 \times 40 = 2000$

   CROSS FRACTION

   $\dfrac{40 \text{ mL}}{50 \text{ mL}} = \dfrac{4 \text{ mg}}{x \text{ mL}}$

   $40x = 50 \times 4 = 200$
   $x = 5$ mL dose

   d. KNOW WANT TO KNOW
   5 mL : 1 dose = 50 mL : x dose

   $5x = 1 \times 50 = 50$
   $x = 10$ doses in the bottle

   PROOF

   $5 \times 10 = 50$
   $1 \times 50 = 50$

   $\dfrac{5 \text{ mL}}{1 \text{ dose}} = \dfrac{50 \text{ mL}}{x \text{ doses}}$

   $5x = 50$
   $x = 10$ doses

7. a. Add 106 mL of water in two portions.
   b. 7500 mg
   KNOW WANT TO KNOW
   250 mg : 5 mL = x mg : 150 mL

   $5x = 250 \times 150 = 37500$
   $x = 7500$ mg

   PROOF
   $250 \times 150 = 37500$
   $5 \times 7500 = 37500$

   CROSS FRACTION
   $\dfrac{250 \text{ mg}}{5} = \dfrac{x}{150}$
   $5x = 37500$
   $x = 7500$

   c. 21.4 doses
   KNOW WANT TO KNOW
   350 mg : 1 dose = 7500 mg : x doses
   $350x = 7500$
   $x = 21.42$ doses

   PROOF
   $1 \times 7500 = 7500$
   $21.42 \times 350 = 7497$

   d. 7 mL
   KNOW WANT TO KNOW
   250 mg : 5 mL = 350 mg : x mL

   $25x = 5 \times 35 = 175$
   $x = 7$ mL

   PROOF
   $5 \times 350 = 1750$
   $7 \times 250 = 1750$

   $\dfrac{25 \text{ mg}}{5 \text{ mL}} = \dfrac{35 \text{ mg}}{x \text{ mL}}$
   $25x = 5 \times 35 = 175$
   $x = 7$ mL

216 Answer Key

8. a. 65 mL total
  b. 9 mL

KNOW	WANT TO KNOW	PROOF	CROSS FRACTION
250 mg : 5 mL = 450 mg : x mL		9 × 250 = 2250	$\dfrac{25}{5} = \dfrac{45}{x}$
25x = 5 × 45 = 225		5 × 450 = 2250	25x = 225
x = 9 mL per dose times 3 doses = 27 mL per day for 24 hr			x = 9 mL

  c. 75 mL total in the bottle
   − 27 mL initial dose for 24 hours
    48 mL left in the bottle
  d. No

KNOW	WANT TO KNOW	PROOF	
250 mg : 5 mL = 450 mg : x mL		25 × 9 = 225	$\dfrac{250 \text{ mg}}{5 \text{ mL}} = \dfrac{450 \text{ mg}}{x \text{ mL}}$
25x = 5 × 45 = 225		5 × 45 = 225	x = 9 mL
x = 9 mL per dose × 2 doses = 18 mL per day × 4 days = 72 mL total			

   48 mL left in the bottle; order another bottle

9. a. Add 26 mL of sterile water.
  b.
  KNOW   WANT TO KNOW   PROOF
  10 mg : 1 mL = 50 mg : x mL   1 × 50 = 50
  10x = 1 × 50 = 50   10 × 5 = 50
    x = 5 mL to administer
  c.
  KNOW   WANT TO KNOW   PROOF
  50 mg : 1 dose = 350 mg : x doses   1 × 350 = 350
  50x = 1 × 350 = 350   50 × 7 = 350
    x = 7 doses in the bottle

10. a. Add 55 mL of water.

  b. KNOW   WANT TO KNOW   PROOF   CROSS FRACTION

125 mg : 5 mL = 200 mg : x mL   5 × 200 = 1000 $\dfrac{125 \text{ mg}}{5 \text{ mL}} = \dfrac{200 \text{ mg}}{x \text{ mL}}$

125x = 5 × 200 = 1000   125 × 8 = 1000   125x = 5 × 200 = 1000

    x = 8 mL to administer x = 8 mL

  c. KNOW   WANT TO KNOW   PROOF

100 mL : x dose = 8 mL : 1 dose   1 × 100 = 100 $\dfrac{100 \text{ mg}}{x \text{ doses}} = \dfrac{8 \text{ mL}}{1 \text{ dose}}$

8x = 1 × 100 = 100   12.5 × 8 = 100   8x = 100

    x = 12.5 doses in the bottle x = 12.5 doses

WORKSHEET 6B (page 193)

1. a. Add 4.0 mL of diluent to yield 250,000 units/mL.

  b. KNOW   WANT TO KNOW

250,000 units : 1 mL = 300,000 units : x mL

25x = 30

   x = 1.2 mL

PROOF

25 × 1.2 = 30

1 × 30 = 30

CROSS FRACTION

$\dfrac{25}{1} = \dfrac{30}{x \text{ mL}}$

25x = 30

x = 112 mL

  c. KNOW   WANT TO KNOW

300,000 units : 1 dose = 1,000,000 units : x dose

3x = 10

3x = 10

   x = 3.3 = 3 full doses in the vial

PROOF

1 × 1,000,000 = 1,000,000

3.3 × 300,000 = 9.9

If the 1.8 mL diluent were used, the resulting dosage would be 0.6 mL, which is concentrated and may create tissue inflammation.

$\dfrac{3}{1} = \dfrac{10}{x \text{ dose}}$

3x = 10

x = 3.3 doses

2. a. 4.2 mL 1% lidocaine
   b. 350 mg per mL
   c. 1.4 mL

KNOW	WANT TO KNOW	PROOF	CROSS FRACTION
350 mg : 1 mL = 500 mg : x mL		500 × 1 = 500	$\dfrac{350}{1} = \dfrac{500}{x\ mL}$
350x = 500		350 × 1.428 = 499.8	350x = 500
x = 1.428 = 1.4 mL			x = 1.4 mL

d. 5.7 doses

KNOW	PROOF	CROSS FRACTION
350 mg : 1 dose = 2000 mg : x mL	1 × 2000 = 2000	$\dfrac{350}{1} = \dfrac{2000}{x\ dose}$
350x = 1 × 2000 = 200	5.71 × 350 = 1998.5 = 2000	350x = 2000
x = 5.7 doses		x = 5.7 doses

3. a. Administer 4 mL.

KNOW	PROOF	CROSS FRACTION
250 mg : 1 mL = 1000 mg : x mL	1 × 1000 = 1000	$\dfrac{25}{1} = \dfrac{100}{x\ mL}$
250x = 1000	250 × 4 = 1000	25x = 100
x = 4 mL		x = 4 mL

b. Give 2 mL in each site = 500 mg per injection.

4. a. Add 5.7 mL sterile water for injection.
b. Administer: 3 mL.

KNOW	PROOF	CROSS FRACTION
1.5 mL : 250 mg = x mL : 500 mg	25 × 3 = 75	$\dfrac{1.5}{250} = \dfrac{x\ mL}{500}$
25x = 1.5 × 50 = 75	1.5 × 50 = 75	25x = 1.5 × 50 = 75
x = 3 mL		x = 3 mL

This can be given in divided doses.

5. Administer entire amount, 2.6 mL.

6. a. Add 1 mL of 1% lidocaine.
  b. 1.3 mL

KNOW	WANT TO KNOW	PROOF	CROSS FRACTION
350 mg : 1 mL = 450 mg : x mL		1 × 45 = 45	$\dfrac{35}{1} = \dfrac{45}{x\ mL}$
35x = 1 × 45 = 45		35 × 1.285 = 44.975	35x = 45
x = 1.285 = 1.3 mL			x = 1.28 = 1.3 mL

7. a. Add 3 mL of sterile water for injection as the diluent.
  b. 280 mg/mL is the concentration.
  c.

KNOW	WANT TO KNOW	PROOF	CROSS FRACTION
280 mg : 1 mL = 250 mg : x mL		1 × 250 = 250	$\dfrac{28}{1} = \dfrac{25}{x\ mL}$
280x = 250		0.892 × 280 = 250	28x = 25
x = 0.892 = 0.9 mL			x = 0.89 mL = 0.9 mL

8. a. Add 1.2 mL of diluent.
  b. 1 hour
  c. 125 mg/mL
  d.

KNOW	WANT TO KNOW	PROOF	CROSS FRACTION
125 mg : 1 mL = 100 mg : x mL		125 × 0.8 = 100	$\dfrac{125}{1} = \dfrac{100}{x\ mL}$
125x = 100		100 × 1 = 100	125x = 100
x = 0.8 mL			x = 0.8 mL

9. a. Administer 1.7 mL.

KNOW	WANT TO KNOW	PROOF	CROSS FRACTION
500 mg : 1.2 mL = 700 mg : x mL		5 × 1.68 = 8.4	$\dfrac{5}{1.2} = \dfrac{7}{x\ mL}$
5x = 1.2 × 7		1.2 × 7 = 8.4	5x = 7 × 1.2 = 8.4
5x = 8.4			x = 1.68 = 1.7 mL
x = 1.68 or 1.7 mL			

b. Patient will receive 2800 mg/day.

KNOW	WANT TO KNOW	PROOF	CROSS FRACTION
700 mg : 1 dose = x mg : 4 doses		700 × 4 = 2800	$\dfrac{700}{1} = \dfrac{x\ mg}{4}$
x = 4 × 700		1 × 2800 = 2800	x = 700 × 4 = 2800
x = 2800 mg/day			x = 2800 mg

c. Need 2.8 or 3 vials per day.

KNOW	WANT TO KNOW	PROOF	CROSS FRACTION
1000 mg : 1 vial = 2800 mg : x vials		1 × 28 = 28	$\dfrac{10}{1} = \dfrac{28}{x\ vials}$
10x = 28 = 2.8 or 3 vials needed for a 24-hr period		10 × 2.8 = 28	10x = 28
			x = 2.8 vials

10. a. Administer 4 mL in first dose.
  b. Divide into two equal injections.
  c. Give deep intramuscularly in the right or left ventrogluteal area.

WORKSHEET 6C (page 198)

1. a. 400 mg per mL.
   b. 1.25 mL

KNOW	WANT TO KNOW	PROOF	CROSS FRACTION
400 mg : 1 mL = 500 mg : x mL		1 × 5 = 5	$\dfrac{4}{1} = \dfrac{5}{x\ mL}$
4x = 1 × 5 = 5		4 × 1.25 = 5	4x = 5
x = 1.25 = 1.3 mL			x = 1.25 = 1.3 mL

2. **a.** Add 2 mL of sterile water.
   b. Have 500 mg/1.2 mL.
   c. Administer 1.2 mL.

3. KNOW   WANT TO KNOW
   250 mg : 1 mL = 500 mg : x mL
   250x = 500
       x = 2 mL
   PROOF
   500 × 1 = 500
   250 × 2 = 500
   OR

KNOW	WANT TO KNOW	PROOF	CROSS FRACTION

   350 mg : 1 mL = 500 mg : x mL   1 × 500 = 500 $\frac{35}{1} = \frac{50}{x\ mL}$

   350x = 1 × 500 = 500   350 × 1.428 = 500   35x = 50
       x = 1.428 = 1.4 mL   x = 1.4 mL

4. If you add 4 mL of diluent

   KNOW   WANT TO KNOW   **PROOF**   **CROSS FRACTION**

   250,000 units : 1 mL = 400,000 units : x mL   25 × 1.6 = 40 $\frac{25}{1} = \frac{40}{x\ mL}$

   25x = 40   1 × 40 = 40   25x = 40
      x = 1.6 mL   x = 1.6 mL

   If you add 1.5 mL of diluent
   KNOW   WANT TO KNOW
   500,000 units : 1 mL = 400,000 units : x mL
   5x = 4
     x = 0.8 mL
   PROOF
   5 × 0.8 = 4
   1 × 4 = 4

222   Answer Key

5. a. Add 16 mL of bacteriostatic water with benzyl alcohol.
   b. 62.5 mg/mL
   c.

KNOW	WANT TO KNOW	PROOF	CROSS FRACTION
62.5 mg : 1 mL = 125 mg : x mL		$1 \times 125 = 125$	$\dfrac{62.5}{1} = \dfrac{125}{x \text{ mL}}$
$62.5x = 1 \times 125 = 125$		$62.5 \times 2 = 125$	$62.5x = 125$
$x = 2$ mL/dose			$x = 2$ mL

   d.

KNOW	WANT TO KNOW	PROOF	CROSS FRACTION
125 mg : 1 dose = 1000 mg : x doses		$1 \times 1000 = 1000$	$\dfrac{125}{1} = \dfrac{1000}{x \text{ doses}}$
$125x = 1 \times 1000$		$125 \times 8 = 1000$	$125x = 1000$
$x = 8$ doses in the vial			$x = 8$ doses

   e. The literature states the medication must be used within 48 hours.

   f.

KNOW	WANT TO KNOW	PROOF	
500 mg : 1 day = 1000 mg : x days		$1 \times 1000 = 1000$	$\dfrac{5}{1} = \dfrac{10}{x \text{ days}}$
$500x = 1000$		$500 \times 2 = 1000$	$5x = 10$
$x = 2$ days to administer the vial.			$x = 2$ days

   The allowed time is 48 hr, which is within the allotted time frame.

6.
   a.

KNOW	WANT TO KNOW	PROOF	CROSS FRACTION
250,000 units : 1 mL = 400,000 units : x mL		$1 \times 40 = 40$	$\dfrac{25}{1} = \dfrac{40}{x \text{ mL}}$
$25x = 1 \times 40 = 40$		$25 \times 1.6 = 40$	$25x = 40$
$x = 1.6$ mL twice a day			$x = 1.6$ mL

KNOW	WANT TO KNOW	PROOF	
500,000 units : 1 mL = 400,000 units : x mL		$5 \times 0.8 = 4$	$\dfrac{5}{1} = \dfrac{4}{x \text{ mL}}$
$5x = 1 \times 4 = 4$		$4 \times 1 = 4$	$5x = 4$
$x = 0.8$ mL twice a day			$x = 0.8$ mL

   b. The muscle mass of your patient will help you decide which dosage to use.

7. **a.** Add 2 mL of sterile water for injection.
   b. The reconstituted medication will yield 1 g/2.6 mL.
   c. Use medication promptly.
   d. 1000 mg or 1 g
   e. Administer 2 mL.

KNOW	WANT TO KNOW	PROOF	CROSS FRACTION
1000 mg : 2.6 mL = 750 mg : x mL		$1000 \times 1.95 = 1950$	$\dfrac{100}{2.6} = \dfrac{75}{x\ mL}$
$1000x = 2.6 \times 750 = 1950$		$2.6 \times 750 = 1950$	$100x = 2.6 \times 75 = 195$
$1000x = 1950$			$x = 1.95 = 2\ mL$
$x = 1.95 = 2\ mL$			

8. **a.** 3.5 mL of diluent
   b. 250 mg per mL
   c. 2 mL
   d. Shelf life is 1 hour

KNOW	WANT TO KNOW	PROOF	CROSS FRACTION
250 mg : 1 mL = 500 mg : x mL		$1 \times 50 = 50$	$\dfrac{25}{1} = \dfrac{50}{x\ mL}$
$25x = 50$		$2 \times 25 = 50$	$25x = 50$
$x = 2\ mL$			$x = 2\ mL$

9. **a.** Add 3.5 mL diluent.
   b. The reconstituted medication will yield 250 mg/mL.
   c. Use within 1 hr, as this is a very unstable medication.
   d. Administer 2 mL.

KNOW	WANT TO KNOW	PROOF	CROSS FRACTION
250 mg : 1 mL = 500 mg : x mL		$1 \times 500 = 500$	$\dfrac{25}{1} = \dfrac{50}{x\ mL}$
$250x = 500$		$250 \times 2 = 500$	$25x = 50$
$x = 2\ mL$			$x = 2\ mL$

Answer Key

10. a. Add 2.7 mL of sterile water for injection.
  b. 1.5 mL/250 mg
  c. Refrigerated, 7 days; room temperature, 3 days
  d. 500 mg
  b. Administer 2.7 mL.

KNOW	WANT TO KNOW	PROOF	CROSS FRACTION
250 mg : 1.5 mL = 450 mg : x mL		250 × 2.7 = 675	$\dfrac{25}{1.5} = \dfrac{45}{x \text{ mL}}$
250x : 1.5 × 450		1.5 × 450 = 675	25x = 1.5 × 45 = 67.5
250x = 67.5		x = 2.7 mL	
x = 2.7 mL			

WORKSHEET 6D (page 203)

1. b.

KNOW	WANT TO KNOW	PROOF	CROSS FRACTION
40 mcg : 1 mL = 60 mcg : x mL		1 × 60 = 60	$\dfrac{40}{1} = \dfrac{60}{x}$
40x = 1 × 60 = 60		40 × 1.5 = 60	40x = 60
x = 1.5 mL			x = 1.5 mL

2. b. Directions read: Add 1.2 mL of diluent to yield 125 mg/mL.
  d.

KNOW	WANT TO KNOW	PROOF	CROSS FRACTION
250 mg : 1 dose = x mg : 2 doses		1 × 500 = 500	$\dfrac{250}{1} = \dfrac{x}{2}$
x = 250 × 2 = 500		250 × 2 = 500	x = 500 mg
x = 500 mg for 2 doses			

KNOW	WANT TO KNOW	PROOF	CROSS FRACTION
125 mg : 1 vial = 500 mg : x vials		1 × 500 = 500	$\dfrac{125}{1} = \dfrac{500}{x}$
125x = 1 × 500 = 500		125 × 4 = 500	125x = 500
x = 4 vials for 24 hr			x = 4 vials for 24 hr

3. d. Add 1.2 mL sterile water.
  d. 0.9 mL.

KNOW	WANT TO KNOW	PROOF	CROSS FRACTION
40 mg : 1 mL = 35 mg : x mL		1 × 35 = 35	$\dfrac{40}{1} = \dfrac{35}{x}$
40x = 1 × 35 = 35		40 × 0.875 = 35	40x = 35
x = 0.875 = 0.9 mL			x = 0.87 = 0.9 mL

4. b.

KNOW	WANT TO KNOW	PROOF	CROSS FRACTION
2 mL : 1 g = x mL : 1.5 g		1 × 3 = 3	$\dfrac{2}{1} = \dfrac{x}{115}$
x = 2 × 1.5 = 3		2 × 1.5 = 3	x = 2 × 1.5 = 3
x = 3 mL divided into 2 doses			x = 3 mL

  d.

KNOW	WANT TO KNOW	PROOF	CROSS FRACTION
1000 mg : 1 vial = 3000 mg : x vials		1000 × 3 = 3000	$\dfrac{1}{1} = \dfrac{3}{x}$
1000x = 3000		1 × 3000 = 3000	x = 3 vials
x = 3 vials needed			

5. c.

KNOW	WANT TO KNOW	PROOF	CROSS FRACTION
4 mL : 2000 mg = x mL : 1000 mg		2000 × 2 = 4000	$\dfrac{4}{2} = \dfrac{x}{1}$
2000x = 4 × 1000 = 4000		4 × 1000 = 4000	2x = 4
2x = 4			x = 2 mL
x = 2 mL			

6. c.

KNOW	WANT TO KNOW	PROOF	CROSS FRACTION
2.6 mL : 1000 mg = x mL : 500 mg		2.6 × 500 = 1300	$\dfrac{2.6}{10} = \dfrac{x}{5}$
10x = 2.6 × 5 = 13		1000 × 1.3 = 1300	10x = 5 × 2.6 = 13
x = 1.3 mL			10x = 13
			x = 1.3 mL

7. c.

KNOW   WANT TO KNOW   PROOF   CROSS FRACTION

500 mg : 1 dose = x mg : 3 doses   500 × 3 = 1500 $\dfrac{500}{1} = \dfrac{x}{3}$

x = 500 × 3 = 1500   1500 × 1 = 1500   x = 500 × 3 = 1500 mg
x = 1500 mg/24 hr

KNOW   WANT TO KNOW   PROOF
1000 mg : 1 vial = 1500 mg : x vials   1 × 1500 = 1500 $\dfrac{1000}{1} = \dfrac{1500}{3}$

1000x = 1500   1000 × 1.5 = 1500   10x = 15
x = 1.5 vials   You will need to have   x = 1.5 vials
                 2 vials on hand for 24 hr.

8. c. Directions read: Add 1.5 mL of diluent = 500,000 units/mL

   d.

KNOW   WANT TO KNOW   PROOF   CROSS FRACTION

500,000 units : 1 mL = 400,000 units : x mL   0.8 × 500,000 = 400,000 $\dfrac{5}{1} = \dfrac{4}{x}$

500,000x = 1 × 400,000 = 400,000   1 × 400,000 = 400,000   5x = 4
5x = 4   x = 0.8 mL
x = 0.8 mL

9. c. Add 9 mL of diluent = 400 mg/mL

   a.

KNOW   WANT TO KNOW   PROOF   CROSS FRACTION

400 mg : 1 mL = 500 mg : x mL   1 × 500 = 500 $\dfrac{4}{1} = \dfrac{5}{x}$

400 x = 1 × 500   400 × 1.25 = 500   4x = 5
4x = 5   x = 1.25 = 1.3 mL
x = 1.25 = 1.3 mL

10. c. 330 mg : 1 mL = 250 mg : x mL   PROOF   CROSS FRACTION

330x = 250   1 × 250 = 250 $\dfrac{300}{1} = \dfrac{250}{x}$
x = 0.757 = 0.8 mL   0.757 × 330 = 249.8   30x = 25
                                              x = 0.8 mL

226   Answer Key

CHAPTER 6 FINAL: MEDICATIONS FROM POWDERS AND CRYSTALS: ORAL AND INTRAMUSCULAR (page 208)

1. a. Add 55 mL of water.
   b. 125 mg per 5 mL
   c. Give 6 mL.

2. a. 700 mg
   b. doxycycline calcium

3. a. Add 3.5 mL diluent.
   b. Administer 1 mL.

4. a. Add 2 mL of sterile water for injection.
   b. Administer 1.3 mL.

5. a. 250,000 units/mL
   b. 1.2 mL
   c. 16.6 doses in the vial

Answer Key   227

6. **a.** Add 9.5 mL of diluent.
   b. Give 1.9 mL IM.

7. **a.** 30 mL of diluent
   b. 280 mg per mL
   c. 1.785 = 1.8 mL
   Give 1.8 mL.

8. **a.** Add 9.6 mL of diluent to make 100,000 units/mL. A more concentrated solution may be caustic to the tissue.
   b. Administer 1 mL.

9. **a.** Add 2.7 mL sterile water for injection.
   b. Administer 1.5 mL.

10. Administer 0.7 mL.

Basic Intravenous Therapy Calculations

Objectives
- Calculate intravenous (IV) flow rates for drops per min, mL per hr, mg per hr, g per hr, and infusion time.
- Interpret IV labels.
- Identify various electronic IV infusion devices.
- Identify IV sets: primary, primary with a port, IVPB extension tubing, transfusion sets, and venous access devices for intermittent use.
- Calculate the amount of saline or heparin for use in keeping venous access patent.
- Calculate the grams of sodium chloride or dextrose in IV infusions.
- Identify osmolarity values for IV solutions.
- Check physician's IV order for type of solution, amount, additives, and rate.
- Understand PCA pump using standard protocol.
- Analyze IV orders for safe administration using critical thinking skills.
- Analyze medication errors using critical thinking skills.

Introduction

It is the nurse's responsibility to calculate the milliliters per hour or drops per minute to regulate an intravenous infusion. Knowledge of electronic infusion devices is required, as is knowledge of basic hand-regulated primary sets. The nurse is responsible for calculating the intravenous piggyback (IVPB) infusions that are timed for shorter periods.

Vocabulary

Bolus: A concentrated form of IV medication given in a short time period, usually given with a syringe into the IV port by a nurse or physician.

Continuous IV Infusion: An IV solution infused at a continuous, prescribed rate.

Drop Factor (DF): The number of drops per milliliter delivered through the size of the needle into the drip chamber.

Electronic Infusion Device (EID): A device that can be programmed to deliver a prescribed rate of solution in milliliters per hour.

Free-Flow: The uncontrolled delivery of an infusion to a patient when a controlled or metered delivery was intended.

Gravity Infusion Device: An IV solution infused by gravity. The height of the IV solution affects the flow of the solution in relation to the drop factor. The IV is manually controlled with a type of roller or clip device.

Hypertonic Solution: A solution that contains more dissolved particles such as Na^+, C^-, and other electrolytes than normal cells; water is pulled out of the cells by osmosis.

Hypotonic Solution: A solution with a lower salt concentration than normal body cells; water flows into the cells across the cell membrane by osmosis.

Isotonic Solution: A solution that has the same concentration of dissolved solutes on each side of the cell membrane.

IV Injection Port: A rubber or latex port on IV infusion tubing to add additional medications. Most ports are needleless, ensuring safety from punctures.

IV Piggyback (IVPB): Small-volume infusions, usually 50, 100, or 250 mL of medication, infused through a port on the existing primary line and delivered over 20 to 60 minutes.

Osmolarity: The total concentration of solutes, both penetrating and nonpenetrating. The mOsm is in the cell and can also pass into the extracellular space. The exchange of mOsms from cellular to extracellular determines the isotonic, hypotonic, or hypertonic value of the solution.

Patient-Controlled Analgesia (PCA): An IV device/pump that is calibrated to deliver a prescribed amount of opioid medication over a set period of time.

Tonicity: The concentration of extracellular, nonpenetrating solutes such as Cl^-, Na^+, and Ca^{++}.

IV Infusions

Intravenous (IV) infusions are used more frequently today than intramuscular (IM) injections. Continuous medication therapy can be delivered via an IV route, minimizing multiple injections via the IM route. Intermittent medication therapy can be delivered through a saline/heparin lock (Figure 7-1), which allows the patient free movement until the next scheduled dose. The saline lock is used for intermittent short-duration therapy in acute care, long-term care, and home care. Intermittent therapy can also be delivered as a piggyback with a continuous infusion. A heparin or saline flush can also be used to keep the port patent per manufacturer's guidelines or facility policy.

FIGURE 7-1 Intermittent lock covered with a transparent shield. (From Perry AG, Potter PA: *Clinical nursing skills and techniques,* ed. 8, St. Louis, 2014, Mosby.)

FIGURE 7-2 **A,** Needleless infusion system. **B,** Connection into an injection port. (From Perry AG, Potter PA, Ostendorf WR: *Clinical nursing skills and techniques,* ed. 8, St. Louis, 2014, Mosby.)

Medications can be added to the IV by the manufacturer, pharmacist, or nurse. The prescriber orders the medication, strength, and amount, and the manufacturer determines the type and amount of diluent. It is important that the person responsible for the IV understand the actions of the medication, flow rate, adverse reactions, and antidotes. IV fluids flow directly into the vein, resulting in immediate action, and cannot be retrieved. Therefore it is imperative that the correct calculations, medications, and flow rate be administered.

An intermittent IV lock (see Figure 7-1) is known by many different terms. The terms most used are saline lock, hep/heparin lock, PRN cap, intermittent IV (INT), and intermittent peripheral infusion device (IPD). Most have needleless resealable valves (Figure 7-2).

CLINICAL ALERT!
For patient safety, before medication is added to an IV infusion, always verify compatibility with the existing IV solution. When the medication and solution are incompatible, precipitation may result, which could harm the patient.

IV Calculations

Check IV orders before beginning calculations. There are two steps in IV calculations. The first step is to find out how many *milliliters per hour* (volume) the IV is ordered to infuse. The second step is to calculate the *drops per minute* needed to infuse the ordered volume.

Analyze your problem. If the order says to infuse the IV for 24 hours, calculate the mL per hr by beginning with Step 1. If the order states to infuse the IV at a specified rate per hour, such as 75 mL per hr, begin with Step 2.

Step 1 mL/hr

RULE When the total volume is given, calculate the mL/hr.

$$\frac{\text{Total volume (TV)}}{\text{Total time (TT) in hours}} = \text{mL per hr}$$

Example Ordered: 2000 mL D5W (dextrose 5% in water) to be infused for 24 hours. The problem is to find out how many mL per hour the patient must receive for the 2000 mL to be infused in 24 hours.

Formula
$$\frac{\text{Total volume (TV)}}{\text{Total time (TT) in hours}} = \text{mL per hr}$$

Calculation
$$\frac{\text{TV}}{\text{TT}} = \frac{2000}{24} = 83 \text{ mL per hr}$$

We now know that to infuse 2000 mL of fluid in 24 hours, the patient must receive 83 mL per hour. Infusion devices are calibrated for milliliters per hour (mL per hr).

Drop Factor Calculations for Gravity Infusions

Step 2 Drops per min

The drop factor is needed to calculate drops per minute. The drop factor is the number of drops in 1 mL. The diameter of the needle where the drop enters the drip chamber varies from one manufacturer to another. The bigger the needle, the fatter the drop (Figure 7-3, *A*); it takes only 10 macrodrops to make a milliliter. The smallest unit is the microdrop (60 drops per mL) (Figure 7-3, *B*). This is used for people who can tolerate only small amounts of fluid, such as pediatric and geriatric patients and patients who require fluid restrictions. Drop factors of 10, 15, 20, and 60 (microdrip) are the most common. The drop factor is determined by the manufacturer and is found on the IV tubing package.

FIGURE 7-3 Drops per minute must be calibrated for gravity flow. **A,** InterLink System Continu-Flo Solution Set with drop factor of 10 (10 drops = 1 mL). **B,** InterLink System Continu-Flo Solution Set with drop factor of 60 (60 drops = 1 mL).

CLINICAL RELEVANCE

Gravity tubing is used by EMTs and in the emergency department, outpatient surgical centers, and long-term care facilities. The nurse will select the calibration of the IV set needed, based on the flow rate ordered. The drops per minute are printed on the IV tubing package (see Figure 7-3). The drops per minute are calculated by the nurse. When using a roller or slide pinch to regulate the IV, the nurse must check the IV rate every hour or more frequently because gravity rates are approximate and positional. The Dial-a-Flo tubing is calibrated in mL per hour (Figure 7-4).

RULE When the mL per hour is given, calculate the drops per minute.

$$\frac{\text{Drop factor or gtt/mL (from IV package)}}{\text{Time in minutes}} \times \text{Total hourly volume (V/hr)} = \text{drops per min}$$

Example Ordered: D5W to infuse at 83 mL per hour. The drop factor (Df) is 10.

$$\frac{\text{Df}}{\text{Time (min)}} \times \text{V/hr} = \frac{10 \text{ (Df)}}{60 \text{ (min)}} \times 83 \text{ (V/hr)}$$

$$\frac{10}{60} \times \frac{83}{1} = \frac{1}{6} \times \frac{83}{1} = \frac{83}{6} = 13.8 \text{ or } 14 \text{ drops per min}$$

Drops cannot be timed in tenths, only in whole numbers. If the decimal is greater than or equal to 0.5, round to the next higher number.

Example Ordered: Antibiotic to infuse at 100 mL in 30 minutes. The drop factor is 15.

$$\frac{\text{Df}}{\text{Time (min)}} \times \text{V/hr} = \frac{15 \text{ (Df)}}{30 \text{ (min)}} \times 100 \text{ (V/hr)}$$

$$\frac{15}{30} \times \frac{100}{1} = \frac{1}{2} \times \frac{100}{1} = \frac{100}{2} = 50 \text{ drops per min}$$

Summary Two-step IV flow rate calculations.

Step 1 $\quad \dfrac{\text{TV}}{\text{TT in hr}} = \text{mL per hr}$

Step 2 $\quad \dfrac{\text{Df}}{\text{Time in min}} \times \text{V per hr} = \text{drops per min}$

The reduced fraction is easier to calculate.

remember Reduce the fraction Df per min *before* multiplying by the volume.

Example Which would you rather calculate?

$$\frac{12}{60} \times 60 \text{ or } \frac{1}{5} \times 60$$

The reduced fraction is easier to calculate.

FIGURE 7-4 Dial-a-Flo extension set with pre-pierced Y-site. Dial-a-Flo provides a range from 5 to 250 mL per hour. (From Hospira, Inc. Lake Forest, Ill.)

CHAPTER 7 Basic Intravenous Therapy Calculations

remember When the IV tubing is microdrip, 60 drops per mL, the drops per minute will be the same as the mL per hour.

Example 1000 mL to infuse in 8 hours with a microdrip set.

Step 1 $\dfrac{TV}{TT \text{ in hr}} = \dfrac{1000}{8} = 125$ mL per hr

Step 2 $\dfrac{Df}{\text{Time in min}} \times V \text{ per hr} = \dfrac{60}{60} \times 125 = 125$ drops per min

IV Delivery Sets

Figure 7-5, *A* shows a primary set. This is the basic set that delivers IV fluids for a short duration. It does not have a port for additions. This is a needleless connector.

Figure 7-5, *B* shows a primary set with a port for adding piggyback medications. This set has a manual dial for the mL per hr rate.

FIGURE 7-5 Primary set with a roller clamp to regulate the IV set.

Needleless IV systems are designed to protect caregivers from accidental punctures by contaminated needles. The BD SafetyGlide™ needle (Figure 7-6) used to inject medication into IV ports is another measure to avoid accidental punctures.

Drops per Minute by Manufacturer

A simple approach to calculate drops per min after you have determined the mL per hr is to memorize the reduced fraction numbers. Manufacturers have established rates for the products (Figure 7-6). Below is an example.

Product Drip Rates	Minutes	Df	=	Reduced Number
60 drops per mL	60	60	=	1
20 drops per mL	60	20	=	3
15 drops per mL	60	15	=	4
10 drops per mL	60	10	=	6

You may have to memorize only one number because most facilities purchase equipment from a single company.

FIGURE 7-6 Various drop rates from different manufacturers.

Example If you know you are using a set that delivers 20 drops per mL, divide 3 into the mL per hr.

$$\frac{125}{3} = 41.6 = 42 \text{ drops per min}$$

As you already know, the formula for calculating drops per min is:

$$\frac{Df}{\text{Time in min}} \times V \text{ per hr} \quad \text{or} \quad \frac{20}{60} \times 125 = \frac{1}{3} \times 125 = 41.6 = 42 \text{ drops per min}$$

Now you know two different methods for calculating drops per min (Figure 7-7).

FIGURE 7-7 Count drops per minute by watching the drip chamber for 1 minute and adjusting the roller clamp as needed to deliver the desired number of drops per minute. (From Potter PA, Perry AG, Stockert P, Hall A: *Essentials for nursing practice,* ed. 8, St. Louis, 2014, Mosby.)

> ### ⊝ CLINICAL ALERT!
> Check the IV every hour, even if an infusion device is used. Recheck drops per minute rate frequently because the IV rate can vary with position. Time taping the IV has become important, as electrical blackouts and brownouts can adversely affect the infusion accuracy (Figure 7-8).

Flo Meter Tape

The order is to infuse 1000 mL in 10 hr (Figure 7-9): The infusion label shows a starting time of 0700 hr and an ending time of 1700 hr. The IV is scheduled to infuse for 10 hr. Use the 10-hr rate per hr on the tape and initial each hour at 100 mL per hour. The ending time will be 1700 hr.

FIGURE 7-8 IV bag with timed tape. (From Potter PA, Perry AG, Stockert P, Hall A: *Essentials for nursing practice*, ed. 8, St. Louis, 2014, Mosby.)

FIGURE 7-9 A FloMeter Tape on a 1000 mL IV bag indicating start time and the hourly rate at 100 mL per hour and initialed hourly.

236   Drug Calculations: *Ratio and Proportion Problems for Clinical Practice*

WORKSHEET 7A: IV Calculations

Answers on page 262

Use either the Step 1 or the Step 2 formula to calculate mL per hr or drop per min to answer the following questions.

Step 1 $\dfrac{TV}{TT \text{ in hr}} = mL \text{ per hr}$

Step 2 $\dfrac{Df}{Time \text{ in min}} \times V \text{ per hr} = \text{drops per min}$ or $\dfrac{mL \text{ per hr}}{\text{reduced drop rate}}$

1. Ordered: 1000 mL to be infused for 8 hr. How many drops per min will be administered if the drop factor is 10?

2. Ordered: 50 mL to be infused for 1 hr. How many drops per min will be administered with microdrip?

3. Ordered: 100 mL to be infused for 30 min. How many drops per min is this if the drop factor is 10?

4. Ordered: 1500 mL to be infused for 12 hr. If the drop factor is 15, how many drops per min is this?

5. Ordered: 200 mL to be infused for 1 hr. If the drop factor is 15, how many drops per min will be administered?

6. Ordered: 1000 mL to be infused at 150 mL per hr. The drop factor is 20. How many drops per min will be infused?

7. Ordered: 75 mL to be infused for 45 min. The drop factor is 10. How many drops per min will be administered?

8. Ordered: 150 mL to be infused for 90 min. The drop factor is microdrip. How many drops per min will be administered?

9. Ordered: 150 mL to be infused for 40 min. The drop factor is 15 drops per mL. How many drops per min is this?

10. Ordered: 1500 mL to be infused for 8 hr. How many mL per hr will be administered?
    a. How many drops per min is this with a drop factor of 10?
    b. How many drops per min is this with a drop factor of 15?

Answers on page 263

WORKSHEET 7B | Additional Practice in IV Calculations

Use either the Step 1 or the Step 2 formula to calculate mL per hr or drops per min to answer the following questions.

1. Ordered: 1000 mL to be infused for 12 hr on microdrip. At how many drops per min will you regulate the infusion?

2. You have 1500 mL normal saline (NS). The drop factor is 15. The solution is to be given for an 8-hr period.
   a. How many mL per hr will be infused?
   b. How many drops per min will be infused?

3. A solution of 3000 mL D5W with 1.5 g carbenicillin is being infused for 24 hr. The drop factor is 15 drops per minute.
   How many drops per min will be infused?

4. You have 500 mL 0.45% NS infusing for 4 hr. The drop factor is 15. How many drops per min will be infused?

5. Ordered: 2000 mL for 24 hr. The drop factor is 15. How many drops per min will be administered?

6. Ordered: 100 mL gentamicin to be infused for 30 min. The drop factor is 20.
   a. With which step will you begin?
   b. How many drops per min will be infused?

7. You have 2000 mL D5W being infused for 24 hr. How many mL per hr will be infused?

8. Ordered: 250 mL D5W is to be infused for 10 hr on a microdrip. How many drops per min will be administered?

9. Ordered: 1500 mL of Ringer's lactate solution to be infused for 12 hr.
   a. How many mL per hr will be infused?
   b. The drop factor is 15. How many drops per min will be infused?

10. Write your two-step formula again.
    Step 1   **Step 2**

Answers on page 264

WORKSHEET 7C | More Practice in IV Calculations

Use either the Step 1 or the Step 2 formula to calculate mL per hr or drops per min to answer the following questions.

1. Ordered: 500 mL for 8 hr by microdrip. How many drops per min is this?

2. Ordered: 50 mL to be infused for 30 min. At how many drops per min will you set the IV rate if the drop factor is 10?

3. Ordered: 1000 mL to be infused for 6 hr. How many drops per min will be administered if the drop factor is 15?

238 Drug Calculations: *Ratio and Proportion Problems for Clinical Practice*

4. Ordered: 100 mL to be infused for 60 min. At how many drops per min will you set the IV rate if a microdrip is used? Is this the same as mL per hr?

5. Ordered: D5W continuous infusion at 85 mL per hr. The drop factor is 20. At how many drops per min will you set the IV rate?

6. Ordered: 100 mL per hr. At how many drops per min will you set the IV rate if the drop factor is 10?

7. Ordered: 1500 mL 0.45% NS for 24 hr. The drop factor is 10. At how many drops per min will you set the IV rate?

8. Ordered: 100 mL to be infused for 30 min. The drop factor is 15. At how many drops per min will you set the IV rate?

9. Ordered: 1000 mL Ringer's lactate solution at 75 mL per hr. The drop factor is 15. How many drops per min will be administered?

10. Ordered: 2000 mL to be infused for 12 hr. The drop factor is 20.
    a. At how many mL per hr will you set the IV rate?
    b. How many drops per min will this be?

Abbreviations for Common IV Solutions

NS	Normal saline; 0.9% sodium chloride (Figure 7-10)
½ NS	Normal saline; 0.45% saline or ½ strength sodium chloride (Figure 7-11)
D5W or 5% D/W	Dextrose 5% in water (Figure 7-12)
D5RL	Dextrose 5% in Ringer's lactate solution (Figure 7-13)
RL, LR, or RLS	Ringer's lactate solution (Figure 7-14)
D5NS	Dextrose 5% in 0.9% normal saline (Figure 7-15)
D5 and ½ NS (0.45% NS)	Dextrose 5% in ½ normal saline or 0.45% sodium chloride (Figure 7-16)

FIGURE 7-10   Normal saline 0.9% (osmolarity range 280-308).

LOT   EXP

2B1313
NDC 0338-0043-03 — 1

0.45% Sodium Chloride Injection USP — 2

500 mL — 3

Each 100 mL contains 450 mg Sodium Chloride USP pH 5.0 (4.5 to 7.0) mEq/L Sodium 77 Chloride 77 Hypotonic Osmolarity 154 mOsmol/L (calc) Sterile Nonpyrogenic Single dose container Additives may be incompatible Consult with pharmacist if available When introducing additives use aseptic technique Mix thoroughly Do not store Dosage Intravenously as directed by a physician See directions Cautions Squeeze and inspect inner bag which maintains product sterility Discard if leaks are found Must not be used in series connections Do not use unless solution is clear Federal (USA) law prohibits dispensing without prescription Store unit in moisture barrier overwrap at room temperature (25°C/77°F) until ready to use Avoid excessive heat See insert — 4

Baxter
Baxter Healthcare Corporation   Viaflex® container
Deerfield IL 60015 USA   PL 146® plastic
Made in USA   For product information
                                 Call 1-800-933-0303

FIGURE 7-11   Normal saline 0.45% (osmolarity 154).

LOT   EXP

2B0064
NDC 0338-0017-04 — 1

5% Dextrose Injection USP — 2

— 3

1000 mL

Each 100 mL contains 5 g Dextrose Hydrous USP — 4
pH 4.0 (3.2 to 6.5) Osmolarity 252 mOsmol/L (calc) Sterile Nonpyrogenic Single dose container Additives may be incompatible Consult with pharmacist if available When introducing additives use aseptic technique Mix thoroughly Do not store Dosage Intravenously as — 5
directed by a physician See directions Cautions Squeeze and inspect inner bag which maintains product sterility Discard if leaks are found Must not be used in series connections Do not administer simultaneously with blood Do not use unless solution is clear Federal (USA) law — 6
prohibits dispensing without prescription Store unit in moisture barrier overwrap at room temperature (25°C/77°F) until ready to use Avoid excessive heat See insert

— 7

Baxter
Baxter Healthcare Corporation   Viaflex® container   — 8
Deerfield IL 60015 USA   PL 146® plastic
Made in USA   For product information
                                 Call 1-800-933-0303

— 9

FIGURE 7-12   5% dextrose.

LOT   EXP

2B2073
NDC 0338-0125-03 — 1

Lactated Ringer's and 5% Dextrose Injection USP — 2

500 mL — 3

Each 100 mL contains   5 g Dextrose Hydrous USP   600 mg Sodium Chloride USP   310 mg Sodium Lactate   30 mg Potassium Chloride USP   20 mg Calcium Chloride USP   pH 5.0 (4.0 to 6.5)   mEq/L Sodium 130   Potassium 4   Calcium 2.7   Chloride 109   Lactate 28   Hypertonic   Osmolarity 525 mOsmol/L (calc)   Sterile   Nonpyrogenic   Single dose container   **Not for use in the treatment of lactic acidosis**   Additives may be incompatible   Consult with pharmacist if available   When introducing additives use aseptic technique   Mix thoroughly   Do not store   Dosage Intravenously as directed by a physician   See insert   Cautions   Squeeze and inspect inner bag which maintains product sterility   Discard if leaks are found   Must not be used in series connections   Do not administer simultaneously with blood   Do not use unless solution is clear   Federal (USA) law prohibits dispensing without prescription   Store unit in moisture barrier overwrap at room temperature (25°C/77°F) until ready to use   Avoid excessive heat   See insert — 4

Baxter
Baxter Healthcare Corporation
Deerfield IL 60015 USA
Made in USA

Viaflex® container
PL 146® plastic
For product information
Call 1-800-933-0303

FIGURE 7-13   Ringer's lactate solution and 5% dextrose.

LOT   EXP

2B2324
NDC 0338-0117-04
DIN 00061085 — 1

Lactated Ringer's Injection USP — 2

— 3

1000 mL

Each 100 mL contains   600 mg Sodium Chloride USP   310 mg Sodium Lactate   30 mg Potassium Chloride USP   20 mg Calcium Chloride USP   pH 6.5 (6.0 to 7.5)   mEq/L Sodium 130   Potassium 4   Calcium 2.7   Chloride 109   Lactate 28   Osmolarity 273 mOsmol/L (calc)   Sterile   Nonpyrogenic   Single dose container   **Not for use in the treatment of lactic acidosis**   Additives may be incompatible   Consult with pharmacist if available   When introducing additives use aseptic technique   Mix thoroughly   Do not store   Dosage   Intravenously as directed by a physician   See directions   Cautions   Squeeze and inspect inner bag which maintains product sterility   Discard if leaks are found   Must not be used in series connections   Do not administer simultaneously with blood   Do not use unless solution is clear   Federal (USA) law prohibits dispensing without prescription   Store unit in moisture barrier overwrap at room temperature (25°C/77°F) until ready to use   Avoid excessive heat   See insert — 4, 5, 6, 7

Baxter — 8
Baxter Healthcare Corporation
Deerfield IL 60015 USA

Made in USA
Distributed in Canada by
Baxter Corporation
Toronto Ontario Canada

Viaflex® container
PL 146® plastic
For product information
Call 1-800-933-0303

— 9

FIGURE 7-14   Ringer's lactate solution.

FIGURE 7-15 5% dextrose in normal saline 0.9%.

FIGURE 7-16 5% dextrose in normal saline 045%.

Percentage of Solute in IV Bags

The percentage numbers of the IV bags indicate the amount of dextrose, sodium chloride, or other constituents in the infusion. The type of IV solution ordered is determined by the diagnosis. Patients with diabetes mellitus, kidney disease, hematologic disorders, or cardiac problems will need different types of solutions. The nurse must be aware of the diagnosis as it relates to the type of IV solution used. To determine the number of milliliters of dextrose or sodium chloride the percentage (%) represents, use the following formula. The dissolved substance or solute (dextrose, sodium chloride) is represented by a weight measurement (g). However, 1 mL of water weighs 1 g. Therefore the solute is weighed in grams per 100 mL of solution. The percentage = g solute per 100 mL solution.

remember Percentage is based on 100.

Example How many g of dextrose are in 1000 mL of D5W?

KNOW

5 g (solute) : 100 mL = x g (solute) : 1000 mL

$1x = 5 \times 1000 = 5000$
$1x = 5000$
$x = 50$ g (solute)
  or mL of dextrose in 1000 mL

OR

FRACTION CROSS PRODUCT

$$\frac{5 \text{ g}}{100 \text{ mL}} = \frac{x \text{g}}{1000}$$

$x = 5 \times 10 = 50$ mL

PROOF $100 \times 50 = 5000$
$5 \times 1000 = 5000$

5% Dextrose Injection USP

1000 mL
EACH 100 mL CONTAINS 5 g DEXTROSE HYDROUS USP pH 4.0 (3.2 TO 6.5) OSMOLARITY 252 mOsmol/L (CALC) STERILE NONPYROGENIC SINGLE DOSE CONTAINER ADDITIVES MAY BE INCOMPATIBLE CONSULT WITH PHARMACIST IF AVAILABLE WHEN INTRODUCING ADDITIVES USE ASEPTIC TECHNIQUE MIX THOROUGHLY DO NOT STORE DOSAGE INTRAVENOUSLY AS DIRECTED BY A PHYSICIAN SEE DIRECTIONS CAUTIONS SQUEEZE AND INSPECT INNER BAG WHICH MAINTAINS PRODUCT STERILITY DISCARD IF LEAKS ARE FOUND MUST NOT BE USED IN SERIES CONNECTIONS DO NOT ADMINISTER SIMULTANEOUSLY WITH BLOOD DO NOT USE UNLESS SOLUTION IS CLEAR FEDERAL (USA) LAW PROHIBITS DISPENSING WITHOUT PRESCRIPTION STORE UNIT IN MOISTURE BARRIER OVERWRAP AT ROOM TEMPERATURE (25°C/77°F) UNTIL READY TO USE AVOID EXCESSIVE HEAT SEE INSERT

Baxter
BAXTER HEALTHCARE CORPORATION   Viaflex® CONTAINER
DEERFIELD IL 60015 USA   PL 146® PLASTIC
MADE IN USA   FOR PRODUCT INFORMATION
CALL 1-800-933-0303

Osmolarity

Osmolarity is a measurement of osmoles (Osm or osmol) that refers to the total concentration of solutes both penetrating and nonpenetrating. This is known as the osmolarity of a solution. The osmol is in the cell but can also pass into the extracellular space (osmosis). Tonicity is the concentration of the nonpenetrating solutes that are extracellular, such as Cl, Na, and Ca, and do not pass into the cell. This exchange of osmols from cellular to extracellular determines the hypotonic, hypertonic, or isotonic value of the solution. All IV labels will show the mOsm/L (milliosmole per liter). Table 7-2 shows the differences among *hypotonic*, *isotonic*, and *hypertonic* solutions according to the mOsm/L content.

Table 7-2 Tonicity of Solutes

Hypotonic (less than 250 mOsm/L)	Isotonic (250-375 mOsm/L)	Hypertonic (greater than 375 mOsm/L)
Fluid shift out of intravascular compartment, hydrating cells	Osmolarity equal to that of serum	Fluid is drawn into the intravascular compartment from the cells
Examples: 0.45% saline (154 mOsm/L) 2.5% dextrose in water	Examples: 0.9% saline (308 mOsm/L) 5% dextrose in water (252 mOsm/L) lactated Ringer's solution (273 mOsm/L)	Examples: 5% dextrose and 0.9% NaCl (560 mOsm/L) 5% dextrose and lactated Ringer's solution (525 mOsm/L) 10% dextrose in water

Answers on page 265

WORKSHEET 7D — IV Solute Calculations

Calculate the grams of NaCl or dextrose in the following IV solutions and state the osmolarity and tonicity: hypotonic, hypertonic, or isotonic solution.

1. **5% Dextrose and 0.9% Sodium Chloride Injection USP — 1000 mL**
   Each 100 mL contains 5 g Dextrose Hydrous USP 900 mg Sodium Chloride USP pH 4.0 (3.2 to 6.5) mEq/L Sodium 154 Chloride 154 Hypertonic Osmolarity 560 mOsmol/L (calc) Sterile Nonpyrogenic Single dose container

   g _____ NaCl
   g _____ dextrose
   osmolarity: _____
   tonicity: _____

2. **5% Dextrose and 0.45% Sodium Chloride Injection USP — 500 mL**
   Each 100 mL contains 5 g Dextrose Hydrous USP 450 mg Sodium Chloride USP pH 4.0 (3.2 to 6.5) mEq/L Sodium 77 Chloride 77 Hypertonic Osmolarity 406 mOsmol/L (calc) Sterile Nonpyrogenic Single dose container

   g _____ dextrose
   g _____ NaCl
   osmolarity: _____
   tonicity: _____

3. **10% Dextrose and 0.9% Sodium Chloride Injection USP — 500 mL**

g _____ dextrose
g _____ NaCl
osmolarity: _____
tonicity: _____

Calculate the g of NaCl in the following intravenous fluids. State the osmolarity.

4. Normal saline 0.9%
   (osmolarity range 280-308)

   0.9% Sodium Chloride Injection USP — 1000 mL

   g _____ NaCl
   osmolarity: _____
   tonicity: _____

5. Normal saline 0.45%
   (osmolarity 154)

   g _____ NaCl
   osmolarity: _____
   tonicity: _____

Calculate the g of dextrose and osmolarity in the following intravenous fluids.

6. Ringer's lactate solution
   and 5% dextrose

   g _____ dextrose
   osmolarity: _____
   tonicity: _____

246 Drug Calculations: *Ratio and Proportion Problems for Clinical Practice*

Calculate the g of NaCl and the osmolarity in the following intravenous fluid.

7. Ringer's lactate solution

Lactated Ringer's Injection USP

1000 mL
Each 100 mL contains 600 mg Sodium Chloride USP 310 mg Sodium Lactate 30 mg Potassium Chloride USP 20 mg Calcium Chloride USP pH 6.5 (6.0 to 7.5) mEq/L Sodium 130 Potassium 4 Calcium 2.7 Chloride 109 Lactate 28 Osmolarity 273 mOsmol/L (calc) Sterile Nonpyrogenic Single dose container Not for use in the treatment of lactic acidosis

g _____ sodium chloride
osmolarity: _____
tonicity: _____

Calculate the g of NaCl and dextrose and osmolarity in the following intravenous fluids.

8. 5% dextrose in normal saline

5% Dextrose and 0.9% Sodium Chloride Injection USP

1000 mL
Each 100 mL contains 5 g Dextrose Hydrous USP 900 mg Sodium Chloride USP pH 4.0 (3.2 to 6.5) mEq/L Sodium 154 Chloride 154 Hypertonic Osmolarity 560 mOsmol/L (calc) Sterile Nonpyrogenic Single dose container

g _____ dextrose
osmolarity: _____
tonicity: _____

CHAPTER 7 Basic Intravenous Therapy Calculations 247

9. Calculate the dextrose, NaCl and osmolarity.

    5% dextrose in ½ normal saline

    g _____ dextrose
    g: _____ NaCl
    osmolarity: _____
    tonicity: _____

Answers on page 267

WORKSHEET 7E — IV Calculations

Directions: Calculate mL per hr, hours to infuse, and completion time when indicated.

1. The patient is receiving an IV of D5W at 125 mL per hr. How many grams of dextrose per hour is the patient receiving?

2. Ordered: 1500 mL D5W to infuse in 4 hr. How many mL per hr should be delivered?

3. Ordered: Magnesium sulfate 2 g over 4 hr for hypomagnesium blood level.
   Available: 500 mL D5W with 2 g of magnesium sulfate.
   How many mL per hr should be infused?

4. Ordered: 5 g Rocephin IV for bronchitis to infuse in 6 hr.
   Available: 5 g Rocephin in 1000 mL of D5W.
   How many mL per hour should infuse?

5. Ordered: 1000 mL of lactated Ringer's solution to infuse at 125 mL per hour. The IV was started at 0900. When will the infusion be completed?

6. Ordered: 500 mg aminophylline in 250 mL normal saline IVPB for emphysema to infuse at 30 mL per hr. The IV started at 1330 hours. When will the infusion be complete?

7. Ordered: 1000 mL normal saline with 500 mg erythromycin for COPD lung infection to infuse in 8 hr. The infusion was started at 0715 hours. How many mL per hour will be infused? When will the infusion be complete?

8. Ordered: Aminophylline 1 g in 500 mL D5W for asthma to infuse at 40 mL per hr.
   Available: 1 g of aminophylline in 500 mL of D5W. The IV was started at 2100 hours. When will the infusion be complete?

9. Ordered: 2 g Keflin in 200 mL normal saline IVPB for infected sinus to infuse in 3 hr. How many mL per hour will the infusion device be set for?

10. Ordered: Rocephin 1 g in 500 mL of normal saline to infuse in 4 hr for endometriosis. At what rate will you set the IV pump?

IV medications must be charted on a flow sheet (Figure 7-17).

IV MEDICATION ADMINISTRATION RECORD

HOSPITAL

DATA FLOW RECORD

NURSING CARE RECORD
Medical/Surgical
Date _____
1-12-16

TIME	0600	1600												
PULSE	84	80												
RESPIRATION	20	22												
BLOOD PRESSURE	150/92	152/90												
COUGH/ DEEP BREATH	✓	✓												
INITIALS	JG	CB												

The IV flow sheet may record the vital signs prior to initiating IV therapy and again on every shift. The IV site and location is recorded along with the time and date it was started. The catheter type and needle size are recorded next to the type and rate of the IV solution. Additional IV solutions are recorded in the date/time inserted column. When the IV is discontinued, the reason is recorded under the comments column.

IV THERAPY

SITE	DATE/TIME INSERTED	SITE LOCATION	CATH TYPE/ SIZE	IV SOLUTION	RATE	DEVICE	TUBING CHANGE	APPEARANCE 7-3	3-11	11-7	SITE D/C'd	COMMENTS
R	1-12-16 0600	LPF	22 angio	1000 D5W	75°			1				
R	1-12-16 1900	LPF	22 angio	1000 D5W	75°		△		1			
R	1-12-16 2200	LPF	22 angio						2		✓	Slight redness noted at site pt denies pain or tenderness.

HEALTH DEVIATION NEEDS

DCP ASSESSED: In Progress ☐   Revise Plan ☐
DCP Conference ☐ _____

REFERRAL MADE: SS ☐ HHC ☐ Dietary ☐ Pharmacy ☐
Other _____

PATIENT/FAMILY TEACHING:
Pt/Other _____

PT/FAMILY TEACHING RESPONSE CODES
1 = Received Literature
2 = Communicates Understanding
3 = Requires Reinforcement
4 = Previous Experience
5 = Return Demonstration
6 = Objective Achieved
7 = Referral Initiated
8 = Refused
9 = Preprinted Teaching Protocol

IV CODES
Site Location
L = Left   AC = Antecubital   UAF = Upper
R = Right   UA = Upper Arm   Anterior
S = Scalp   UPF = Upper   Forearm
Ft = Foot   Posterior   LAF = Lower
F = Femoral   Forearm   Anterior
H = Hand   LPF = Lower   Forearm
W = Wrist   Posterior   IJ = Internal
                              Forearm   Jugular
                                                SC = Subclavian

Catheter
S.G. = Swan Ganz
H.D. = Hemodialysis
Hick = Hickman
G = Groshong
Port = Port-A-Cath or other implanted port
I = Introducer
PP = Pace Port

Appearance
1 = Asymptomatic
2 = Red
3 = Swollen
4 = Ecchymotic
5 = Warm
6 = Cool
7 = Draining
8 = Leaking

Lumen
d = distal
m = middle
p = proximal

EMOTIONAL SUPPORT CODES
1 = Active Listening
2 = Reassurance/Comfort
3 = Relaxation
    A = Breathing
    B = Visualization/Imagery
4 = Coping Skills Review

△ = Change

PROCEDURES

TIME	DEPT.	MODE	TRANSPORTER	RETURN

INITIAL	SIGNATURE/TITLE	INITIAL	SIGNATURE/TITLE
mj	J Jackie, RN		

FIGURE 7-17 Example of an IV therapy medication administration record (MAR).

CLINICAL RELEVANCE

When IVPBs are added to an existing IV solution, the nurse must ensure that the additive medication is compatible. When IVPBs are added to an existing IV line, the ports must be cleansed with antiseptic before puncturing.

Gravity Piggyback Infusions

The acronym for intravenous piggyback is IVPB (Figure 7-18). When special medications are ordered intermittently, the primary IV can be bypassed by introducing the medication through a special entry or portal. Piggyback (PB) medications are infused intermittently via the existing IV line. A secondary IV tube with a needleless attachment is inserted into the portal or entry site. The PB infusion amount is usually 50 to 250 mL of medicated solution.

Elevating the IVPB 12 inches above the existing IV allows the PB to infuse by **gravity** (Figure 7-19). When all of the medication has been infused, the existing IV will resume to the rate set for the PB infusion. The nurse must remember to regulate the primary IV to the previous rate. If an infusion device is used, the IV can be programmed to resume to the primary infusion rate at the completion of the PB.

FIGURE 7-18 50 mL of solution for IV piggyback infusion.

FIGURE 7-19 Gravity-flow IV piggyback. The IV piggyback is elevated above the existing IV, allowing it to infuse by gravity.

Piggyback medications are premixed by the pharmacy, drug manufacturer, or nurse. The manufacturer's insert provides recommended times for IVPBs to infuse if the physician does not state the rate in the order.

remember Gravity-flow sets are delivered in drops per minute.

Piggyback Premixed IVs

Piggyback IV additions are premixed by the pharmacy or the manufacturer. The medication is diluted in 50 to 250 mL of an iso-osmotic sterile solution. The amount of solution used depends on the type of medication, the presence of fluid restrictions, and the weight of the patient.

FIGURE 7-20 50 mL of dextrose. Medication can be added for infusion as an IV piggyback.

IVPB admixtures (Figure 7-20) are usually prepared in bulk by the pharmacist for more efficient use of time. If more than one day's supply is prepared, the IVPB can be frozen without altering its stability.

Premixed frozen IVPBs should be thawed in the refrigerator or at room temperature. Never thaw in a microwave oven or in hot or warm water.

All IVPB admixtures must be visually inspected before starting. Check the order, label, medication, strength, and quantity. Make sure that the admixture is clear and free from particles and that the expiration date has not passed.

CLINICAL RELEVANCE

Medication added to an IV bag in an upright position will cause the drug to be concentrated in the lower part of the bag. Disperse the medication by inverting the bag to avoid a concentrated dose, which could harm the patient.

Nurse-Activated Piggyback Systems

The Hospira ADD-Vantage and the Baxter Mini-Bag Plus (Figure 7-21) are used in home care as well as in hospitals and long-term care centers. The IVPB mini-bag has a vial of medication attached to a special port. The pharmacy dispenses the IVPB with the unreconstituted drug vial attached to the

FIGURE 7-21 A, Hospira ADD-Vantage with a drug vial of vancomycin. **B,** The Mini-Bag Plus Container has a built-in vial adapter that fits standard powdered drug vials. The system can be assembled without immediately mixing the drug and diluent. The drug admixture is prepared by breaking the seal between the vial and the IV solution container. The vial remains attached to the Mini-Bag™ Plus Container, which reduces the potential for medication errors. (A, From Hospira, Inc., Lake Forest, IL. B, From Baxter Healthcare Corp., Deerfield, Ill.)

FIGURE 7-22 Hospira ADD-Vantage® System. From Hospira, Inc., Lake Forest, IL.

mini-bag. At the time of delivery, the nurse breaks the seal between the vial and the mini-bag. This allows the medication to flow into the mini-bag. The medication vial remains attached to the mini-bag, which is a safety feature created to decrease potential medication errors. Figure 7-22 shows the steps for assembling and using the ADD-Vantage system.

Electronic Infusion Devices (EIDs)

Electronic infusion devices are used in hospitals, extended-care facilities, home care, and ambulatory care settings. They deliver a set amount of intravenous solution per hour. Some examples of electronic infusion devices are shown in Figure 7-23. They are individually programmed to deliver a set amount of IV solution per hour.

CADD-Prizm (see Figure 7-23, *A*) is a battery-operated pump that provides IV medications to confined or ambulatory patients. There are four delivery modes:
- Patient-controlled analgesia (PCA)
- Continuous infusion
- Intermittent infusion
- Total parenteral nutrition

CLINICAL ALERT!

There is a wide variety of infusion devices/pumps. Make sure you understand how to program the pumps to avoid medication errors. Some institutions require another nurse to verify the setting. Adhere to hospital policy for IV device protocol.

FIGURE 7-23 Electronic infusion devices. **A,** CADD® -Solls pain management pump. **B,** Alaris® PC System. **C,** Patient-controlled analgesia (PCA) ambulatory infusion pump. (**A,** From Smiths Medical ASD, Inc., St. Paul, Minn. **B,** From CareFusion, San Diego, Calif. **C,** From Perry AG, Potter PA, Elkin MK: *Nursing interventions and clinical skills,* ed. 5, St. Louis, 2012, Mosby.)

CLINICAL RELEVANCE

It is the nurses' responsibility to check the ordered IV rate for accuracy (mL per hr) and time or completion factor. If the IV is infusing too slowly, the rate can be adjusted, depending on the medication and the patient's condition. Check the hospital's protocol for discretionary adjustments. If the flow rate is too rapid, return to the ordered rate and notify the prescriber if deemed necessary.

Blood Transfusions

Packed RBCs (250 to 300 mL) are derived from whole blood with two thirds of the plasma removed. Packed cells increase the oxygen-carrying capacity of the blood.

Whole blood (500 mL) is used to replace volume. It contains O_2-carrying cells as well as RBCs, plasma, proteins, and clotting factors that are needed for hypovolemic shock.

Frozen RBCs can be frozen for 3 years, but this product is infrequently used.

Fresh frozen plasma (FFP) (200 to 300 mL) improves the PT and PTT.

CLINICAL RELEVANCE

- Check the physician's order.
- Ensure that consent is signed.
- Check patient ID.
- Check and record patient's blood pressure.
- Ensure IV access with a large-bore catheter (18- to 20-gauge).
- Use a Y-tubing blood administration set with a filter.
- Start the IV with 0.9% normal saline solution and infusion pump.
- Two nurses must verify the numbers on the blood with the laboratory's type and cross-match.
- Blood should be completed within 3 to 4 hours after it is received from the blood bank or a chance of bacterial contamination may occur.

CLINICAL ALERT!

The rate for the first 15 minutes of blood administration should be set at 25 to 50 mL per hour. The nurse stays at the bedside during that time to monitor for an adverse reaction (Figure 7-24). If no adverse reactions present, the EID flow rate is usually set at 100 to 120 mL per hour. Physicians may order an antihistamine to be given to the patient before blood administration. If a reaction occurs, **stop** the transfusion and follow facility protocols.

FIGURE 7-24 **A,** Filter used for blood administration. **B,** Blood administration with Y tubing and normal saline. (From Mulholland J, Turner S: *The nurse, the math, the meds: Drug calculations using dimensional analysis*, ed. 3, St. Louis, 2015, Mosby.)

PCA Protocol

The patient-controlled analgesia (PCA) device allows a prespecified amount of narcotic to be available to the patient upon demand. This provides a more constant blood level of analgesia and better pain control (Figure 7-25, *A*). The patient can control the pain level by pushing the control button (Figure 7-25, *B*). An opioid such as morphine is usually the medication of choice. The nurse programs the amount and frequency of the ordered medication as well as the safety lockout time. The usual programmed amount is minimal effective analgesic concentration (MEAC), which can be *1 mg with a 6-minute lockout; 1.5 mg with a 9-minute lockout;* or *2 mg with a 12-minute lockout*. The device also stores information about how frequently the patient pushed the button during the lockout phase. This information allows the nurse to adjust the medication level or lockout time to achieve the MEAC after consulting with the physician. Evaluation of the patient's pain and respiratory status must be monitored every half hour when using opioid analgesia due to possible respiratory suppression.

FIGURE 7-25 A, Lifecare® Patient-controlled analgesia 3 Infusion System. (From Hospira, Inc., Lake Forest, IL.) **B,** The nurse instructs the patient on the use of a PCA infusion pump for pain control. (**A,** From Hospira, Inc., Lake Forest, Ill. **B,** From Perry AG, Potter PA, Ostendorf WR: *Clinical nursing skills and techniques,* ed. 8, St. Louis, 2014, Mosby.)

CLINICAL RELEVANCE

There are many types of PCA pumps with different syringe calculations. Errors can result from incorrect programming. It is best to have another nurse check the ordered medication, the ordered dose, and the program setting. The Joint Commission on Accreditation of Healthcare Organizations (JCAHO) and a statement of National Patient Safety Goals (NPSG) have established goals to improve client safety when using PCA devices and IV infusion pumps. All IV pumps must have safety alerts when the IV is not infusing properly. Unregulated flow can be delivered if the pump tubing is improperly attached, disarming the mechanism to prevent free-flow as well as disarming the alarm. The institute for Safe Medication Practices (ISMP) reports that administration sets now have integral antisiphon valves to prevent a free-flow event if a pump is improperly loaded.

Pressure-Flow Infusion Device

The ambulatory infusion device system was developed for ambulatory use. It can be put in a pocket, inside a shirt, or in any other convenient place where it can be concealed. The flow rate is preset. Figure 7-26 shows an example of an ambulatory infusion device.

FIGURE 7-26 MedFlo postoperative pain management system, an ambulatory infusion device (Smith & Nephew Endoscopy, Andover, Mass.)

Piggyback Infusions

Examples
- Ordered: Cefazolin 1 g IV in 50 mL for 30 min. At how many mL per hr should the infusion pump be set?

KNOW | WANT TO KNOW | FRACTION CROSS PRODUCT

50 mL : 30 min = x mL : 60   OR $\dfrac{50 \text{ mL}}{30 \text{ min}} = \dfrac{x}{60 \text{ min}} = \dfrac{300}{3} = 100$ mL per hr

30 x = 50 × 6 = 300   3x = 6 × 50 = 300   **PROOF** 30 × 100 = 30
x = 100 mL per hr   x = 100 mL per hr   50 × 60 = 30

Set the infusion pump for 100 mL per hr.

- Ordered: Ampicillin 500 mg IV in 100 mL NS for 45 min. At how many mL per hr should the infusion pump be set?

KNOW | WANT TO KNOW | FRACTION CROSS PRODUCT

100 mL : 45 min = x mL : 60 min   OR $\dfrac{100}{45} = \dfrac{x}{60}$

45 x = 100 × 60 = 6000   45x = 100 × 60 = 6000
45 x = 6000   x = 133.3 = 133 mL per hr
x = 133.3 = 133 mL per hr

PROOF 45 × 133.3 = 5998.5   Convert minutes into a decimal
          60 × 100 = 6000   45 min ÷ 60 = 0.75
                                       100 mL ÷ 0.75 = 133 mL per hr

Set the infusion pump at 133 mL per hr.

CLINICAL ALERT!

Potassium chloride as an additive to an IV can be dangerous. The IV solution must be clamped when the KCl is added. The IV bag must then be inverted or gently shaken for thorough mixing to avoid a bolus dose of potassium that could be lethal to the patient.

CLINICAL ALERT!

When using an EID that infuses mL per hour, the device must be set at mL per hour when infusing an IVPB medication in less than 1 hour. Be aware that smart pumps can deliver different rates such as mL per hour, mg per kg, mg per kg per min, mg per min, mcg per min, and mcg per hour. It is the nurse's responsibility to be knowledgeable of the different types of EIDs and program the infusion depending on the device.

Answers on page 268

WORKSHEET 7F | Infusion Device and Solute g/mL and gtt/min Calculations

Use the two-step formula to answer the following questions.

1. **Ordered:** 100 mL IVPB to be infused for 1 hr. At how many mL per hr will you set the infusion device?

2. **Ordered:** 250 mL NS to be infused at 150 mL per hr. The drop factor is 15 drops per mL. How long will it take to infuse?

3. **Ordered:** 100 mL to be infused for 30 min by microdrip (microdrip = 60 drops per min).
   a. How many drops per min will be infused on a gravity flow if the drop factor is used?
   b. At how many mL per hr will you set the infusion device?

4. **Ordered:** 50 mL IVPB ADD-Vantage® System to be infused for 20 min.
   a. At how many mL per hr would you set the infusion device?
   b. How many drops per min will be administered on a gravity flow if the drop factor is 15?

5. **Ordered:** 100 mL IVPB to be infused for 1 hr. The drop factor is 15. How many drops per min is this? At how many mL per hr will you set the infusion device?

6. **Ordered:** 50 mL IVPB to be infused for 30 min.
   a. At how many mL per hr will you set an infusion device?
   b. How many drops per min will infuse for a gravity flow if the drop factor is 60?

7. **Ordered:** 200 mL to infuse for 90 min. The drop factor is microdrip.
   a. How many drops per min will infuse?
   b. At how many mL per hr will you set the infusion pump?

8. **Ordered:** 1000 mL 0.9% saline to infuse for 12 hr. The drop factor is 15 drops per mL.
   a. How many drops per min will infuse?
   b. At how many mL per hr will you set the infusion pump?
   c. How many milliliters of sodium chloride will the patient receive?

9. **Ordered:** 2000 mL D5W to be infused for 8 hr. The drop factor is 15 drops per mL.
   a. How many mL per hr will infuse?
   b. How many drops per min will infuse?
   c. How many milliliters of dextrose will the patient receive in 8 hours?

10. **Ordered:** 150 mL IVPB. Label reads to infuse for 40 to 60 min. The drop factor is microdrip.
    a. What is the fastest rate for the IVPB to infuse? At what rate will you set the infusion device?
    b. What is the slowest rate for the IVPB to infuse? At what rate will you set the device?

Answers on page 269

WORKSHEET 7G | Multiple-Choice Practice

Circle the letter of the correct answer in the following problems. Remember: To convert tenths of an hour into minutes, multiply by 60. Example: 0.65 hr × 60 = 39 min

1. Calculate the infusion time for an IV of 1000 mL of D5W infusing at 25 drops per min with a drop factor of 10 drops per mL.
   - **a.** 6 hr, 40 min
   - **b.** 6 hr, 10 min
   - **c.** 5 hr, 57 min
   - **d.** 4 hr, 17 min

2. Administer 50 mL of an IV antibiotic for 15 min. The IV set is calibrated at 15 drops per mL. At how many drops per min will you set the rate?
   - **a.** 100 drops per min
   - **b.** 50 drops per min
   - **c.** 25 drops per min
   - **d.** 60 drops per min

3. **Ordered:** 50 mL piggyback to be infused for 30 min. The drop factor is 20. At how many drops per min will you set the rate?
   - **a.** 17 drops per min
   - **b.** 100 drops per min
   - **c.** 20 drops per min
   - **d.** 33 drops per min

4. **Ordered:** 300 mL of 0.9% NS for 6 hr. The IV set is microdrip. At how many drops per min will you set the rate?
   - **a.** 60 drops per min
   - **b.** 50 drops per min
   - **c.** 30 drops per min
   - **d.** 45 drops per min

5. **Ordered:** Dobutrex 150 mg in 150 mL Ringer's lactate (RL). The infusion device is set at 12 mL per hr. How long will it take to infuse?
   - **a.** 6 hr, 15 min
   - **b.** 12 hr, 50 min
   - **c.** 8 hr, 15 min
   - **d.** 12 hr, 30 min

6. The IV is infusing at 30 drops per min. The drop factor is 20 drops per mL. The IV bag label reads 500 mL of 0.45% NS. How many hours will it take to infuse?
   - **a.** 5 hr, 50 min
   - **b.** 3 hr, 36 min
   - **c.** 4 hr, 40 min
   - **d.** 5 hr, 30 min

7. **Ordered:** 2500 mL to be infused for 24 hr. Available: An IV tubing with 15 drops per mL. At what rate will you set the IV device?
   - **a.** 26 drops per min
   - **b.** 35 drops per min
   - **c.** 52 drops per min
   - **d.** 104 drops per min

8. A pint of blood (500 mL) is hung at 1100 hours. The flow rate is 42 drops per min. The drop factor on the administration set is 10 drops per mL. When will the infusion be complete?
   - **a.** 1733 hours
   - **b.** 1920 hours
   - **c.** 1300 hours
   - **d.** 1654 hours

9. Tridil is infusing at 30 mL per hr. The IV label reads: *500 mL D5W with Tridil 5 mcg per 3 mL*. How many hours will it take to infuse?
   - **a.** 15 hr, 10 min
   - **b.** 18 hr, 45 min
   - **c.** 16 hr, 40 min
   - **d.** 12 hr, 48 min

10. **Ordered:** Amicar 5 g in 250 mL for 2 hr. At how many mL per hr should the infusion device be set?
    - **a.** 150 mL per hr
    - **b.** 100 mL per hr
    - **c.** 175 mL per hr
    - **d.** 125 mL per hr

Drug Calculations: *Ratio and Proportion Problems for Clinical Practice*

Critical Thinking Exercises

Critical Thinking Exercises provide math and medication-related patient safety issues for student discussion. Answers are not provided.

Analyze the following scenarios.

1. It is the change of shift. The patient with congestive heart failure (CHF) is being infused with an IV of 1000 mL D5W. The patient complains of being very short of breath. After checking the IV rate, you find that it is infusing at 175 mL per hr. Taking into consideration the patient's diagnosis, you check the IV order and it reads 500 mL D5W in 24 hr.

   Ordered:

   Given:

   Error(s):

   Potential adverse drug event:

   Preventive measures:

   ### Discussion
   - What would be your first action?
   - What are the serious effects that might jeopordize the patient's safety?
   - At what rate should the IV be infusing?
   - How can this type of error be reconciled to reduce potential risks?

2. Mr. K. has been transferred from the PACU to the surgical floor at 1400 hr after having a pneumonectomy. An IV with 1 gram of Rocephin in 500 mL of D5W is infusing at 42 mL per hr. The PACU nurse indicated on the chart that she had given Mr. K. 4 mg of morphine IV push about 10 minutes ago. Orders are to continue the Rocephin and start a PCA with 1 mg of morphine with a 6-minute lockout. At 1800 hr you notice that Mr. K. has pushed the lockout button three times, which indicated that the dose of 1 mg every 6 minutes was not adequate. The physician gave a verbal order to increase the dosage to 1.5 mg. You increase the morphine to 1.5 mg. At 2200 hr the evening nurse reports that Mr. K.'s respirations were 10 per min.

   ### Discussion
   - What will be your first action?
   - What is the potential risk to the patient?
   - Was the physician's order incomplete?
   - How frequently should a patient on a PCA be checked?
   - What is the protocol for a lockout time for 1.5 mg of morphine?
   - To promote safety using a PCA, how would you reconcile this error?

3. A 75-year old patient, Mrs. J., has an IV of ampicillin 1 g in 500 mL D5W to be infused in 6 hours. The IV was started at 0730 hr. At 0830 hr when you check the IV, you notice that Mrs. J.'s face is flushed. You ask if she feels OK and she answers yes. You ask Mrs. J. if she has any allergies and she replies that a long time ago when she was little she had a rash when she was given what she thought was penicillin but never thought anything more about it because it was so long ago. You check Mrs. J.'s chart and find that penicillin was listed as an allergy. At 1030 hr Mrs. J. reports feeling frightened and that she was having a hard time breathing and feels as if her throat is closing. At this time, you stop the IV, notify the physican, and give the patient epinephrine, which is the protocol for allergy emergencies. You notice that the IV has 150 mL left to be infused.

Discussion
- Do you think you acted prudently?
- What was the correct rate for the IV? At what rate was it infusing?
- What was the potential risk to the patient?
- How can a situation like this be reconciled for patient safety?

CHAPTER 7 Final

1. **Ordered:** 250 mL to infuse for 90 min. How many mL per hr will infuse if the electronic infusion device is used? How many drops per min will infuse using a drop factor of 15?

   $\dfrac{250 \text{ mL}}{90 \text{ min}} \times \dfrac{60 \text{ min}}{1 \text{ hr}}$

   $\boxed{166.7 \text{ mL/hr}}$

   $\dfrac{250 \text{ mL}}{90 \text{ min}} \times \dfrac{15 \text{ gtt}}{1 \text{ mL}}$

   $\boxed{42 \text{ gtt/min}}$

2. **Ordered:** 3000 mL D5W to infuse for 24 hr with 0.5 g of penicillin in each 1000 mL. The drop factor is 20, ~~by microdrip~~. How many mL per hr will infuse? How many drops per min will be administered?

   $\boxed{125 \text{ mL/hr}}$ $\dfrac{125 \text{ mL}}{60 \text{ min}} \times \dfrac{20 \text{ gtt}}{1 \text{ mL}}$ $\boxed{42 \text{ gtt/min}}$

3. **Ordered:** 1000 mL to be infused for 12 hr IV. At how many mL per hr will you set the infusion device? How many drops per min will be administered via a gravity device if the drop factor is 20?

   $\boxed{83.3 \text{ mL/hr}}$ $\dfrac{83.3 \text{ mL}}{1 \text{ hr}/60 \text{ min}} \times \dfrac{20 \text{ gtt}}{1 \text{ mL}}$ $\boxed{28 \text{ gtt/min}}$

4. **Ordered:** 1200 mL to be infused for 8 hr. The drop factor is microdrip. How many drops per min will infuse using a gravity device?

   $\dfrac{180 \text{ mL/hr}}{60 \text{ min}} \times \dfrac{60 \text{ gtt}}{\text{mL}} = \boxed{180 \text{ gtt/min}}$

5. **Ordered:** Infuse 2000 mL D5W for 24 hr. The drop factor is 10. At how many mL per hr will you set the infusion device? How many drops per min will be administered using a gravity device?

   $\boxed{83 \text{ mL/hr}}$ $\dfrac{83 \text{ mL}}{60 \text{ min}} \times \dfrac{10 \text{ gtt}}{1 \text{ mL}}$ $\boxed{14 \text{ gtt/min}}$

6. **Ordered:** 1500 mL NS to infuse for 12 hr. The drop factor is 15. How many mL per hr will be administered? How many drops per min will infuse?

   $\dfrac{125 \text{ mL}}{60 \text{ min}} \times \dfrac{15 \text{ gtt}}{1 \text{ mL}}$ $\boxed{125 \text{ mL/hr}}$ $\boxed{31 \text{ gtt/min}}$

7. **Ordered:** 75 mL to be infused for 45 min. The drop factor is 10. At how many mL per hr will you set the infusion device? How many drops per min will infuse via a gravity device if the drop factor is 10?

   $\dfrac{75 \text{ mL}}{45 \text{ min}} \times \dfrac{10 \text{ gtt}}{1 \text{ mL}}$ $\boxed{17 \text{ gtt/min}}$ $\boxed{100 \text{ mL/hr}}$

8. **Ordered:** 200 mL cefazolin to infuse for 45 min via the infusion device. At how many mL per hr will you set the infusion device?

   $\dfrac{200 \text{ mL}}{45 \text{ min}} \times \dfrac{60 \text{ min}}{1 \text{ hr}}$ $\boxed{267 \text{ mL/hr}}$

9. **Ordered:** 1000 mL to run for 12 hr on microdrip. At how many drops per min will you regulate the flow?

   $\dfrac{83.3 \text{ mL}}{60 \text{ min}} \times 60$ $\boxed{83 \text{ gtt/min}}$

10. **Ordered:** 3000 mL for 24 hr. The drop factor is 15. How many drops per min will infuse via a gravity device?

    $\dfrac{125 \text{ mL}}{60 \text{ min}} \times \dfrac{15 \text{ gtt}}{1 \text{ mL}}$ $\boxed{31 \text{ gtt/min}}$

evolve **Refer to the Intravenous Calculations section of Drug Calculations Companion, version 5 on Evolve for additional practice problems.**

Answer Key

7 Basic Intravenous Therapy Calculations

WORKSHEET **7A** (page 237)

remember
1. $\dfrac{TV}{TT \text{ in hr}} = mL \text{ per hr}$

2. $\dfrac{Df}{\text{Time in min}} \times V \text{ per hr} = \text{drops per min}$

1. Step 1: $\dfrac{TV}{TT} = \dfrac{1000}{8} = 125$ mL per hr

   Step 2: $\dfrac{10}{60} \times \dfrac{125 \text{ mL}}{1} = \dfrac{1}{6} \times \dfrac{125}{1} = \dfrac{125}{6} = 20.8$ or 21 drops per min

2. Step 2: $\dfrac{60}{60} \times \dfrac{50}{1} = \dfrac{1}{1} \times \dfrac{50}{1} = \dfrac{50}{1} = 50$ drops per min

3. Step 2: $\dfrac{10}{30} \times \dfrac{100}{1} = \dfrac{1}{3} \times \dfrac{100}{1} = \dfrac{100}{3} = 33.3$ or 33 drops per min

4. Step 1: $\dfrac{1500}{12} = 125$ mL per hr

   Step 2: $\dfrac{15}{60} \times \dfrac{125}{1} = \dfrac{1}{4} \times \dfrac{125}{1} = 31.25$ or 31 drops per min

5. Step 2: $\dfrac{15}{60} \times \dfrac{200}{1} = \dfrac{1}{4} \times \dfrac{200}{1} = \dfrac{200}{4} = 50$ drops per min

6. Step 2: $\dfrac{\cancel{20}^{1}}{\cancel{60}_{3}} \times 150 = \dfrac{1}{3} \times \dfrac{150}{1} = \dfrac{150}{3} = 50$ drops per min

7. Step 2: $\dfrac{10}{45} \times \dfrac{75}{1} = \dfrac{750}{45} = 16.6$ or 17 drops per min

8. Step 2: $\dfrac{\cancel{60}^{2}}{\cancel{90}_{3}} \times \dfrac{150}{1} = \dfrac{300}{3} = 100$ drops per min

9. Step 2: $\dfrac{\cancel{15}^{3}}{\cancel{40}_{8}} \times 150 = \dfrac{3}{8} \times \dfrac{150}{1} = \dfrac{450}{8} = 56.25$ or 56 drops per min

10. Step 1: $\dfrac{1500}{8} = 188$ mL per hr

    Step 2: a. $\dfrac{10}{60} \times \dfrac{188}{1} = \dfrac{1}{6} \times \dfrac{188}{1} = \dfrac{188}{6} = 31.3$ or 31 drops per min

    b. $\dfrac{15}{60} = \dfrac{1}{4} \times \dfrac{188}{1} = 47$ drops per min

WORKSHEET 7B (page 238)

remember

1. $\dfrac{TV}{TT \text{ in hr}} = \text{mL per hr}$

2. $\dfrac{Df}{\text{Time in min}} \times V \text{ per hr} = \text{drops per min}$

1. Step 1: $\dfrac{TV}{TT} = \dfrac{1000}{12} = 83.3 \text{ or } 83 \text{ mL per hr}$

Step 2: $\dfrac{\cancel{60}^{1}}{\cancel{60}_{1}} \times \dfrac{83}{1} = \dfrac{83}{1} = 83 \text{ drops per min}$

2. Step 1: $\dfrac{TV}{TT} = \dfrac{1500}{8} = 187.5 \text{ or } 188 \text{ mL per hr}$

Step 2: $\dfrac{\cancel{15}^{1}}{\cancel{60}_{4}} \times \dfrac{188}{1} = 47 \text{ drops per min}$

3. Step 1: $\dfrac{TV}{TT} = \dfrac{3000}{24} = 125 \text{ mL per hr}$

Step 2: $\dfrac{\cancel{15}^{1}}{\cancel{60}_{4}} \times \dfrac{125}{1} = \dfrac{125}{4} = 31 \text{ drops per min}$

4. Step 1: $\dfrac{TV}{TT} = \dfrac{500}{4} = 125 \text{ mL per hr}$

Step 2: $\dfrac{\cancel{15}^{1}}{\cancel{60}_{4}} \times \dfrac{125}{1} = \dfrac{125}{4} = 31.2 \text{ or } 31 \text{ drops per min}$

5. Step 1: $\dfrac{TV}{TT} = \dfrac{2000}{24} = 83.3 \text{ or } 83 \text{ mL per hr}$

Step 2: $\dfrac{\cancel{15}^{1}}{\cancel{60}_{4}} \times \dfrac{83}{1} = \dfrac{83}{4} = 20.75 \text{ or } 21 \text{ drops per min}$

6. Start with Step 2 because we already know how many milliliters per 30 minutes.

Step 2: $\dfrac{\cancel{20}^{2}}{\cancel{30}_{3}} \times \dfrac{100}{1} = \dfrac{200}{3} = 67 \text{ drops per min}$

7. Step 1: $\dfrac{TV}{TT} = \dfrac{2000}{24} = 83.3 \text{ or } 83 \text{ mL per hr}$

8. Step 1: $\dfrac{TV}{TT} = \dfrac{250}{10} = 25 \text{ mL per hr}$

Step 2: $\dfrac{\cancel{60}^{1}}{\cancel{60}_{1}} \times \dfrac{25}{1} = 25 \text{ drops per min}$

9. Step 1: $\dfrac{TV}{TT} = \dfrac{1500}{12} = 125$ mL per hr

   Step 2: $\dfrac{\cancel{15}^{1}}{\cancel{60}_{4}} \times \dfrac{125}{1} = \dfrac{125}{4} = 31.25$ or 31 drops per min

10. **MEMORIZE** * Step 1: $\dfrac{TV}{TT \text{ in hr}} = $ mL per hr

    Step 2: $\dfrac{Df}{\text{Time in min}} \times V \text{ per hr} = $ drops per min

WORKSHEET 7C (page 238)

remember
1. $\dfrac{TV}{TT \text{ in hr}} = $ mL per hr
2. $\dfrac{Df}{\text{Time in min}} \times V \text{ per hr} = $ drops per min

1. Step 1: $\dfrac{TV}{TT} = \dfrac{500}{8} = 62.5$ or 63 mL per hr

   Step 2: $\dfrac{\cancel{60}^{1}}{\cancel{60}_{1}} \times \dfrac{63}{1} = 63$ drops per min

2. Step 2: $\dfrac{\cancel{10}}{\cancel{30}} \times \dfrac{50}{1} = \dfrac{50}{3} = 16.6$ or 17 drops per min

3. Step 1: $\dfrac{TV}{TT} = \dfrac{1000}{6} = 166.6$ or 167 mL per hr

   Step 2: $\dfrac{\cancel{15}^{1}}{\cancel{60}_{4}} \times \dfrac{167}{1} = \dfrac{167}{4} = 41.75$ or 42 drops per min

4. Step 2: $\dfrac{\cancel{60}^{1}}{\cancel{60}_{1}} \times \dfrac{100}{1} = 100$ drops per min   Yes, the mL per hr is the same as the drops per min rate.

5. Step 2: $\dfrac{20}{60} \times 85 = \dfrac{1}{3} \times \dfrac{85}{1} = \dfrac{85}{3} = 28.3$ or 28 drops per min

6. Step 2: $\dfrac{\cancel{10}}{\cancel{60}} \times 100 = \dfrac{100}{6} = 16.6$ or 17 drops per min

7. Step 1: $\dfrac{TV}{TT} = \dfrac{1500}{24} = 62.5$ or 63 mL per hr

   Step 2: $\dfrac{\cancel{10}^{1}}{\cancel{60}_{6}} \times \dfrac{63}{1} = \dfrac{63}{6} \times 10.5 = 11$ drops per min

8. Step 2: $\dfrac{15}{30} \times \dfrac{100}{1} = \dfrac{1}{2} \times \dfrac{100}{1} = \dfrac{100}{2} = 50$ drops per min

9. Step 2: $\dfrac{\cancel{15}^{1}}{\cancel{60}_{4}} \times \dfrac{75}{1} = \dfrac{75}{4} = 18.7$ or 19 drops per min

10. Step 1: $\dfrac{TV}{TT} = \dfrac{2000}{12} = 166.6$ or 167 mL per hr

Step 2: $\dfrac{\cancel{20}^{1}}{\cancel{60}_{3}} \times \dfrac{167}{1} = \dfrac{167}{3} = 55.6 = 56$ drops per min

WORKSHEET 7D (page 244)

1.
KNOW	WANT TO KNOW
5 g : 100 mL	= x g : 1000 mL

$x = 5 \times 10 = 50$
$x = 50$ g or mL dextrose

FRACTION CROSS PRODUCT

$\dfrac{5 \text{ g}}{100 \text{ mL}} = \dfrac{x \text{ g}}{1000 \text{ mL}}$

$x = 5 \times 10 = 50$
$x = 5$ g

PROOF
$5 \times 1000 = 5000$
$100 \times 50 = 5000$

KNOW	WANT TO KNOW
0.9 g : 100 mL	= x g : 1000 mL

$x = 0.9 \times 10 = 9$
$x = 9$ g of sodium chloride

PROOF
$0.9 \times 1000 = 900$
$100 \times 9 = 900$
Osmolarity: 560 Osmol/L
Tonicity: Hypertonic

2.
KNOW	WANT TO KNOW
5 g : 100 mL	= x g : 500 mL

$x = 5 \times 5 = 25$
$x = 25$ g or mL of dextrose

PROOF
$5 \times 500 = 2500$
$100 \times 25 = 2500$

KNOW	WANT TO KNOW
0.45 g : 100 mL	= x g : 500 mL

$x = 0.45 \times 5 = 2.25$
$x = 2.25$ g of sodium chloride

PROOF
$0.45 \times 500 = 225$
$100 \times 2.25 = 225$
Osmolarity: 406 Osmol/L
Tonicity: Hypertonic

3. KNOW   WANT TO KNOW
10 g : 100 mL = x g : 500 mL
x = 10 × 5 = 50
x = 50 g or mL of dextrose
PROOF
10 × 500 = 5000
100 × 50 = 5000
   KNOW   WANT TO KNOW
0.9 g : 100 mL = x g : 500 mL
x = 0.9 × 5
x = 4.5 g or mL of sodium chloride
PROOF
0.9 × 500 = 450
4.5 × 100 = 450
Osmolarity: 813 Osmol/L
Tonicity: Hypertonic

5. KNOW   WANT TO KNOW
0.45 g : 100 mL = x g : 500 mL
x = 0.45 × 5 = 2.25
x = 2.25 g or mL of sodium chloride
PROOF
0.45 × 500 = 225
100 × 2.25 = 225
Osmolarity: 154 mOsmol/L
Tonicity: Hypotonic

7. KNOW   WANT TO KNOW
600 mg : 100 mL = x mg : 1000 mL
x = 10 × 600 = 6000
x = 6000 mg of sodium chloride in 1000 mL
PROOF
600 × 1000 = 600,000
100 × 6000 = 600,000
   KNOW   WANT TO KNOW
1 g : 1000 mg = x g : 6000 mg
x = 6 × 1 = 6
x = 6 g of sodium chloride in 1000 mL
PROOF
1 × 6000 = 6000
6 × 1000 = 6000
Osmolarity: 273 Osmol/L
Tonicity: Isotonic

4. KNOW   WANT TO KNOW
0.9 g : 100 mL = x g : 1000 mL
x = 0.9 × 10 = 9
x = 9 g or mL of sodium chloride
PROOF
0.9 × 1000 = 900
9 × 100 = 900
Osmolarity: 308 Osmol/L
Tonicity: Isotonic

6. KNOW   WANT TO KNOW
5 g : 100 mL = x g : 500 mL
x = 5 × 5 = 25
x = 25 g or mL of dextrose
PROOF
100 × 25 = 2500
5 × 500 = 2500
Osmolarity: 525 Osmol/L
Tonicity: Hypertonic

8. KNOW   WANT TO KNOW
5 g : 100 mL = x g : 1000 mL
x = 5 × 10 = 50
x = 50 g or mL of dextrose
PROOF
5 × 1000 = 5000
100 × 50 = 5000
   KNOW   WANT TO KNOW
0.9 g : 100 mL = x g : 1000 mL
x = 0.9 × 10 = 9
x = 9 g or mL of sodium chloride
PROOF
100 × 9 = 900
0.9 × 1000 = 900
Osmolarity: 560 Osmol/L
Tonicity: Hypertonic

9. KNOW   WANT TO KNOW
5 g : 100 mL = x g : 500 mL
x = 5 × 5 = 25
x = 25 g or mL of dextrose
PROOF
5 × 500 = 2500
100 × 25 = 2500
KNOW   WANT TO KNOW
0.45 g : 100 mL = x g : 500 mL
x = 0.45 × 5 = 2.25
x = 2.25 g or mL of sodium chloride
PROOF
0.45 × 500 = 225
100 × 2.25 = 225
Osmolarity: 406 Osmol/L
Tonicity: Hypertonic

WORKSHEET 7E (page 248)

1. KNOW   WANT TO KNOW
5 g : 100 = x g : 125 mL
100x = 5 × 125 = 625
x = 6.25 g per hr
PROOF
5 × 125 = 625
100 × 6.25 = 625

2. $\dfrac{\text{Total volume}}{\text{Total time}}$ = mL per hr

$\dfrac{1500 \text{ mL}}{4 \text{ hr}}$ = 375 mL per hr

3. HAVE   WANT TO HAVE
500 mL : 4 hr = x mL : 1 hr
4x = 500 × 1 = 500
x = 125 mL per hr
PROOF
500 × 1 = 500
4 × 125 = 500

4. HAVE   WANT TO HAVE
1000 mL : 6 hr = x mL : 1 hr
6x = 1000
x = 166.6 = 167 mL per hr
PROOF
1000 × 1 = 1000
6 × 166.6 = 999

5. KNOW   WANT TO KNOW
125 mL : 1 hr = 1000 mL : x hr
125x = 1000
x = 8 hr
The IV will be completed by 1700 hours.
PROOF
1 × 1000 = 1000
125 × 8 = 1000

6. HAVE   WANT TO HAVE
30 mL : 1 hr = 250 mL : x hr
30x = 250
x = 8.33 hr
Convert 0.33 × 60 min = 19.8 = 20 min
The IV will take 8 hr and 20 min to infuse.
The IVPB was started at 1330 hr + 8 hr
20 min = 2150 for the hour of completion.
PROOF
1 × 250 = 250
8.33 × 30 = 249.9

7. $\dfrac{\text{Total volume}}{\text{Total time}}$ = mL per hr

$\dfrac{1000 \text{ mL}}{8 \text{ hr}}$ = 125 mL per hr

The IV was started at 0715 + 8 = 1515 for the hour of completion.

8. HAVE   WANT TO HAVE
40 mL : 1 hr = 500 mL : x hr
40x = 500
x = 12.5 hr
IV started at 2100 hr + 12.5 hr (12 hr
30 min) = 0930 for the hour of completion.
PROOF
1 × 500 = 500
40 × 12.5 = 500

Answer Key   **267**

9. HAVE　　　　　　WANT TO HAVE
200 mL : 3 hr = x mL : 1 hr
$3x = 200$
$x = 66.66 = 67$ mL per hr
OR

$\dfrac{\text{Total volume}}{\text{Total time}} =$ mL per hr

$\dfrac{200 \text{ mL}}{3 \text{ hr}} = 66.66 = 67$ mL per hr

PROOF
$200 \times 1 = 200$
$3 \times 66.66 = 199.98$

10. $\dfrac{\text{Total volume}}{\text{Total time}} =$ vol per hr

$\dfrac{500 \text{ mL}}{4 \text{ hr}} = 125$ mL per hr

WORKSHEET 7F (page 257)

1. KNOW　　　　　　WANT TO KNOW
100 mL : 60 min = x mL : 60 min
$60x = 6000$
$x = 100$ mL per hr
PROOF
$100 \times 60 = 6000$
$60 \times 100 = 6000$

2. KNOW　　　　　　WANT TO KNOW
150 mL : 60 min = 250 mL : x min
$150x = 250 \times 60 = 15{,}000$
$x = 100$ min = 1.6 hr = 1 hr 40 min
PROOF
$100 \times 150 = 15{,}000$
$250 \times 60 = 15{,}000$

3. a. $\dfrac{\cancel{60}^{2}}{\cancel{30}_{1}} \times 100 = 200$ drops per min

b. The infusion device will be set at 200 mL per hr.
　　KNOW　　　　　　WANT TO KNOW
100 mL : 30 min = x mL : 60 min
$30x = 100 \times 60 = 6000$
$30x = 6000$
$x = 200$ mL per hr

4. a. KNOW　　　　　　WANT TO KNOW
50 mL : 20 min = x mL : 60 min
$20x = 50 \times 60 = 3000$
$x = 150$ mL per hr
PROOF
$20 \times 150 = 3000$
$50 \times 60 = 3000$

b. $\dfrac{15}{20} \times \dfrac{50}{1} = \dfrac{\cancel{15}^{3}}{\cancel{20}_{4}} \times \dfrac{50}{1} = \dfrac{150}{4}$
$= 37.5$ or 38 drops per min

5. a. $\dfrac{15}{60} \times \dfrac{100}{1} = \dfrac{1}{4} \times \dfrac{100}{1} = \dfrac{100}{4} = 25$ drops per min

b. 100 mL : 60 min = x mL : 60 min
$60x = 100 \times 60 = 6000$
$60x = 6000$
$x = 100$ mL per hr
PROOF
$100 \times 60 = 6000$
$60 \times 100 = 6000$

6. a. KNOW　　　　　　WANT TO KNOW
50 mL : 30 min = x mL : 60 min
$30x = 50 \times 60 = 3000$
$x = 100$ mL per hr
PROOF
$30 \times 100 = 3000$
$50 \times 60 = 3000$

b. $\dfrac{60}{30} \times \dfrac{50}{1} = \dfrac{\cancel{60}^{2}}{\cancel{30}_{1}} \times \dfrac{50}{1} = 100$ drops per min

7. a. $\dfrac{\cancel{60}^{2}}{\cancel{90}_{3}} \times 200 = \dfrac{400}{3} = 133$ drops per min

   OR

   b. 200 mL : 90 min = x mL : 60 min
   90x = 200 × 60 = 12,000
   90x = 12,000
   x = 133 mL per hr
   Set infusion device for 133 mL per hr.

8. Step 1: $\dfrac{1000}{12} = 83.3$ or 83 mL per hr

   a. Step 2: $\dfrac{\cancel{15}^{1}}{\cancel{60}_{4}} \times 83 = \dfrac{83}{4}$

   = 20.8 or 21 drops per min

   b. The infusion device will be set at 83 mL per hr.

   KNOW   WANT TO KNOW

   c. 0.9 g : 100 mL = x g : 1000 mL
   x = 0.9 × 10 = 9
   x = 9 g of sodium chloride (solute)
   PROOF
   0.9 × 1000 = 900
   100 × 9 = 900

9. a. Step 1: $\dfrac{TV}{TT} = \dfrac{2000}{8} = 250$ mL per hr

   b. Step 2: $\dfrac{\cancel{15}^{1}}{\cancel{60}_{4}} \times 250 = \dfrac{250}{4}$

   = 62.5 or 63 drops per min

   KNOW   WANT TO KNOW

   c. 5 g : 100 mL = x g : 2000 mL
   x = 5 × 20 = 100
   x = 100 g of dextrose
   PROOF
   5 × 2000 = 10,000
   100 × 100 = 10,000

10. a. $\dfrac{\cancel{60}^{3}}{\cancel{40}_{2}} \times 150 = \dfrac{450}{2}$

    = 225 drops per min is the fastest rate. Set infusion device for 225 mL per hr using the microdrip formula.

    b. $\dfrac{60}{60} \times 150 = 150$ drops per min is the slowest rate. Set infusion device for 150 mL per hr using the microdrip formula.

WORKSHEET 7G (page 258)

1. a. KNOW   WANT TO KNOW
   25 drops : 1 min = 10 drops : x min
   25x = 10
   x = 0.4 min = 1 mL
   PROOF
   25 × 0.4 = 10
   1 × 10 = 10
   KNOW   WANT TO KNOW
   1 mL : 0.4 min = 1000 mL : x min
   x = 0.4 × 1000 = 400
   x = 400 min divided by 60
   = 6.66 hr = 6 hr 40 min

2. b. $\dfrac{15}{15} \times 50 = 50$ drops per min

3. d. $\dfrac{20 \text{ gtt}}{30 \text{ min}} \times 50 = \dfrac{100}{3} = 33$ drops per min

4. b. KNOW   WANT TO KNOW
300 mL : 6 hr = x mL : 1 hr
6x = 300 × 1 = 300
  x = 50 mL per hr. mL per hr and microdrip
     drops per min are the same, so
     50 drops per min is correct
PROOF
300 × 1 = 300
6 × 50 = 300
OR

$\dfrac{\overset{1}{\cancel{60}} \text{ gtt}}{\underset{6}{\cancel{360} \text{ min}}} \times 300 \text{ mL} = \dfrac{300}{6} = 50$ drops per min and 50 mL per hr

5. d. KNOW   WANT TO KNOW
12 mL : 1 hr = 150 mL : x hr
12x = 150
  x = 12.5 = 12 hr 30 min
PROOF
1 × 150 = 150
12.5 × 12 = 150

6. d. KNOW   WANT TO KNOW
30 drops : 1 min = 20 drops : x min
30x = 20
  x = 0.66 min
PROOF
1 × 20 = 20
30 × 0.66 = 20
KNOW   WANT TO KNOW
1 mL : 0.66 min = 500 mL : x min
x = 0.66 × 500 = 330
x = 330 min ÷ 60 = 5.5 hr = 5 hr 30 min
PROOF
1 × 330 = 330
0.66 × 500 = 330

7. a. KNOW   WANT TO KNOW
2500 mL : 24 hr = x mL : 1 hr
24x = 2500
  x = 104.16 mL per hr
PROOF
2500 × 1 = 2500
24 × 104.16 = 2500 = 104 mL per hr
KNOW   WANT TO KNOW
15 gtt : 1 mL = x gtt : 104.16 mL
OR
$\dfrac{15}{60} \times 104 = \dfrac{1560}{60} = 26$ drops per min
x = 15 × 104.16 = 1562
x = 1562 divided by 60 min = 26 drops per min
PROOF
15 × 104.16 = 1562
1 × 1562 = 1562

8. c. KNOW   WANT TO KNOW
42 gtt : 1 min = 10 drops : x min
42x = 1 × 10 = 10
  x = 0.238 = 0.24 min per mL
PROOF
1 × 10 = 10
42 × 0.24 = 10.08 = 10
KNOW   WANT TO KNOW
1 mL : 0.24 min = 500 mL : x min
x = 0.24 × 500 = 120
x = 120 min divided by 60 = 2 hr
PROOF
1 × 120 = 120
0.24 × 500 = 120
The transfusion was started at 1100 hours. The completion time will be 1300 hours.

9. c.   KNOW   WANT TO KNOW
30 mL : 1 hr = 500 mL : x hr
$30x = 500$
$x = 16.66$ hr = 16 hr 40 min
PROOF
$30 \times 16.6 = 499.8 = 500$
$1 \times 500 = 500$

10. d. $\dfrac{250}{2} = 125$ mL per hr

CHAPTER 7 FINAL: BASIC INTRAVENOUS THERAPY CALCULATIONS (page 261)

1. 42 drops per min or 167 mL per hr if infusion device is used

2. 125 mL per hr
    42 drops per min

3. 83 mL per hr
    28 drops per min

4. 150 drops per min

5. 83 mL per hr
    14 drops per min

6. 125 mL per hr
    31 drops per min

7. 100 mL per hr
    17 drops per min

8. Set infusion device at 267 mL per hr.

9. 83 drops per min

10. 31 drops per min

Advanced Intravenous Calculations

Objectives
- Calculate time and dose intervals for direct IV push (bolus) medications administered by a syringe.
- Calculate hourly drug dose and hourly flow rate for IV solutions.
- Calculate milligrams per kilogram and micrograms per kilogram per minute and per hour.
- Estimate and calculate infusion rates and drug doses using ratio and proportion.
- Evaluate existing infusions for correct flow rate and/or drug dose.
- Analyze IV medication errors using critical thinking.

Introduction

This chapter builds on the basic IV calculations taught in Chapter 7. The problems cover single-dose intravenous medication administration and weight-based intravenous dosing in mcg per minute and per hour in solutions using ratio and proportion. The difference between basic IV calculations and more complex calculations is that there are more questions to be answered and sequenced to arrive at correct drug dosing, flow rates, and safe technique. Pharmacy, flow-rate charts, and IV pump equipment provide flow rates, but the nurse must be able to independently calculate and verify that they reflect the provider's order and that they will be diluted with compatible solutions. IV errors do occur, and because the medication is delivered directly into circulation, errors are more serious. Many of the problems involve ISMP-identified high-alert medications. Many practice problems to simplify the math as well as clinically-relevant safety alerts are provided.

Vocabulary

Half-life ($t_{1/2}$): Amount of time for one half of a drug's concentration to be cleared from the plasma.

IV Flush: Injection of sterile normal saline for injection (preservative-free) into an existing vascular access device (VAD) to clear the line of existing medications or solutions that may be incompatible with subsequent products and to maintain patency of the device.*

---

*Always check compatibility of the medication to be administered with diluents, and any other IV medications the patient is receiving.

Peak and Trough Levels: IV measurement of levels of specific medications in the blood at *specific* time intervals to determine the highest (peak) and lowest (trough) levels of drug concentration in the blood so that adequate medication dosing and dosing intervals can be maintained in circulation.

SAS (Saline, Administer [medication], Saline): A flush of a *specified* amount of sterile normal saline for injection (preservative–free) in a vascular access device (VAD) before and after administration to prevent the mixture of the medication with prior or subsequent substances and/or maintain patency of the line.

SASH (Saline, Administer [medication], Saline, Heparin): A flush to maintain patency of a vascular access device with a very small amount of heparin and to prevent the mixture of heparin with any existing incompatible substances in the line.

Sepsis: A grave complication of an infection that spreads into circulation and affects all parts of the body.

Titration: The gradual adjustment of a drug dose to reach a *desired response,* such as lowering a blood pressure, raising a pulse, or easing respiratory difficulty. Intravenous medications are titrated by adjusting flow rate to increase or decrease a drug dose.

VAD (Vascular Access Device): An indwelling catheter, port, or other device in a vein or artery to give medications or monitor pressures.

Direct IV (Bolus) (IV Push)

IV push medications are used to administer small amounts of a medication in a single procedure to bring a drug level to a certain desired concentration. They may be prepared in relatively small amounts with a specific amount of compatible diluent to be administered over a specific limited amount of time. They often deliver more concentrated drug mixtures and are smaller volumes than IV infusions.

CLINICAL ALERT!

Whenever the word "concentrate" is seen on any medication label, look for dilution directions.

CLINICAL ALERT!

Before administering any IV medication, including bolus injections, the following checks *must* be made to avoid an adverse drug event:
- A comparison of the order with the supplied drug, dose, and solutions.
- Compatibility and interaction of the ordered drug with diluents, flushes, and with any other solutions with which the ordered drug may come in contact, for example, those infusing or recently infused in an existing line.
- Agency policies pertaining to flush volumes and safe syringe sizes for various sites and lines (see *Clinical Alert*).
- Recommended rates of flow—usually per minute—for the specific drug, dose, and purpose

Preservative-free solutions need to be used for intravenous flushes and bolus preparations. Because the appearance of the solutions is similar, check the labels carefully for the terms "preservative free" versus "bacteriostatic," which contains a preservative. Preferably the flush materials are single-use preparations to avoid the introduction of bacterial contaminants. If using multidose vials, check agency policy for discard dates—usually 24 hours—and examine for particulates and cloudiness before using. Multidose vials are needed for larger-volume diluents.

FIGURE 8-1 Hospira flush solutions. (From Hospira, Inc., Lake Forest, Ill.)

CLINICAL ALERT!

The words "direct" and "push" erroneously suggest push hard at a fast rate directly into a vein. Only a few emergency drugs are to be pushed very fast. Always check the recommended safe flow rate. Pushing any bolus injection (direct IV) (IV push) *hard and/or fast,* particularly against resistance, increases the chance of damaging the line, vein, or port and/or having the syringe disengage from the connection, causing medication loss. Pushing faster than recommended can result in serious adverse drug events (ADE).

Check a current, reliable IV drug reference and/or pharmacist for the recommended rate limits and dilutions for all IV medications (Figure 8-2). It is also recommended to administer boluses via a VAD if available so that countermeasures can be taken promptly if complications arise.

FIGURE 8-2 IV push. (From Potter PA, Perry AG, Stockert P, Hall A: *Fundamentals of nursing,* ed. 8, St. Louis, 2013, Mosby.)

CHAPTER 8 Advanced Intravenous Calculations

Boluses may be delivered with a syringe, a syringe pump, or a volume-control device, or they may be connected to an IV as a piggyback (Figures 8-3, 8-4, and 8-5).

FIGURE 8-3 Using watch time to time an IV push medication. **A,** IV catheter with saline lock adapter. **B,** Syringe inserted into injection port. (From Potter PA, Perry AG, Stockert P, Hall A: *Essentials for nursing practice*, ed. 8, St. Louis, 2014, Mosby.)

FIGURE 8-4 Syringe pump. (From Clayton BD, Willihnganz M: *Basic pharmacology for nurses*, ed. 16, St. Louis, 2013, Mosby.)

FIGURE 8-5 Volume-control device. **A,** Inject medication into device. **B,** Prepared dose. (From Potter PA, Perry AG, Stockert P, Hall A: *Essentials for nursing practice*, ed. 8, St. Louis, 2014, Mosby.)

⚑ CLINICAL ALERT!

There has been controversy about syringe size for bolus injections. A syringe with a wider barrel delivers less pressure and reduces the chance of damaging a vein or VAD. 10-mL syringes have been reported to cause less accurate doses and rates for small amounts because of their narrow calibrations. Smaller syringes deliver more accurate doses for small amounts because the calibrations are farther apart and easier to read, but they deliver more pressure because of their narrow diameter. Before selecting a syringe for IV bolus administrations, check agency policies and procedures.

⚑ CLINICAL ALERT!

Certain types of ports on central lines and most central lines require a wide-barreled 10-mL syringe.

To reduce needlestick injuries, the trend is to use infusion systems with safety features (Figure 8-6).

FIGURE 8-6 Shielded needle infusion system. Connection into an injection port. (From Perry AG, Potter PA: *Clinical nursing skills and techniques,* ed 8, St Louis, 2014, Mosby.)

There are two ways to time IV push medications for direct administration of medication through a syringe. Regardless of the method you select, the first step is always to calculate and prepare the correct volume.

Timing IV Push Medications: Method 1 (mL per Minute)

This method calculates the amount in milliliters to be slowly and gradually pushed over each minute.

Formula TV : TM = x mL : 1 minute $\left(\dfrac{TV}{TM} = \dfrac{XV}{1 \text{ Minute}} \right)$
Total volume : Total minutes = x volume (mL) : 1 minute

Example Ordered: Digoxin 0.5 mg IV over 5 min. Dilute to 4 mL with sterile water for injection.
TV : TM = x mL : 1 minute $\left(\dfrac{4}{5} = \dfrac{x}{1} \right)$
4 mL : 5 min = mL : 1 minute

$\dfrac{\cancel{5}}{\cancel{5}} x = \dfrac{4}{5}$

$x = 0.8$ mL to be pushed slowly each minute

PROOF 4 × 1 = 4
5 × 0.8 = 4

Schedule
1600 : 00   4 mL in syringe
1601   3.2 mL remaining
1602   2.4 mL remaining
1603   1.6 mL remaining
1604   0.8 mL remaining
1605   0 remaining

Time/mL
Remaining
- 1604/0.8 — 1
- 1603/1.6 — 2
- 1602/2.4 — 3
- 1601/3.2
Start 1600/4 — 4
5, 6, 7, 8, 9, 10 mL

The schedule above reflects a start time of 1600 hours. It is helpful to write your start time and a schedule of "markers" (increments of time and volume) when you need to push over several minutes. Write this before beginning to inject and have it in front of you to avoid errors caused by distraction.

Timing IV Push Medications: Method 2 (Seconds per Calibration)

Many IV push medications have dilutions that permit 1 mL per minute so that the timing is easy to maintain. Occasionally, when the timing is to be very slow and is not 1 mL per minute, counting seconds per calibration permits more precise timing of the injection.

RULE Divide the number of seconds of total time of administration by the number of calibrated increments in a syringe prepared with medication (lines on the syringe within each milliliter). This will yield the seconds per increment to be pushed.

Formula $\dfrac{\text{Total seconds}}{\text{Total increments}} = $ Seconds to deliver each increment

Example Give 0.5 mg digoxin IV over 5 min. Directions say to dilute to 4 mL with sterile water for injection. There are 20 calibrations in 4 mL on this syringe.

$$\frac{300 \text{ seconds}}{20 \text{ calibrations } (0.2 \text{ mL ea})} = 1 \text{ calibration } (0.2 \text{ mL}) \text{ every 15 seconds}$$

PROOF 300 × 1 = 300
15 × 20 = 300

Use the second hand on your watch and/or count each cycle (1 to 15) as you administer the medication, 1 calibration (0.2 mL) every 15 seconds.
Tip: start count when the second hand is on 12.

4 mL occupies
20 calibrated lines
5 minutes = 300 seconds

Answers on page 299

WORKSHEET 8A | IV Push Calculations

Solve the following problems using the syringes shown to calculate the seconds per calibration, if applicable, and mL/min to be administered.

1. Ordered: 10% calcium chloride (5 mL) over 5 min for a patient with hypocalcemia.
   a. For how many seconds will you administer each calibration?
   b. How many mL/min will be injected?

2. Ordered: Digoxin 0.5 mg IV over 10 min for a patient with heart failure. (The literature specifies a minimum of 5 min for administration.) Available: Digoxin 250 mcg per mL.
   a. Total mL you will inject:
   b. Total minutes for injection:
   c. mL per min to be injected:
   d. minutes per calibration:

3. Ordered: Phenytoin sodium IV loading dose of 900 mg at 50 mg per min on an infusion device for a patient with seizures (Figure 8-7). Available: Phenytoin 100 mg per mL.
   a. Total mL to be injected:
   b. Total time for injection:
   c. mL per min to be administered:

FIGURE 8-7 Freedom 60 infusion syringe pump. This portable reusable manual infusion uses standard 60 mL syringes and can be filled from 1 to 60 mL. It offers flow rates with rate-controlled tubing from 0.5 to 1200 mL per hr. It does not permit free flow. (From Repro-Med Systems, Inc., Chester, NY.)

4. Ordered: Furosemide 20 mg IV undiluted over 2 min for a patient with fluid retention. Available: Furosemide 10 mg per mL.
   a. Total mL to be injected:
   b. Total time in seconds:
   c. Seconds per calibration:
   d. mL per min to be administered:

5. Ordered: Morphine sulfate 4 mg IV injection for a patient with severe pain. The literature states that a single dose should be administered over 4 to 5 min and that the dose may be diluted in 4 to 5 mL with sterile water or normal saline for injection. The nurse dilutes it to 5 mL with NS.
   a. Total mL to be injected:
   b. Total time in minutes:
   c. mL per min to be administered:

Calculating Intravenous Medicated Infusion Flow Rates and Drug Rates From the Order and Total Volume and Total Drug Supplied

Nursing responsibilities include independent calculation of flow rates of medication solutions in mg, mcg, g, or units per hour, and/or per minute and/or per kg of weight, depending on the prescriber order and the supplied solution and medication. Once the hourly volume and drug rates are known, variations such as the rate per minute and per kg are derived with simple arithmetic.

Steps for Calculating Hourly Volume Rate or Hourly Drug Rate

The first steps are always the same:
1. After checking the complete order with the supplied drug amount and solution volume, identify the on-hand total drug (TD) : total volume (TV) ratio (e.g., 250 mg : 1000 mL).
2. Reduce the ratio to lowest terms and place this on the *left* side of the equation (What you have) as in previous ratio and proportion problems.

Example

$$TD : TV = \left(\frac{250}{1000}\right)$$

250 mg : 1000 mL

TD : TV (Reduced ratio)
1 mg : 4 mL =

3. Place the hourly drug (HD) ordered or volume per hr (HV) on the right side of the equation, estimate the unknown (*x*) quantity, and solve the equation.

Check your answer with the estimate. Reducing the TD : TV ratio makes it easy to estimate a correct answer.

Example Hourly Drug and Flow Rate Formula for Medicated Infusions

HAVE		WANT TO HAVE	FRACTION CROSS PRODUCT
TD : TV	=	HD : HV	$\left(\dfrac{TD}{TV} = \dfrac{HD}{HV}\right)$
Total drug : Total volume	=	Hourly drug : Hourly volume	

$\underbrace{\text{Total drug : Total volume}}_{\text{in Lowest reduced ratio}}$ $\underbrace{\text{Hourly drug : Hourly volume}}_{\substack{\text{One of these will be } x. \\ \text{One of these will be known.}}}$

Example Ordered: A drug to infuse at 20 mg per hr IV
Available: An IV solution of 400 mg of a drug in 500 mL

Calculate an hourly flow rate (HV) after reducing the total drug/total volume ratio to lowest terms.

HAVE   WANT TO HAVE
TD : TV   =   HD : HV
400 mg : 500 mL = 20 mg : x mL $\left(\dfrac{4}{5} = \dfrac{20}{x}\right) \rightarrow$ Make an estimate of x.
    4 : 5   =   20 : x
    x = 25 mL per hr

Set the flow rate on the IV infusion device to 25 mL/hr.

Example Existing IV infusing at 25 mL per hr

Calculate the hourly drug amount (HD) being infused.*

HAVE   WANT TO HAVE
TD : TV = HD : HV
400 mg : 500 mL = x mg : 25 mL $\left(\dfrac{4}{5} = \dfrac{x}{25}\right) \rightarrow$ Make an estimate of x.
(reduced ratio) 4 : 5 = x : 25
5x = 100 x = 20 mg per hr of drug being infused

remember When three quantities are known, the fourth can be obtained. The supply and the order provide three of the four quantities for the equation just as they did for basic calculations. The brief worksheets that follow provide stepped practice to increase your understanding and to help you master the calculations.

Answers on page 299

WORKSHEET 8B — Medicated IV Calculations

1. Reduce the **T**otal **D**rug/**T**otal **V**olume ratio to lowest terms as shown in example 1a.

TD : TV	Lowest Ratio
a. 250 mg : 1000 mL	1 : 4 $\left(\dfrac{1}{4}\right)$
b. 500 mg : 500 mL	_____
c. 100 mg : 1000 mL	_____
d. 250 mg : 500 mL	_____
e. 500 mg : 1000 mL	_____

RULE To find the mL per hr for the order, reduce the ratio of total drug to total volume. Enter the known ordered mg per hour (HD). Enter x mL (HV) for the unknown. TD : TV = HD : x HV. Estimate the mL per hr.

---

*This can be evaluated at the bedside to verify that it matches the order.

2. Estimate the value of x (hourly volume) after reducing the ratio of total drug to total volume. The ratio of hourly drug to hourly volume will be the same as total drug to total volume.

        TD : TV = HD : HV   ANSWER

Example
- a. 250 mg : 1000 mL = 10 mg : x mL   1 : 4 = 10 : <u>40</u> mL per hr $\left(\dfrac{1}{4} = \dfrac{10}{40}\right)$
- b. 500 mg : 500 mL = 30 mg : x mL   _____ mL per hr
- c. 100 mg : 1000 mL = 5 mg : x mL   _____ mL per hr
- d. 250 mg : 500 mL = 3 mg : x mL   _____ mL per hr
- e. 500 mg : 250 mL = 10 mg : x mL   _____ mL per hr

RULE   To find the drug per hour being delivered in an existing infusion: Enter the existing IV solution concentration flow rate. Enter x for the drug per hr. Enter the existing flow rate to see if the rate is delivering the correct ordered amount of drug per hr.

Note: x will either be the ordered drug rate or the flow rate. (TD : TV : x HD : HV)

3. Estimate the hourly drug (x).

        TD : TV = HD : HV   ANSWER

Example
- a. 250 mg : 250 mL = x mg : 20 mL   1 : 1 = <u>20</u> : 20 <u>20</u> mg per hr $\left(\dfrac{250}{250} = \dfrac{x}{20}\right)$
- b. 1000 mg : 500 mL = x mg : 6 mL   _____ mg per hr
- c. 250 mg : 500 mL = x mg : 18 mL   _____ mg per hr
- d. 400 mg : 1000 mL = x mg : 10 mL   _____ mg per hr
- e. 500 mg : 250 mL = x mg : 18 mL   _____ mg per hr

4. Calculate the IV drug order per hour based on the patient kg weight.

- a. 2 mcg per kg per hr   Wt 60 kg   2 mcg × 60 kg = 120 mcg per hr
- b. 10 mg per kg per hr   Wt 110 lb   _____
- c. 0.5 mcg per kg per hr   Wt 120 lb   _____
- d. 1.5 mg per kg per hr   Wt 68 kg   _____
- e. 6 mcg per kg per hr   Wt 60 kg   _____

5. Change micrograms to milligrams by moving the decimal three places to the left. Reduce the total drug/total volume ratio to the lowest terms. Finally, estimate the hourly volume. (The hourly drug must always be calculated in the same terms as the total drug.)

        TD : TV = HD : HV   ANSWER

Example
- a. 250 mg : 1000 mL = (4000 mcg) <u>4</u> mg : x mL   1 : 4 = 4 : <u>16</u> mL per hr
- b. 500 mg : 500 mL = (9000 mcg) __ mg : x mL   _____ mL per hr
- c. 1000 mg : 500 mL = (20,000 mcg) __ mg : x mL   _____ mL per hr
- d. 250 mg : 500 mL = (15,000 mcg) __ mg : x mL   _____ mL per hr
- e. 400 mg : 250 mL = (8000 mcg) __ mg : x mL   _____ mL per hr

Calculations for Various Types of IV Medication Orders

Once you understand the ratio of total drug to total volume and dose order per hour, variations on the calculations involve only metric conversions and basic arithmetic—multiplication or division. Medication orders based on weight are common and must be in terms of kg.

Medication orders based on mcg need to be changed to mg if the total drug available in the IV solution (Total Volume, or TV) is based in mg.

WORKSHEET 8C: Equivalent Measurements for IV Medication Orders and Existing Infusions

Use a calculator where needed to solve the problems. Always enter calculator data twice for verification. Examine the relationships between minute and hour, and mg and mcg.

Formulas: 1000 mcg = 1 mg   60 minutes = 1 hr   1000 milliunits = 1 Unit   Patient wt: 80 kg

1. Ordered: 2 mg per minute. How many mcg per minute are ordered? mg per hr ordered?

2. Ordered: 300 mcg per minute. How many mg per minute would be needed? mg per hr?

3. Ordered: 0.2 mg per kg per minute. How many mg per minute would be needed? mg per hr?

4. Ordered: 5 mcg per kg per minute. How many mg per minute would be needed? mg per hr?

5. Ordered: 600 milliunits per hr. How many milliunits per minute?

6. *Infusing: 0.1 mg per hour. How many mcg are flowing per hr?

7. Infusing: 10 mg per hr. How many mg per minute are infusing?

8. Infusing: 100 mg per hr. How many mg per kg per hr are infusing?

9. Infusing: 2.5 mg per hr. How many mcg per minute are infusing?

10. Infusing: 3 units per hr. How many milliunits per minute are infusing?

*Note: Distinguish the need to multiply and the need to divide.

WORKSHEET 8D: IV Drug/Flow Rates

Tip: Being able to convert drug, weight, time, and volume parameters within the metric system with ease facilitates advanced IV calculations.

1. Fill in the table by using a calculator and/or by moving decimals.

	mg per hr	mcg per hr	mg per min	mcg per min
Example a.	0.050.	50	0.050 ÷ 60 = 0.0008	0.8
b.			0.4	
c.	30			
d.				20
e.	7.5			

2. Fill in the table using a calculator.

	kg	mg per hr	mg per kg per min	mcg per kg per min
a.	85	25	25 ÷ 85 ÷ 60 = 0.005	5
b.	70		10	
c.	62			0.1
d.	55	75		
e.	48			50

3. Fill in the table for these IV drug/flow rate calculations using the TD : TV = HD : HV formula.

IV Contents	TD : TV Reduced Ratio	HD (mg per hr)	HV (mL per hr)	mg per mL
a. 500 mg per 1000 mL	1 : 2	5	10	500 ÷ 1000 = 0.5
b. 250 mg per 500 mL			30	
c. 400 mg per 250 mL		24		
d. 500 mg per 500 mL			75	
e. 500 mg per 250 mL		16		

CLINICAL ALERT!

Remember that the difference between a microgram (mcg) and a milligram (mg) is "× 1000." The difference between drug per minute and hourly drug is "× 60."

The difference between mcg per kg per minute and mcg per minute is based on "the weight in kilograms." Manipulating these differences is critical for safe medication administration.

Answers on page 301

WORKSHEET 8E | Medication Doses Infusing in Existing Solutions

It is often necessary to verify the amount of drug being delivered in an existing solution. The amount of drug in the IV solution is frequently a milligram dose, whereas the amount of drug the patient is receiving is a microgram dose or a microgram per kilogram dose.

Note the example in Problem 1 and do the following in the remaining problems:
- Set up the ratios and determine mg per hr. Prove your answer.
- Move decimals to change milligrams to micrograms (× 1000).
- Use a calculator to change hourly drug (HD) to drug per minute (divide by 60).
- Use a calculator to determine kilograms, and divide micrograms by kilogram weight to obtain mcg per kg per minute. Enter all calculator data *twice* for verification.

Example

1. An IV drug 100 mg in 1000 mL is infusing at 20 mL per hr. The physician asks, "How many *mg per hr* is the patient receiving? How many *mcg per minute*? How many *mcg per kg per minute*? The patient weighs 143 lb today.
   a. TD : TV reduced ratio: 100 : 1000 = 1 : 10 $\left(\frac{100}{1000} = \frac{1}{10}\right)$
   b. TD : TV = HD : HV 1 mg : 10 mL = 2 mg : 20 mL
   c. mg per hour infusing: 2 mg per hr
   d. mcg per hour infusing: 2 × 1000 = 2000 mcg per hr
   e. mcg per minute infusing: 2000 ÷ 60 = 33.3 mcg per minute
   f. mcg per kg per minute infusing: 33.3 ÷ 65 kg = 0.5 mcg per kg per minute

   PROOF 1 × 20 = 20
   10 × 2 = 20

2. An IV drug 250 mg in 500 mL is infusing at 15 mL per hr. The patient weighs 110 lb today.
   a. TD : TV = HD : HV reduced ratio:
   b. mcg per hour infusing:
   c. mcg per minute infusing:
   d. mcg per kg per minute infusing:

   PROOF

3. An IV drug 400 mg in 1000 mL is infusing at 5 mL per hr. The patient weighs 121 lb today.
   a. TD : TV = HD : HV reduced ratio:
   b. mcg per hour infusing:
   c. mcg per minute infusing:
   d. mcg per kg per minute infusing:

   PROOF

4. An IV drug 1000 mg in 250 mL is infusing at 10 mL per hr. The patient weighs 132 lb today.
   a. TD : TV = HD : HV reduced ratio:
   b. mcg per hour infusing:
   c. mcg per minute infusing:
   d. mcg per kg per minute infusing:

   PROOF

5. An IV drug 500 mg in 250 mL is infusing at 8 mL per hr. The patient weighs 175 lb today. (Calculate kilograms to nearest tenth.)
   a. TD : TV = HD : HV reduced ratio:
   b. mcg per hr infusing:
   c. mcg per minute infusing:
   d. mcg per kg per minute infusing:

   PROOF

High-Tech Infusion Devices

A variety of sophisticated infusion pump devices have been developed to reduce IV medication errors. Known as "smart pumps," they may have capability to be connected to several different IV solutions and a mixture of IVs, syringes, and syringe pumps. Very small doses can be programmed in mcg per kg per minute up to very large doses in mL per hour (Figure 8-8). Flushes can be programmed, as can intermittent infusions. Alarms are programmed to warn of an overdose *(soft alert)* or to block the dose *(hard alert)*.

FIGURE 8-8 Sigma Spectrum Infusion Smart Pump has a master drug library that helps minimize the risk of pump-related programming medication errors. (From Mulholland J, Turner S: *The nurse, the math, the meds: Drug calculations using dimensional analysis,* ed. 3, St. Louis, 2015, Mosby.)

CLINICAL ALERT!

Most ISMP-identified high-alert medications must be administered on infusion pumps (Table 8-1). Check agency policies.

Table 8-1 ISMP's List of *High-Alert* Medications

Institute for Safe Medication Practices

ISMP's List of *High-Alert* Medications

High-alert medications are drugs that bear a heightened risk of causing significant patient harm when they are used in error. Although mistakes may or may not be more common with these drugs, the consequences of an error are clearly more devastating to patients. We hope you will use this list to determine which medications require special safeguards to reduce the risk of errors. This may include strategies like improving access to information about these drugs; limiting access to high-alert medications; using auxiliary labels and automated alerts; standardizing the ordering, storage, preparation, and administration of these products; and employing redundancies such as automated or independent double-checks when necessary. (Note: manual independent double-checks are not always the optimal error-reduction strategy and may not be practical for all of the medications on the list).

Classes/Categories of Medications
adrenergic agonists, IV (e.g., epinephrine, phenylephrine, norepinephrine)
adrenergic antagonists, IV (e.g., propranolol, metoprolol, labetalol)
anesthetic agents, general, inhaled and IV (e.g., propofol, ketamine)
antiarrhythmics, IV (e.g., lidocaine, amiodarone)
antithrombotic agents (anticoagulants), including warfarin, low-molecular-weight heparin, IV unfractionated heparin, Factor Xa inhibitors (fondaparinux), direct thrombin inhibitors (e.g., argatroban, lepirudin, bivalirudin), thrombolytics (e.g., alteplase, reteplase, tenecteplase), and glycoprotein IIb/IIIa inhibitors (e.g., eptifibatide)
cardioplegic solutions
chemotherapeutic agents, parenteral and oral
dextrose, hypertonic, 20% or greater
dialysis solutions, peritoneal and hemodialysis
epidural or intrathecal medications
hypoglycemics, oral
inotropic medications, IV (e.g., digoxin, milrinone)
liposomal forms of drugs (e.g., liposomal amphotericin B)
moderate sedation agents, IV (e.g., midazolam)
moderate sedation agents, oral, for children (e.g., chloral hydrate)
narcotics/opiates, IV, transdermal, and oral (including liquid concentrates, immediate and sustained-release formulations)
neuromuscular blocking agents (e.g., succinylcholine, rocuronium, vecuronium)
radiocontrast agents, IV
total parenteral nutrition solutions

Specific Medications
epoprostenol (Flolan), IV
insulin, subcutaneous and IV
magnesium sulfate injection
methotrexate, oral, non-oncologic use
opium tincture
oxytocin, IV
nitroprusside sodium for injection
potassium chloride for injection concentrate
potassium phosphates injection
promethazine, IV
sodium chloride for injection, hypertonic (greater than 0.9% concentration)
sterile water for injection, inhalation, and irrigation (excluding pour bottles) in containers of 100 mL or more

Background

Based on error reports submitted to the USP-ISMP Medication Errors Reporting Program, reports of harmful errors in the literature, and input from practitioners and safety experts, ISMP created and periodically updates a list of potential high-alert medications. During February-April 2007, 770 practitioners responded to an ISMP survey designed to identify which medications were most frequently considered high-alert drugs by individuals and organizations. Further, to assure relevance and completeness, the clinical staff at ISMP, members of our advisory board, and safety experts throughout the US were asked to review the potential list. This list of drugs and drug categories reflects the collective thinking of all who provided input.

© ISMP 2008

➔ CLINICAL ALERT!

It has been recommended that all high-alert drug calculations and preparations be double-checked independently by a second, licensed person.

© ISMP 2008. Permission is granted to reproduce material for internal newsletters or communications with proper attribution. Other reproduction is prohibited without written permission. Unless noted, reports were received through the USP-ISMP Medication Errors Reporting Program (MERP). Report actual and potential medication errors to the MERP via the web at www.ismp.org or by calling 1-800-FAIL-SAF(E). ISMP guarantees confidentiality of information received and respects reporters' wishes as to the level of detail included in publications.

Institute for Safe Medication Practices
www.ismp.org

Hospital pharmacies often manage the multiple sources of preprogrammed software information, including drug libraries and types of safe dose parameters of specific medications for specific target populations. These parameters include doses based on age, weight, diagnosis, and other variables, with alerts if the data entered exceed the safe dose limits for the target population. Some smart pumps will alert if the same drug is being infused on another line. All infusions administered and alerts are logged to permit audits as needed.

CLINICAL ALERT!

Although these pumps can reduce errors, the nurse cannot be overly reliant on infusion alerts. The alerts depend upon the accuracy and scope of preprogrammed information as well as the function of the pump. Also, errors have been reported due to overrides of soft alerts. *Carefully research soft alerts and consult with pharmacy before overriding.

CLINICAL ALERT!

When entering data on an electronic IV device (EID), beware of decimal errors and of substituting mcg for mg or vice versa. Lack of familiarity with equipment function or equipment malfunction can cause medication errors. The nurse needs to confirm all the data with the order before initiating the flow of the drug and to ask for help if there is any question about the medication or the equipment.

CLINICAL ALERT!

Never override an IV alarm without rechecking the order. Consult a supervisor, pharmacist, or the prescriber before changing a program.

---

*The QSEN Institute (Quality and Safety Education for Nurses) Patient Goal No. 4 is: "Use Alarms Safely." www.jointcommission.org

Answers on page 301

WORKSHEET 8F | Advanced IV Flow Rate and Dose Evaluation

Perform the requested calculations. Use a calculator for long division or multiplication. Evaluate flow rates. Refer to ISMP's List of High-Alert Medications.

Example 1. Nitroprusside sodium infusion is ordered at 0.3 mcg per kg per minute IV and is being infused on a patient with hypertension in a pharmacy-prepared solution of 50 mg in 500 mL of D5W. Pharmacy directions instruct to set a flow rate of 12.6 mL an hr for this patient and administer on an IV pump. The patient's weight is 70 kg.

   a. Hourly drug order in mcg: a. $0.3 \times 70 \times 60 = 1269$ mcg per hr
   b. Hourly drug order in mg: b. 1.26 mg per hr (decimal moved 3 places to left)
   c. TD : TV reduced ratio: c. 1:10 (50:500)
   d. Hourly flow rate ordered to nearest tenth of a mL: d. 12.6 mL per hr (1 mg:10 mL=1.26 mg:12.6 mL per hr)
   e. Is the pharmacy direction correct? e. Yes

2. Azithromycin 500 mg IV is ordered for a patient with pelvic inflammatory disease. Directions state that each 500 mg vial must be reconstituted first with 4.8 mL SW to give 100 mg per mL. Further dilute each 500 mg to 250 mL with D5W or other compatible solutions. Give over 1 hr. The nurse you are replacing on shift has set the flow at 500 mL per hour.
   a. Mg per mL final dilution:
   b. Is flow rate correct?
   c. If not, what should it be?

3. Cefepime HCl 1 g is ordered IV q12h for a patient with severe pneumonia. Supplied is an ADD Vantage vial. 1 g vial to be diluted to 50 mL with NS in an ADD Vantage infusion container. Dose concentrations between 1 mg per mL and 40 mg per mL are acceptable. Current IV drug reference text for intermittent infusions states, "Infuse over 30 minutes."
   a. Mg per mL concentration after dilution:
   b. Is the concentration safe to administer?
   c. Flow rate to administer over 30 minutes:

4. Pantroprazole sodium 40 mg IV infusion once daily for 10 days is ordered for a patient with severe gastroesophageal reflux disease (GERD). A 40-mg dose is reconstituted first with 10 mL NS and further diluted to total volume of 100 mL with D5W and infused over at least 15 minutes, per label instructions. The IV is programmed when you come on duty for 6.7 mL per minute on a pump.
   a. Mg per mL after first dilution:
   b. Mg per mL after final dilution:
   c. Is the IV program approximately correct?
   d. IV flow rate per hr (to the nearest tenth of a mL):

5. Cytoxan* 5 mg per kg IV two times a week is ordered for an adult patient with malignant disease. The patient's weight is 50 kg. The pharmacy has sent a diluted solution of 250 mg in 250 mL NS. This order is to infuse over 90 minutes. When you arrive on duty, the IV is infusing at 100 mL per hr.
   a. Drug order in mg:
   b. TD : TV reduced ratio:
   c. Hr equivalent of 90 min:
   d. Flow rate on pump in tenth of a mL per hr:
   e. Is current infusion rate correct?

   *Nurses need certification to administer this drug.

CLINICAL ALERT!

Patient Safety Issue: Each nurse needs to refer to manufacturer instructions, current drug references, and personal calculations to protect the patient from prescriber, pharmacy, and prior caretaker IV drug dose errors and/or flow rate errors and ADE or sentinel events.

Beware of programming and mechanical errors with IV pumps.

Answers on page 302

WORKSHEET 8G | Critical Care IV Practice

Evaluate the following orders and infusions for safety. Use a calculator to determine kilogram weights to the nearest tenth. Change micrograms to milligrams, when applicable, by moving decimals. Use a calculator to determine the Safe Dose Range (SDR) when needed. Double-check and label all calculations. Prove the hourly flow-rate calculation. If requested, decide whether the order/infusion is:

1. Safe/Correct

2. Unsafe/Incorrect. Consult with physician.

Example 1. Ordered: Dopamine HCl (Intropin) 4 mcg per kg per minute IV for a 110-lb patient with hypotension. The literature states that the usual dose is 2 to 5 mcg per kg per min. Available: Dopamine 200 mg in 250 mL D5W.

    a. Patient's weight in kg: 110 ÷ 2.2 = 50

    b. SDR per minute: 100 – 250 mcg per minute
                                (2 mcg × 50 kg : 5 mcg × 50 kg)

    c. Is the order safe?   Yes. 4 mcg × 50 = 200 mcg per minute.
                                200 mcg per minute is within the SDR

    d. Hourly drug order in mcg: 12,000 (200 mcg × 60 minute)

    e. Hourly drug order in mg*:   12 (decimal moved 3 places to left)

    f. TD : TV reduced ratio: 4 : 5 (200 mg : 250 mL)

    g. Hourly flow rate to be set on infusion device: 15 mL per hr (4 : 5 : 12 : x)
                                4x = 60
                                x = 15 mL per hr

PROOF   4 × 15 = 60
              5 × 12 = 60

2. Ordered: Dobutamine HCl (Dobutrex) 5 mcg per kg per minute IV for a 132-lb patient in cardiogenic shock. Available: Dobutamine 250 mg in 250 mL D5W. The flow rate is currently infusing at 36 mL per hr.

    a. Patient's weight in kg:
    b. Hourly drug order in mcg:
    c. Hourly drug order in mg*:
    d. TD : TV reduced ratio:
    e. Hourly flow rate to be set on infusion device:
    f. Is current infusion correct?
    g. Evaluation and decision:

PROOF

3. Ordered: Lidocaine 4 mg per minute to treat a patient with ventricular tachycardia. Available: 1 g of lidocaine in 500 mL of D5W.

    a. TD : TV reduced ratio (mg : mL):
    b. Hourly drug ordered:
    c. Hourly flow rate to be set on infusion device:

PROOF

4. Ordered: Isuprel (isoproterenol hydrochloride) 5 mcg per minute to treat a patient in shock. Available: Isoproterenol hydrochloride 1 mg in 250 mL D5W.

    a. TD : TV reduced ratio:
    b. Hourly drug ordered in mcg and in mg:
    c. TD : TV = HD : HV ratio:
    d. Hourly flow rate to be set on infusion device:

PROOF

*Because the available drug (250 mg) is in mg, the hourly drug order must also be entered in mg.

290   Drug Calculations: *Ratio and Proportion Problems for Clinical Practice*

5. Conversion: 1000 milliunits = 1 unit
Ordered: Initial dose: oxytocin, a uterine stimulant, 1 milliunit per minute to induce uterine contractions for a patient in labor. On hand: IV of 10 units of oxytocin in 1000 mL D5W. *Titrate* in 30 minutes by additional 1 milliunit per minute until there are two contractions every 10 minutes. Then call for orders and gradually decrease rate. Monitor fetal heart rate and uterine contractions continuously.
   a. How many total milliunits of oxytocin are in the IV?
   b. How many mL in the IV?
   c. How many milliunits per mL?
   d. What is ordered dose in milliunits per hr now that the terms are the same?
   e. Flow rate in mL per hr on the pump?

   The patient in Problem 1 needed to have the dose increased 30 minutes later:
   f. What would the new dose be in milliunits per minute?
   g. How many ordered milliunits per hr needed to infuse?
   h. How many mL per hr should be set on the pump?

CLINICAL ALERT!
Document IVs carefully according to hospital policies. Consult the prescriber if the flow rate needs adjustment.

CLINICAL RELEVANCE
Titration orders do not require new methods of calculation. To get the desired response, the ordered dose starts low and the dose is gradually increased or lowered in a series of similar equations.

Example Initial: 0.1 mg per minute. Titrate every 15 minutes by additional 0.1 mg per minute until systolic BP is less than 160. Solution 10 mg in IV 5% DW 250 mL.

The total volume (TV) and the total drug supplied (TD) stay the same. A changed titrated drug order based on patient response is recalculated for a changed hourly dose (HD), which sets up the equation for the new hourly flow rate (HV). If the titrated dose is increased, the HV should increase. If the dose is decreased, the HV should decrease.

Note: If the blood pressure requires another dose, the only *entry* that needs to be recalculated is the hourly drug (HD), based on the increased new dose to be given.

CLINICAL ALERT!
If the supplied medicated IV solution is changed, the entire equation changes and must be recalculated. Assessment for expected responses, potential known side effects, and complications of the varying doses must be done frequently.

Answers on page 303

WORKSHEET 8H — IV Calculations for Obstetrics

Calculate and evaluate the following orders. Remember that the terms must be the same in your TD : TV = HD : HV ratio and proportion.

Example 1. Ordered: Magnesium sulfate 2 g to be infused over 60 minutes for a patient with eclampsia infusion IV. Available: Magnesium sulfate 4 g per 250 mL Ringer's lactate solution on an infusion device infusing at 125 mL per hr.
   a. TD : TV = HD : HV   4 g : 250 mL = 2 g : x mL $\left(\dfrac{4}{250} = \dfrac{2}{x}\right)$
   b. mL per hr ordered (HV):   4x = 500, x = 125 mL per hr
   c. mL per hr infusing: 125 mL per hr
   d. Evaluation and decision: Rate is correct.

   PROOF 4 × 125 = 500
              250 × 2 = 500

2. Ordered: Pitocin (oxytocin) 10 milliunits per minute to induce labor in a full-term pregnant female. Available: 1000 mL D5NS with 1 unit of Pitocin (1000 milliunits = 1 unit). The IV is infusing at 100 mL per hr. (Hint: Change units to milliunits to obtain the total drug equivalent for the equation.)
   a. TD : TV reduced ratio:
   b. TD (milliunits) : TV = HD (milliunits) : HV ordered:
   c. Evaluation and decision:

   PROOF

3. Ordered: Stadol (butorphanol tartrate) 1 mg slow IV push to reduce pain in a patient with a full-term pregnancy in early labor. Available is a Stadol ampule 2 mg per mL. Directions state to deliver the medication over 3 to 5 minutes. It may be repeated every 4 hours prn pain but *not* within 4 hours of anticipated delivery. To give it slowly, the nurse adds 3.5 mL of sterile 0.9% NaCl solution preservative free in a 5- or 10-mL syringe and plans to deliver it in a vascular access device over 4 minutes. Monitor mental status, BP, and respirations.

```
1 mL                       NDC 0409-1626-01
Single-dose  Rx only       Usual dosage:
                           See insert.
BUTORPHANOL                Store at 20 to
TARTRATE Inj., USP         25°C (68 to
                           77°F).
 2 mg   (2 mg/mL)          Hospira
For I.M. or I.V. use       RL-0547 (9/16)
HOSPIRA, INC., LAKE FOREST, IL 60045 USA
```

   a. How many total mL will there be in the syringe?
   b. At how many mL per minute will the medication be administered?
   c. How many seconds per calibration should the nurse count in order to push each mL at a fairly even rate?

   Note: It is difficult to give 1 mL evenly over 1 minute. It is better to count the seconds for each calibration.

4. Ordered: Magnesium sulfate 25 mL per hr for a patient with eclampsia. Call the doctor when 2 g have been infused. Available: 500 mL D5W with 20 g of magnesium sulfate on infusion device.
   a. TD (g) : TV reduced ratio:
   b. TD : TV = HD : HV (existing infusion):
   c. g per hr ordered at 25 mL per hr:
   d. Length of time 2 g to be infused:

   PROOF

5. Ordered: Pitocin (oxytocin) 2 milliunits per minute. Available: 10 units Pitocin in 1000 mL of D5NS.
   a. milliunits per mL of Pitocin in IV container:
   b. TD : TV reduced ratio:
   c. Hourly drug ordered:
   d. TD : TV = HD : HV ratio:
   e. Flow rate on infusion device to be set:

   PROOF

Answers on page 303

WORKSHEET 8I | Multiple-Choice Practice

1. Ordered: Isoproterenol at 5 mcg per minute. How many mg per hr would be infused?
   a. 0.5 mg
   b. 50 mg
   c. 0.3 mg
   d. 300 mg

2. Available 2 g of lidocaine in 500 mL of D5W. What is the mg per mL ratio?
   a. 4 : 1
   b. 2 : 1
   c. 1 : 4
   d. 1 : 2

3. Why do the ISMP-identified High-Alert Medications need special attention?
   a. They can result in significant harm if given in error because they are powerful drugs.
   b. They are new drugs on the market and the manufacturers need feedback.
   c. They are expensive medications and must not be wasted.
   d. They are in clinical testing and can only be given to those patients who have signed up to be part of the study

4. Which diluent is isotonic and often (but not always) specified for intravenous medication IVP dilutions?
   a. 0.9% sodium chloride (NaCl) solution
   b. 0.9% bacteriostatic (NaCl) solution
   c. 10% NaCl solution
   d. Bacteriostatic sterile water for injection

5. Ordered: Levophed (norepinephrine bitartrate) IV infusion bolus for a patient with severe hypotension. Titrate every 10 to 15 minutes to maintain blood pressure of 90/60. Initial 0.1 mg per dose to 0.5 mg per dose. The patient's blood pressure is 70/30. Which diluted dose would you give this patient first?
   a. 0.5 mg
   b. 0.4 mg
   c. 0.3 mg
   d. 0.1 mg

> **CLINICAL ALERT!**
> Never leave the patient unattended. Monitor the BP continuously. Levophed bitartrate is for IV use. Norepinephrine base is for other routes. 2 mg of norepinephrine bitartrate is equal to 1 mg of norepinephrine base. They are *not* interchangeable. Recheck labels and orders. Contact pharmacy if there is a question about the solution provided.

6. What size syringe is recommended for central lines?
   a. 1 mL because it is easier to manipulate
   b. 20 mL because it can deliver higher pressure to the line
   c. 10 mL because the wider barrel delivers lower pressure
   d. 3 mL because they are almost always available

7. What is the main reason for the recommendation to deliver a bolus medication into a vascular access device, such as a port or an existing infusion line?
   a. It avoids the trauma of a separate puncture for direct access to a vein.
   b. It reduces the risk of infection.
   c. It permits quick countermeasures if an adverse reaction occurs.
   d. It is easier to count the rate that is required for the medication IV push delivery.

8. Which statement about bolus, direct IV, and IV push is true?
   a. They are concentrated, and directions for rate vary and are specified.
   b. They need to be given very quickly directly into a vein.
   c. They are used only for emergencies.
   d. They are used to determine peak and trough levels.

9. Which sterile IV solution must be administered with blood?
   a. D5W
   b. Sterile water for injection
   c. Normal saline
   d. Lactated Ringer's solution

10. Ordered: An IV solution at 60 mg per hr on an infusion pump. Available 1 g in 1000 mL D5W. What flow rate should be programmed on the infusion pump?
    a. 30 mL per hr
    b. 60 mL per hr
    c. 100 mL per hr
    d. 120 mL per hr

Analyzing IV Medication Errors for Safe Nurse Practice

IV errors are not infrequent and have the potential to do serious damage because of immediate entry of drugs into circulation. As you review this list of errors, think about preventive methods.

1. Wrong patient
2. Wrong drug
3. Wrong dose
4. Wrong time
5. Incompatible mixtures (medications and/or diluents)
6. Piggyback solutions' timing and compatibility errors
7. Infusion volume and rate errors
8. Bolus rate and dilution errors

9. Technique problems and site infections
10. Wrong route
11. Incorrect or lack of dilution of concentrated solutions
12. Delayed or omitted documentation
13. Lack of nursing experience with assignment
14. Unnoticed side effects
15. Subtle significant patient statements

Notes:

Critical Thinking Exercises

Critical Thinking Exercises provide math and medication-related patient safety issues for student discussion. Answers are not provided.

Analyze the following scenarios.

1. One night during a bedside emergency for a patient with ventricular fibrillation, a physician called for potassium chloride (KCl) 20 mEq to be added to an IV line of D5W and for Amiodarone to be given by direct push into a second, separate IV line. Pharmacy prepared all KCl known ordered infusions but was closed for the night. The nurse obtained KCl 20 mEq concentrate from a locked cabinet. As the orders were called out, one nurse prepared the medications and handed them to the nurse who was assisting, who then administered the medications. At one point, the nurse was handed two syringes of medication. She was told that one was Amiodarone and that the other syringe contained KCl 20 mEq. The KCl was administered undiluted to the patient by direct push, and the Amiodarone was placed in D5W. Refer to current drug reference for preparation of KCl IV and complications if given undiluted.

Error(s):

Causes of error(s):

Potential injuries:

Nursing actions:

Preventive measures:

2. A patient in the ICU weighing 60 kg was to receive an IV infusion of Dobutrex ordered to start at 3 mcg per kg per min. The nurse programmed the IV pump to infuse at 3 mg per kg per minute.

   Error(s):

   Amount of error:

   Causes of error(s):

   Potential injuries:

   Nursing interventions:

   Recommendations for the patient safety committee to prevent this type of error:

3. A patient was admitted with seizures. Phenobarbital 130 mg IV push stat at 65 mg per minute was ordered. The nurse diluted the medication in 3 mL of sterile water for injection. It was administered over 1 minute.

   Phenobarbital Sodium Injection, USP
   130 mg/mL R only
   FOR IM OR SLOW IV USE
   25 x 1 mL Vials
   DO NOT USE IF DISCOLORED OR CONTAINS A PRECIPITATE
   Manufactured by: WEST-WARD
   Eatontown, NJ 07724 USA
   NDC 0641-0477-25

   Error:

   Cause(s) of error:

   Potential adverse drug event(s) (ADE):
   (Refer to side effects of phenobarbital IV in current IV drug reference)

   Nursing interventions and antidotes needed:
   (Refer to current IV drug reference)

   Recommendations for the patient safety committee to prevent this type of error:

CHAPTER 8 Final

Answers on page 304

Solve the following problems by using a calculator, moving decimals, reducing ratios, and labeling your answers. Prove your work.

Make a decision:

A. Safe to give   B. Unsafe; consult with physician

1. Ordered: Dobutamine HCl IV infusion 5 mcg per kg per min. Available: Dobutamine HCl 2000 mcg/mL in an infusion device. Patient's weight is 50 kg.
   a. mcg/hr needed: **15,000 mcg/hr**
   b. Flow rate to be set on IV infusion device: **7.5 mL/hr** hr

   $\dfrac{2000\,mcg}{1\,mL} \times \dfrac{hr}{15,000\,mcg}$

2. Ordered: Potassium chloride IV infusion 10 mEq to be administered to a 44-lb child with hypokalemia. Administer over 4 hr. Available: D5W 100 mL including 10 mEq KCl prepared by pharmacy. The literature states that the rate should not exceed 3 mEq per kg per 24 hr for a child.
   a. Patient's weight in kg: **20 kg**
   b. SDR for this child per 24 hr: **60 mEq/24hr. or less**
   c. Total drug ordered: **10 mEq**
   d. Decision (Safe/Unsafe): **Safe**
   e. Amount of drug in mL in IV (refer to label for mEq per mL): **2 mEq/mL**
   f. Hourly flow rate on infusion device in mL:

   $\dfrac{2.5\,mEq/hr}{}$ $\dfrac{10\,mEq}{4\,hr} = \dfrac{60\,mEq}{24\,hr}$

   $\dfrac{2\,mEq}{1\,mL} \quad \dfrac{10\,mEq}{5\,mL}$

   $\dfrac{5\,mL}{4\,hr} = \dfrac{1 X}{1\,hr}$ → **1.25 mL/hr**

   25 mL of D5W

   Label: 20 mEq Potassium Chloride for Inj. Concentrate, USP (2 mEq/mL) — 10 mL, NDC 0409-3907-03. Hospira.

3. Ordered: An IV of Adrenalin (epinephrine) of 1 mg in 250 mL to be infused at 1 mcg per minute. The IV is infusing at 15 mL per hr for a patient in shock.
   a. Total drug amount in the solution in mcg (TD): **1000 mcg**
   b. Total volume of the solution (TV): **250 mL**
   c. TD : TV ratio: **4 : 1**
   d. Hourly drug (HD) order in mcg: **60 mcg/hr**
   e. mL per hour needed for order? **15 mL/hr**
   f. Is the existing hourly mL (HV) correct for the order? **yes**

   $\dfrac{4\,mcg}{1\,mL} \times \dfrac{1\,min}{1\,mcg}$ = 0.25 mL/min

4. Ordered: Dopamine IV at 4 mcg per kg per min for a patient in septic shock who weighs 110 lb today. The SDR is 2 to 10 mcg per kg per min. The IV is flowing at 15 mL per hr when you enter the room.
   a. Patient's weight in kg: **50 kg**
   b. SDR for this patient: **100 – 500 mcg/min**
   c. Ordered drug rate per min: **200 mcg/min**
   d. Decision (Safe/Unsafe): **safe**
   e. TD : TV ratio: **800 mcg/1 mL**
   f. mg per hr of drug ordered: **12 mg/hr**

g. Hourly flow rate needed:
h. Decision (correct or needs order for change):

$$\frac{12 \text{ mg}}{1 \text{ hr}} \times \frac{1 \text{ mL}}{0.8 \text{ mg}} = \boxed{15 \text{ mL/hr}}$$

correct decision

5. Ordered: Dilaudid (hydromorphone HCl) 3 mg IV push for a patient with severe pain. Directions state it may be given undiluted slowly or diluted up to 5 mL with SW or NS to facilitate titration. It may be administered over 2 to 5 minutes slowly. The nurse dilutes it to 3 mL and plans to administer it over 3 minutes.*

a. Total amount of Dilaudid to be prepared (in mL, round to nearest tenth):
b. Total amount of diluted volume to be administered in mL: 3 mL
c. Total number of minutes for injection: 3 min
d. Amount in mL per minute to be administered: 1 mL / 1 min

4 mg = 1 mL → 3 mL

CLINICAL ALERT!

*When small amounts of medication are ordered, dilution makes it easier to control the rate of injection. This nurse wants to administer 1 mL per minute for ease of administration. There were other options. Always read the directions for dilution and rate of administration. If the patient begins to have side effects, the medication will be withdrawn. It is safer and always preferable to inject into an existing IV port or line so that side effects can be countered quickly when necessary.

evolve Refer to the Advanced Calculation section of Drug Calculations Companion, version 5 on Evolve for additional practice problems.

Answer Key

8 Advanced Intravenous Calculations

WORKSHEET 8A (page 279)

1. **a.** 5 × 60 = 300 sec
      300 ÷ 25 lines = 12 sec per line
   b. 5 mL : 5 min = x mL : 1 minute
      5x = 5
      x = 1 mL per minute

2. **a.** 250 mcg : 1 mL = 500 mcg : x mL
      (x = 2 mL)
   b. 10 minutes
   c. 2 mL : 10 minutes = x mL : 1 minute
      x = 0.2 mL per minute
   d. 1 minute per line (10 ÷ 10)

3. **a.** 100 mg : 1 mL = 900 mg : x mL
      (x = 9 mL)
   b. 50 mg : 1 minute = 900 mg : x minute
      50x = 900
      x = 18 minutes
   c. 9 mL : 18 minutes = x mL : 1 minute
      18x = 9
      x = 0.5 mL per minute

4. **a.** 10 mg : 1 mL = 20 mg : x mL
      (x = 2 mL)
   b. 2 × 60 = 120 sec
   c. 120 ÷ 10 = 12 sec per line
   d. 2 mL : 2 minute = x mL : 1 minute
      2x = 2
      x = 1 mL per minute

5. **a.** 5 mL
   b. 5 minutes
   c. 5 mL : 5 minutes = x mL : 1 minute
      5x = 5
      x = 1 mL per minute

WORKSHEET 8B (page 282)

1. **b.** 1 : 1
   c. 1 : 10
   d. 1 : 2
   e. 1 : 2

2. **b.** x = 30 mL per hr (1 : 1 = 30 : 30)
   c. x = 50 mL per hr (1 : 10 = 5 : 50)
   d. x = 6 mL per hr (1 : 2 = 3 : 6)
   e. x = 5 mL per hr (2 : 1 = 10 : 5)

299

3. **b.** (2 : 1 = 12 : 6) 12 mg per hr
   c. (1 : 2 = 9 : 18) 9 mg per hr
   d. (4 : 10 = 4 : 10) 4 mg per hr
   e. (2 : 1 = 36 : 18) 36 mg per hr

4. **a.** 2 × 60 = 120 mcg per hr
   b. 10 × 50 = 500 mg per hr
   c. $\frac{120}{2.2}$ = 54.5 kg
   0.5 × 54.5 = 27.3 mcg per hr
   d. 1.5 × 68 = 102 mg per hr
   e. 6 × 60 = 360 mcg per hr

5. **b.** (1 : 1 = 9 : 9) 9 mL per hr
   c. (2 : 1 = 20 : 10) 10 mL per hr
   d. (1 : 2 = 15 : 30) 30 mL per hr
   e. (8 : 5 = 8 : 5) 5 mL per hr

WORKSHEET 8C (page 284)

1. 2000 mcg per minute (2 × 1000); 120,000 mcg per hr (2000 × 60)

2. 0.3 mg per minute (300 ÷ 1000); (0.3 × 60) 18 mg per hr

3. 16 mg per minute (0.2 × 80) 960 mg per hr (16 × 60)

4. 5 mcg × 80 kg ÷ 1000 = 0.4 mg per minute; 0.4 mg × 60 minutes = 24 mg per hr

5. 10 milliunits per minute (600 ÷ 60 = 10)

6. 100 mcg per hr (0.1 × 1000)

7. 0.167 mg rounded to 0.17 mg per minute (10 ÷ 60)

8. 1.25 mg per kg per hr (100 mg ÷ 80 kg = 1.25 mg per kg)

9. 41.66 rounded to 41.7 mcg per minute (2.5 × 1000 ÷ 60)

10. 50 milliunits per minute (3 × 1000 ÷ 60)

WORKSHEET 8D (page 284)

1.
		mg per hour	mcg per hr	mg per min	mcg per min
	a.	0.050	50	0.050 ÷ 60 = 0.0008	0.8
	b.	24	24,000	0.4	400
	c.	30	30,000	0.5	500
	d.	1.2	1200	0.02	20
	e.	7.5	7500	0.125	125

2.
		kg	mg per hr	mg per kg per min	mcg per kg per min
	a.	85	25	25 ÷ 85 ÷ 60 = 0.005	5
	b.	70	10 × 70 × 60 = 42,000*	10	10,000
	c.	62	0.37	0.0001	0.1
	d.	55	75	0.02	20
	e.	48	144	0.05	50

*4.2 g per hour.

	IV Contents	TD : TV Reduced Ratio	HD (mg per hr)	HV (mL per hr)	mg per mL
3. a.	500 mg/1000 mL	1 : 2	5	10	0.5
b.	250 mg/500 mL	1 : 2	15	30	0.5
c.	400 mg/250 mL	8 : 5	24	15	1.6
d.	500 mg/500 mL	1 : 1	75	75	1
e.	500 mg/250 mL	2 : 1	16	8	2

WORKSHEET 8E (page 285)

2. a. $1 : 2 = x$ mg : 15 mL   ($x = 7.5$ mg per hr)
   PROOF
   $1 \times 15 = 15$
   $2 \times 7.5 = 15$
   b. 7.5 mg $\times$ 1000 = 7500 mcg per hr
   c. 7500 mcg $\div$ 60 = 125 mcg per minute
   d. 125 mcg per minute $\div$ 50 kg = 2.5 mcg per kg per minute

4. a. $4 : 1 = x$ mg per hr : 10 mL per hr   ($x = 40$ mg)
   PROOF
   $4 \times 10 = 40$
   $1 \times 40 = 40$
   b. 40 $\times$ 1000 = 40,000 mcg per hr
   c. 40,000 mcg $\div$ 60 = 667 mcg per minute
   d. 667 mcg per minute $\div$ 60 kg = 11.1 mcg per kg per minute

3. a. $2 : 5 = x$ mg : 5 mL   ($x = 2$ mg per hr)
   PROOF
   $2 \times 5 = 10$
   $5 \times 2 = 10$
   b. 2 mg per hr $\times$ 1000 = 2000 mcg per hr
   c. 2000 mcg per hr $\div$ 60 = 33.3 mcg per minute
   d. 33.3 mcg per minute $\div$ 55 kg = 0.605 or 0.6 mcg per kg per minute

5. a. $2 : 1 = x$ mg : 8 mL per hr   ($x = 16$ mg per hr)
   PROOF
   $2 \times 8 = 16$
   $1 \times 16 = 16$
   b. 16 mg $\times$ 1000 = 16,000 mcg per hr
   c. 16,000 mcg per hr $\div$ 60 = 266.7 mcg per minute
   d. 266.7 mcg per minute $\div$ 79.5 kg = 3.4 mcg per kg per minute

WORKSHEET 8F (page 288)

2. a. 2 mg per mL (500 mg : 250 mL) = 2 : 1 ratio
   b. No. The nurse is incorrect. The nurse does not understand the mg to mL ratio.
   c. 250 mL per hr*
       TD   TV   HD   HV
   500 mg : 250 mL = 500 mg : 250 mL
       2   :   1   =   2   :   1

4. a. 4 mg per mL (40 mg : 10 mL = x mg : 1 mL)
   PROOF: $40 \times 1 = 40$; $10 \times 4 = 40$
   b. 0.4 mg per mL (40 mg : 100 mL = x mg : 1 mL)
   PROOF: $40 \times 1 = 40$; $100 \times 0.4 = 40$
   c. Yes. (0.4 mg $\times$ 6.7 mL per minute $\times$ 15 minute = 40.2 mg total dose infused per label instructions)
   d. 402 mL per hr (6.7 mg per minute $\times$ 60 min) or approximately 100.5 mL in 15 minutes
   Recheck high-rate calculations and check with pharmacy if needed.

3. a. 20 mg per mL (1000 mg : 50 mL = 20 mg : 1 mL
   PROOF: $1000 \times 1 = 1000$; $50 \times 20 = 1000$
   b. Yes. Safe.
   c. 100 mL per hr (50 mL : 30 minute = x mL : 60 minute)
   PROOF: $50 \times 60 = 3000$
               $30 \times 100 = 3000$

5. a. 250 mg (5 mg $\times$ 50 kg)
   b. 1 : 1 (250 mg : 250 mL)
   c. 1.5 hr (60 minute : 1 hr = 90 minute : 1.5 hr)
   PROOF: $60 \times 1.5 = 90$; $1 \times 90 = 90$
   d. 166.6 mL per hr (250 mL : 1.5 hr = x mL : 1 hr)
   PROOF: $250 \times 1 = 250$; $166.6 \times 1.5 = 249.9$ rounded to approximately 250
   e. Current rate is too slow.
   f. Assess patient; contact prescriber promptly for appropriate rate change if any. Report and document assessment, prescriber order and nurse action. Perform frequent follow-up assessments.

---

*Recheck the 250 mL per hr rate with current IV drug reference and pharmacist. It is very rapid but may be indicated for this patient.

WORKSHEET 8G (page 290)

2.
 a. 60 (132 ÷ 2.2)
 b. 300 mcg per minute × 60 = 18,000 mcg per hr
 c. 18 mg per hr (decimal moved 3 places to left)
 d. 250 : 250 = 1 : 1
 e. 18 mL per hr (1 : 1 = 18 : x)
  PROOF
  1 × 18 = 18
  1 × 18 = 18
 f. Incorrect flow rate. Should be 18 mL per hr, not 36 mL per hr.
 g. Unsafe. Assess patient's vital signs, report per hospital policy, and contact physician for orders.

4.
 a. 1 mg : 250 mL
 b. 5 mcg × 60 = 300 mcg per hr or 0.3 mg per hr
 c. 1 : 250 mL = 0.3 mg : x mL
 d. 0.3 × 250 = 75.0 mL per hr
  PROOF
  1 × 75 = 75
  0.3 × 250 = 75

3.
 a. 1000 mg : 500 mL = 2 mg : 1 mL
 b. 4 mg × 60 = 240 mg per hr
 c. 2 : 1 = 240 : x = 120 mL per hr
  PROOF
  2 × 120 = 240
  1 × 240 = 240

5.
 a. 10 units = 10,000 milliunits
  1000 milliunits = 1 unit
 b. 1000 mL
 c. 10 milliunits per 1 mL (10,000 mU per 1000 mL)
 d. 60 milliunits per hour (1 milliunit per minute × 60 minutes)
  HAVE WANT TO HAVE
  TD : TV = HD : HV
 e. 6 mL per hour   10 milliunits : 1 mL = 60 milliunits : x mL
  10x = 60
  x = 6 mL per hour
 f. 2 milliunits per minute
 g. 120 milliunits per hour (2 milliunits per minute × 60 minutes)
  TD : TV = HD : HV
 h. 12 mL per hour   10 milliunits : 1 mL = 120 milliunits : x mL
  10x = 120
  x = 12 mL per hour

Note: The total drug, total volume did not change. The drug per hour changed. Total Drug : Total Volume is a "staple" of IV dose calculations and verification. When the ratio is reduced, the math becomes very simple. Titrated doses are a series of separate similar problems with a similar setup.

WORKSHEET 8H (page 292)

2. a. 10,000 milliunits : 1000 mL = 10 : 1
  b. 10 milliunits : 1 mL = 1200 milliunits
  (hr) : x mL (120) (hr)
  PROOF
  $10 \times 120 = 1200$
  $1 \times 1200 = 1200$
  c. Rate should be 120 mL per hr; obtain order to increase.

3. a. 4 mL
  b. 1 mL per minute (5 calibrations per minute)
  c. 1 calibration every 12 seconds

4. a. 20 : 500 = 1 : 25
  b. 1 g : 25 mL = x g : 25 mL per hr
  PROOF
  $1 \times 25 = 25$
  $25 \times 1 = 25$
  c. x = 1 g per hr
  d. 2 hr

5. a. 10,000 milliunits : 1000 mL
  b. 10 milliunits : 1 mL
  c. 2 milliunits $\times$ 60 = 120 milliunits per hr
  d. 10 : 1 = 120 : x
  PROOF
  $10 \times 12 = 120$
  $1 \times 120 = 120$
  e. x = 12 mL per hr

WORKSHEET 8I (page 293)

1. c. Finding mg per mL requires that mg is in the numerator and mL is in the denominator.

2. a. 2 g = 2000 mg to 500 mL. Ratio = 4 : 1

3. a.

4. a.

5. d. 0.1 mg; always start with the lowest dose unless otherwise ordered.

6. c. 10 mL. Smaller syringes need more pressure applied against resistance and can disengage and/or damage the line or blood vessel.

7. c. Side effects show up quickly with intravenous medications. Bolus medications are more concentrated (smaller volume, less dilution) and often are high-alert medications.

8. a. The three names convey speed. Many bolus medications are specified to be given *slowly*. Serious ADE have resulted from giving them at the wrong rate.

9. c. NS is administered with blood unless an order is received for another solution, which the nurse would check. Solutions with dextrose can cause hemolysis (breaking of the blood cells within or outside of the blood vessels). Blood should not be administered with IV products that contain calcium such as Lactated Ringer's. Checking any 2 or more IV mixtures for compatibility is critical for patient safety.

10. b. 60 mL per hr. The total drug, total volume is 1 g, or 1000 mg, and 1000 mL, a 1 : 1 ratio. Therefore the mL rate = mg amount.

CHAPTER 8 FINAL: ADVANCED INTRAVENOUS CALCULATIONS (page 297)

1. a. 15,000 mcg (5 mcg × 50 kg × 60 min)
   b. 7.5 mL (2000 mcg : 1 mL = 15,000 mcg : x mL)

2. a. 20 kg
   b. 60 mEq maximum per 24 hours
   c. 10 mEq
   d. Safe
   e. 5 mL
   f. 100 ÷ 4 = 25 mL per hr (95 mL D5W plus 5 mL KCl)

3. a. 1000 mcg
   b. 250 mL
   c. 4 : 1
   d. 60 mcg per hour
   e. 15 mL per hour $\quad \dfrac{TD}{TV} = \dfrac{HD}{HV}$
   f. Yes
   Both drug measurements had to be in mcg or mg. The volume is always in mL.

4. a. 50 kg
   b. 100 to 500 mcg per minute   (2 to 10 mcg per kg per minute)
   c. 200 mcg per minute   (4 mcg per kg per minute)
   d. Safe
   e. 4 : 5 (200 mg : 250 mL)
   f. 12 mg per hr (4 mcg × 50 kg × 60 minutes) ÷ 1000
   g. TD   TV   HD   HV
      4 : 5 = 12 : x   (x = 15 mL per hr)
   h. Correct

5. a. 0.75 mL prepared in 1-mL syringe
   b. 3 mL
   c. 3 min
   d. 1 mL per minute

Insulin Administration and Type 2 Diabetes Medications

Objectives
- Identify sites for insulin injections.
- Identify the different types of insulin labels.
- Compare the actions of fast-, intermediate-, and long-acting insulins.
- Read calibrations on 30-, 50-, and 100-unit insulin syringes.
- Prepare single- and mixed-dose insulin injections.
- Calculate units of insulin based on CHO grams.
- Interpret the sliding scale using the BMBG method.
- Use electronic intravenous devices to administer insulin dosages.
- Calculate IC insulin for units per hr and mL per hr and duration.
- Analyze medication errors using critical thinking.

Introduction

According to the USP and the ISMP, insulin is the drug most commonly involved in errors. Insulin has been given as an overdose or confused with other unit-measured medications such as heparin. The importance of measuring the correct amount of insulin is vital. Different types of insulin syringes are shown for the practice of selecting the most appropriate syringe for the ordered dose. Mixing two types of insulin is shown in drawings. The bedside monitor blood glucose (BMBG) flow sheet shows how to use the sliding scale to chart hourly insulin needs. IV infusions are calculated for units per hour based on the BMBG level.

Vocabulary

Basal Rate: Based on carbohydrate intake, weight, and exercise, A low continuous dose of insulin units needed to cover the glucose output of the liver.

BGL: Blood glucose level; measures the glucose level in blood.

Bolus Dose: A rapid-acting insulin injection to keep the blood glucose level under control following a meal or if the blood sugar level is too high.

Diabetes Mellitus (DM): A chronic metabolic disorder resulting in hyperglycemia due to inadequate production of insulin by the islets of Langerhans in the pancreas.

Diabetic Ketoacidosis (DKA): A complication of diabetes diagnosed by elevated blood glucose (above 250 mg per dL), elevated ketones in the blood and urine, and a blood pH below 7.3. This condition is an emergency because it may result in death.

Glucagon: A hormone produced by the beta cells of the islets of Langerhans in the pancreas. This hormone increases the blood glucose level by stimulating the liver to change stored glycogen to glucose.

Hyperglycemia: Blood glucose levels above the basic normal values of 80 to 120 mg per dL.

Hypoglycemia: A decreased level of blood glucose (below 70 mg per dL).

Incretin Mimetics: A group of metabolic hormones that stimulate a decrease in insulin release from the islets of Langerhans in the pancreas.

Insulin Shock: Blood sugar level below 60 mg per dL (hypoglycemia) caused by too much insulin in the blood. Treated by giving glucose orally or intravenously, depending on the patient's condition.

Postprandial: Blood glucose measurement taken after a meal.

Preprandial: Blood glucose measurement taken before a meal.

Type 1 DM: Failure of the pancreas to produce insulin.

Type 2 DM: Insulin resistance or inadequate insulin secretion due to a decrease in sensitivity of muscle cells to uptake insulin.

Insulin

Insulin is an aqueous solution of the principal hormone of the pancreas. Insulin affects metabolism by allowing glucose to leave the blood and enter the body cells, preventing hyperglycemia or hypoglycemia.

Diabetes Mellitus

Diabetes mellitus (DM) is a deficiency of insulin and is classified according to its cause. Type 1 DM usually affects people before the age of 30 years. The pancreatic cells do not produce insulin. Insulin injections must be taken every day to control the blood glucose level.

The onset of type 2 diabetes usually occurs after 30 years of age; however, obesity has contributed to a rise in the diagnosis of type 2 diabetes in children and young adults. The pancreas produces some insulin but not enough to metabolize the glucose. In some cases, the insulin that is produced is not effective; this is known as insulin resistance. Of people with diabetes, 95% have type 2, and 40% of people with type 2 diabetes take insulin injections in conjunction with oral diabetes medications and the noninsulin incretin and amylin mimetic injections.

The most common complication of insulin therapy is hypoglycemia. This may be caused by injecting too much insulin (a risk in home care), by missing or delaying meals, or by being involved in more physical activity than usual. To treat hypoglycemia, a patient should always carry sugar in some form. The treatment of choice, if the patient can swallow, is glucose tablets (4 to 5 g carbohydrate [CHO] per tablet). Wait 15 minutes to retest the blood glucose. A glucose gel of 15 g is also available for the treatment of hypoglycemia. The glucose gel is to be used if the person cannot swallow but is still conscious. Put gel in the cheek along the gumline and rub vigorously. If the blood glucose level gets very low, unconsciousness may occur. At that point, the patient will need a glucagon injection. Emergency kits are available for home use (Figure 9-1). For patients weighing over 20 kg, use 1 mg. For patients weighing less than 20 kg, use 0.5 mg of glucagon. For unconscious patients, an IV of 50% dextrose solution should be administered.

FIGURE 9-1 **A,** Glucagon emergency kit for home use. **B,** Dextrose 50% (**A,** Copyright Eli Lilly and Company. All rights reserved. Used with permission.)

Injection Sites

The abdomen is the preferred site for insulin injections. When insulin injections are required on a daily basis, it is important to rotate within that site to prevent lipodystrophy (Figure 9-2). The abdomen absorbs insulin more rapidly and is safer as an injection site than the upper arm, back, or thigh. If use of the abdomen is medically contraindicated, alternative sites may be used.

FIGURE 9-2 Insulin injection areas.

CHAPTER 9 Insulin Administration and Type 2 Diabetes Medications

U-100 Insulins

Table 9-1 Insulin Comparison Chart

Insulin Name (Trade Name)	When Does It Start Working? (Onset)	When Will the Effect Be the Greatest? (Peak)	How Long Will It Lower Blood Glucose? (Duration)	Notes for Use
Ultra-Rapid Inhalation				
AFREZZA (insulin human)	10-12 minutes	1 hour	2.5-3 hours	AFREZZA® is a rapid-acting inhaled powder and can be taken at mealtime with long-acting insulin.
Rapid Acting Analogs				
Aspart (Novolog)	<15 minutes	30-90 minutes	3-5 hours	If mixing with NPH, rapid-acting insulin (clear formulation) should be drawn into syringe first. Mixture should be given immediately to avoid effects on peak action.
Lispro (Humalog)	<15 minutes	30-90 minutes	3-5 hours	
Glulisine (Apidra)	<15 minutes	30-90 minutes	3-5 hours	
Short Acting				
Regular (Novolin R or Humulin R)	0.5-1 hour	2-4 hours	4-8 hours	If mixing with NPH, short-acting insulin (clear formulation) should be drawn into syringe first. Mixture should be given immediately to avoid effects on peak action.
Intermediate Acting				
NPH (NovoLIN N or HumuLIN N)	1-2 hours	4-10 hours	10-18 hours	Cloudy formulation.
Long Acting Analogs				
Glargine (Lantus)	1-2 hours	No peak	20-24 hours	Do not mix with other insulin formulations. Both Glargine and Detemir are clear formulations.
Detemir (Levemir)	1-2 hours	Relatively flat	Up to 24 hours (dose-dependent)	
Combinations				
NovoLIN 70/30 or HumuLIN 70/30	0.5-1 hour	2-10 hours	10-18 hours	70% NPH +30% regular insulin. Insulin action includes two peaks (one from each formulation). Cloudy formulation.
Novolog Mix 70/30 or Humalog Mix 75/25 or 50/50	<15 minutes	1-2 hours	10-18 hours	Insulin action includes two peaks (one from each formulation). Novolog mix (cloudy formulation): 70% Aspart protamine + 30% Aspart Humalog mix (cloudy formulation): 75/25 = 75% Lispro protamine + 25% Lispro 50/50 = 50% Lispro protamine + 50% Lispro

*All insulin preparations are 100 units per mL except concentrated regular insulin U500 containing 500 units per mL. Onset, peak, and duration may vary considerably in different people.

Table 9-2 Non-Insulin Injectables for Diabetes Management

Generic Name (Brand Name)	Dosing	Action	When to Take
Amylin Mimetics			
Pramlintide acetate (Symlin)	Given subcutaneously. Prefilled pen.	Works with insulin to help maintain normal glucose concentrations. It has three actions: (1) helps control blood glucose levels by reducing the post-meal release of glucose from the liver; (2) slows the absorption of carbohydrate by slowing the rate of stomach emptying; (3) reduces appetite.	Taken with meals or snacks when more than 30 g of carbohydrates are eaten.

GLP-1 Agonist Medications Chart

Generic Name (Brand Name)	Dosing Schedule	Mixing Required	Preinjection Waiting Time	Dosing
Incretin Mimetics				
Exenatide (Byetta)	BID	No	None	5, 10 mcg
Exenatide extended release (Bydureon Kit)	QW	Yes	None	2 mg
Exenatide extended release (Bydureon Pen)	QW	Yes	None	2 mg
Albiglutide (Tanzeum)	QW	Yes	Yes, 15-30 minutes	30, 50 mg
Dulaglutide (Trulicity)	QW	No	None	0.75, 1.5 mg
Liraglutide (Victoza)	QD	No	None	0.6, 1.2, 1.8 mg

CLINICAL RELEVANCE

Humalog, Novolog, and Apidra may be taken 15 minutes before eating and can be mixed with NPH. Afrezza inhalation insulin can be taken 12 to 15 minutes before eating.

Incretin Mimetics for Type 2 Diabetes Mellitus

Incretin is a natural hormone the body makes to signal the release of insulin from the pancreas after eating to lower blood sugar. Incretin mimetics act like or mimic the action of the incretins the body creates to lower blood sugar after eating.

The Action of Incretin Mimetics

- Signals the pancreas to release insulin when blood sugar level rises
- Prevents the pancreas from releasing too much glucose, which would cause the liver to release stored sugar into the bloodstream
- Helps to slow the rate at which the stomach empties, which may reduce hunger and increase feeling satisfied after a meal
- Helps keep blood sugar level in target range without causing low blood sugar or weight gain
- Incretin mimetics may lower hemoglobin A1c by 0.5% to 1%

Insulin Syringes and Pens

Insulin is usually given in a 1-mL or 0.5-mL insulin syringe calibrated to U-100 insulin. The 0.5-mL insulin syringe is used for smaller doses because the calibrations are larger and easier to read.

Types of U-100 Insulin Syringes

Each calibration in the syringe shown in Figure 9-3 represents 1 unit. This syringe is used for small doses of 30 units or less and as a safety feature for people with diabetes who have vision problems (a Magni-Guide may also be useful for those people [Figure 9-4]) or for children who require small doses of insulin. This syringe is for use with U-100 insulin only.

FIGURE 9-3 30-unit syringes.

FIGURE 9-4 BD Magni-Guide. (From Becton, Dickinson, and Company, Franklin Lakes, N.J.)

CLINICAL ALERT!

Tuberculin syringes are calibrated in tenths and must never be substituted for insulin syringes, which are calibrated from 1 to 100 units.

CLINICAL RELEVANCE

Loss of vision is a complication of diabetes. U-30 and U-50 syringes have large numbers and are easier to read than the U-100 (1-mL) syringes. Tactile insulin measuring devices such as the Jordan Medical Count-a-Dose enable nonvisual insulin measurement and mixing.

Each calibration in the syringe shown in Figure 9–5 represents 1 unit. This syringe is used for small doses of 50 units or less and is used with U-100 insulin only. Needles are usually 24- to 26-gauge for subcutaneous injections. Clip-on magnifiers for syringes are available to enlarge the calibrations and numbers. The most commonly used insulin syringes are 30-, 50-, and 100-unit syringes.

FIGURE 9-5 50-unit syringe.

Each calibration in the syringe shown in Figure 9-6 equals two units. This syringe is for use with U-100 insulin only.

FIGURE 9-6 100-unit syringe.

FIGURE 9-7 Insulin syringes. **A,** 100-unit syringes with odd and even numbers. **B,** 50- and 30-unit syringes. (From Becton, Dickinson and Company, Franklin Lakes, N.J.)

Insulin Orders

A typical order for insulin must include the following:
1. The *name* of the insulin: Humulin, Novolin, Lantus.
2. The *type* of the insulin: regular, lispro, aspart, N, detemir, or glargine.
3. The *number* of units or amount the patient will receive: 10 units.
4. The *time* to be given: AM, ½ hr before a meal.
5. The *route* is subcutaneous unless IV is specified.

Example Prepare 30 units of Humulin R insulin subcutaneously ½ hr before a meal. Using a 100-unit syringe, 50-unit syringe, or 30-unit syringe, fill the syringe to the 30 units calibration (Figure 9-8). (All insulins come in U-100, so orders no longer specify U-100.)

FIGURE 9-8 From left to right: 30 units measured on a 100-unit syringe (each calibration is 2 units), a 50-unit syringe (each calibration is 1 unit), and a 30-unit syringe (each calibration is 1 unit). (From Macklin D, Chernecky C, Infortuna H: *Math for clinical practice,* ed 2, St Louis, 2011, Mosby.)

CLINICAL RELEVANCE

Units must be spelled out (not abbreviated by a U) because abbreviating can be a source of medication errors (e.g., mistaking the U for a zero). Insulin dosages require two licensed nurses to double-check for accuracy.

Dial   The prefilled, disposable Victoza pen can be dialed to the prescribed dose.

Dose   Once a day, at any time, independent of meals, Victoza can be injected with a 32G Tip (6-mm) needle in the abdomen, thigh, or upper arm.

Types of Insulin

The source of insulin is either human or animal. This is known as the species of the insulin. Human insulin is manufactured to be the same as insulin produced by the body. Human insulin is made in one of two ways:
- By recombinant DNA technology, a chemical process used to produce unlimited amounts of human insulin
- By a process that chemically changes animal insulin into human insulin

Humalog insulin (lispro) is recombinant DNA insulin with a rapid action of 5 to 15 minutes, allowing patients to dose and eat. Recombinant DNA insulins cause fewer allergies than those from animal sources.

All insulin is supplied in units denoting strength. Insulin is given via special insulin syringes (Figure 9-9) and pens. Byetta stimulates glucose-dependent insulin from pancreatic beta cells (GLP-1 and GIP) and decreases glucoagon production when glucose levels are elevated. Byetta is not insulin.

A

B

C

D

E

FIGURE 9-9 A, Humulin 70/30 short- and intermediate-acting insulins. **B,** Humulin N intermediate-acting insulin. Prefilled insulin pens. **C,** Novolog rapid-acting insulin. **D,** Novolog 70/30 short- and intermediate-acting insulin. **E,** Levemir long-acting insulin. (**A** and **B** Copyright Eli Lilly and Company. All rights reserved. Used with permission. **C-E,** from Novo Nordisk Inc., Princeton, N.J.)

Insulin is sometimes supplied in 10-mL vials labeled U-100, which means there are 100 units per mL (Figure 9-10). Insulin is also supplied in 10-mL vials of U-500, which means there are 500 units per mL. This strength is used for those whose blood glucose levels fluctuate to very high levels. This type of insulin is rarely used and rarely kept on the nursing unit. Table 9-1 lists the duration of activity of various types of insulins and other injectables. See examples of various U-100 insulins below and on the following pages.

FIGURE 9-10 **A,** Lantus (insulin glargine). The Lantus vial is taller and narrower than the NPH, Regular, and Humalog vials. Lantus is written in purple letters. **B,** Various insulin vials. HUMULIN and HUMALOG are registered trademarks of Eli Lilly and Company. **C,** Rapid-acting Apidra. **D,** Long-acting Levemir. (**A** and **C,** Product images and trademarks are the property of and used with the permission of sanofi-aventis U.S. LLC, Bridgewater, N.J. **B,** Copyright Eli Lilly and Company. All rights reserved. Used with permission. **D** from Novo Nordisk Inc., Princeton, N.J.)

U-100 Insulin Labels

Short-Acting

Rapid-Acting

From Novo Nordisk Inc., Princeton, N.J.

Product images and trademarks are the property of and used with the permission of sanofi-aventis U.S. LLC, Bridgewater, N.J.

Afrezza® inhaled insulin. From sanofi-aventis U.S. LLC, Bridgewater, N.J.

CLINICAL ALERT!

Fast-acting and regular insulin should always be clear. Discard if unclear.

Mix insulins only with those of the **same name** because they may have differing amounts of preservatives. For example, Humulin R should be combined only with Humulin L or N. Humulin is a brand name.

Intermediate-Acting

CHAPTER 9 Insulin Administration and Type 2 Diabetes Medications

Intermediate- and Rapid-Acting Mixtures

The insulin combination of NPH and Regular is used to give a 24-hour effect.

In 1 mL of Humulin 70/30, there are 70 units of intermediate-acting insulin and 30 units of rapid-acting insulin. In 1 mL of Humulin 50/50, there are 50 units of intermediate-acting insulin and 50 units of rapid-acting insulin. The first number in the combination is always the intermediate-acting insulin. The second number and the smaller amount is rapid-acting insulin.

Note: Mix before administration by rolling *gently* between the palms. Never shake because this creates bubbles in the suspension, decreasing accuracy when withdrawing the insulin.

CLINICAL ALERT!
Insulin is available in various strengths: rapid-acting, regular, intermediate-acting, long-acting, and combinations of rapid- and intermediate-acting. READ LABELS CAREFULLY TO AVOID GIVING THE WRONG STRENGTH.

Long-Acting

Product images and trademarks are the property of and used with the permission of sanofi-aventis U.S. LLC, Bridgewater, N.J.

From Novo Nordisk Inc., Princeton, NJ.

CLINICAL ALERT!
Lantus must NOT be mixed in the same syringe with any other insulin or be diluted. It is NOT intended for IV administration. Caution: Lantus is clear like Regular Humalog. Lantus is given anytime for 24-hour coverage without a peak. Consistency in administration is necessary.

Answers on page 346

WORKSHEET 9A | Single-Dose Measures

Read the syringes and write your answers in the spaces provided.

1. Units measured: _____

2. Units measured: _____

3. Units measured: _____

4. Units measured: _____

5. Units measured: _____

6. Units measured: _____

7. Units measured: _____

8. Units measured: _____

9. Units measured: _____

10. Units measured: _____

AM/PM INSULIN SHOT RECORD

NAME: John Doe

Date		Time	Blood Sugar Level	Insulin Injected	Quantity	Site Where Injected
3/16	AM	0630	190 SMBG	Humulin R / Humulin N	3 units / 20 units	AB Ⓡ
	PM	1530	150 SMBG	Humulin R / Humulin N	2 units / 20 units	AB Ⓛ
Date		Time	Blood Sugar Level	Insulin Injected	Quantity	Site Where Injected
	AM					
	PM					
Date		Time	Blood Sugar Level	Insulin Injected	Quantity	Site Where Injected
	AM					
	PM					
Date		Time	Blood Sugar Level	Insulin Injected	Quantity	Site Where Injected
	AM					
	PM					
Date		Time	Blood Sugar Level	Insulin Injected	Quantity	Site Where Injected
	AM					
	PM					
Date		Time	Blood Sugar Level	Insulin Injected	Quantity	Site Where Injected
	AM					
	PM					
Date		Time	Blood Sugar Level	Insulin Injected	Quantity	Site Where Injected
	AM					
	PM					

BGM blood glucose monitor (capillary sample) performed by nurse
SMBG self blood glucose monitoring (by patient) (capillary sample)
Serum FBS fasting blood sugar (by lab or RN) (venous [serum] sample)

RA = Right Arm
LA = Left Arm
RT = Right Thigh
AB - Right abdomen
AB - Left abdomen

Copyright © 2015 by Mosby, an imprint of Elsevier Inc. All rights reserved.

Answers on page 346

WORKSHEET 9B: Additional Practice in Single-Dose Measures

Circle the letter of the syringe with the correct ordered amount.

1. Ordered: 13 units of Humulin NPH subcutaneous at 1100 hr.

   NDC 0002-8315-01
   10 mL HI-310
   100 units per mL
   Humulin® N
   NPH
   human insulin
   (rDNA origin)
   isophane suspension
   U-100

   a.

   b.

2. Ordered: 6 units of Humulin Regular subcutaneous ½ hr before a meal.

   NDC 0002-8215-01
   10 mL HI-210
   100 units per mL
   Humulin® R
   REGULAR
   insulin human
   injection, USP
   (rDNA origin)
   Neutral
   U-100

   a.

   b.

CHAPTER 9 Insulin Administration and Type 2 Diabetes Medications   319

3. Ordered: 12 units of Novolin Regular subcutaneous 30 min before a meal.

   a.

   b.

4. Ordered: 12 units of Lantus subcutaneous at 2200 hr.

   a.

   b.

5. Ordered: 40 units of detemir subcutaneous at 0930.

(From Novo Nordisk Inc., Princeton, N.J.)

a.

b.

Mixing Insulin

Insulin dosages are drawn up *exactly* as ordered. An incorrect dosage could be devastating to the patient. Frequently, regular or rapid-acting insulin is combined with an intermediate-acting insulin. This gives insulin coverage (glucose control) within 15 to 60 minutes and lasts 10 to 16 hours. This technique of combining the two types of insulin is important for the nurse, patient, and family to master. The regular insulin vial should *not* be contaminated with the longer-acting insulin; therefore, the regular insulin should be drawn up first. The mixing procedure is illustrated in Figures 9-11 and 9-12.

Example   Ordered: 10 units of Humulin Regular and 40 units of Humulin N.
Total units: 50 units
Source: DNA and DNA
Which insulin will you draw up first? *Regular* (see Figure 9-11)

FIGURE 9-11   Order: Give 10 units of Humulin R and 40 units of Humulin N via subcutaneous injection. **A,** Inject 40 units of air into Humulin N first. Do **not** allow needle to touch insulin. Withdraw needle. **B,** Inject 10 units of air into Humulin R. **C,** With needle still in place, invert vial and withdraw 10 units of R. Withdraw needle. **D,** Insert needle into vial of Humulin N, invert vial and withdraw 40 units. Total amount in syringe equals 50 units.

FIGURE 9-12   100-unit syringe showing the mixing of two insulins. Remember: **clear to cloudy when drawing up insulins.**

Example Ordered: 10 units of Novolin Regular and 20 units of Novolin N

Nov N 20 units — 10
— 20
Nov R 10 units
— 30
— 40
— 50
— 60
— 70
— 80
— 90
— 100 units

🚩 Novolin® R — U 100, NDC 0169-1833-11, 10 ml 100 units/ml, Regular, Human Insulin Injection (recombinant DNA origin) USP

🚩 Novolin® N — U 100, NDC 0169-1834-11, 10 ml 100 units/ml, NPH, Human Insulin Isophane Suspension (recombinant DNA origin)

Insulin will not stay separated as pictured in the syringe.

⊖ CLINICAL ALERT!

Draw up regular (clear) insulin first before N (cloudy) is added (see Figure 9–11).

Regular insulin should not be contaminated with Humulin N or any N insulin. A multiple-dose vial of regular insulin can be used for IV infusion, and contamination with intermediate-acting insulin could be fatal.

Answers on page 346

WORKSHEET 9C | Mixing Insulin

Calculate the total number of units in the following problems. Circle the letter of the syringe with the correct amount.

1. Ordered: Lispro insulin 8 units and Humulin N 60 units ½ hr before breakfast.
   Total units: _____

   a.

   (syringe showing Hum N filled to ~60 with Lispro to ~68)

   b.

   (syringe showing Lispro to ~8 with Hum N to ~68)

2. Ordered: Humalog R 14 units and Humulin N 25 units. Total units: _____

   a.

   (syringe showing Hum N to 25 with Humalog to ~39)

   b.

   (syringe showing Hum N to ~25 with Humalog to ~39)

324 Drug Calculations: *Ratio and Proportion Problems for Clinical Practice*

3. Ordered: Novolin R 8 units and Novolin N 15 units. Total units: _____
   a.
   b.

4. Ordered: Novolin 8 units and Novolin N 30 units. Total units: _____
   a.
   b.

CHAPTER 9 Insulin Administration and Type 2 Diabetes Medications   325

5. Ordered: 10 units of Humalog and 38 units Humulin N ½ hr before breakfast.
Total units: _____

a.

Humalog / Hum N syringe

b.

Humalog / Hum N syringe

Shade in insulin dose on syringe. All orders are for U-100 insulin.

6. Ordered: Humulin R insulin 12 units and Humulin N 30 units every AM before breakfast. How many total units will you give? When will this peak? What is the duration?

7. Ordered: 10 units of Apidra before meals. Available: Apidra U-100. How many units will you give? When will the action begin (onset)?

8. Ordered: Fixed combination of Humulin 70/30, 44 units daily. Available: Humulin Fixed 70/30. How many units will you give? When will it peak? What is the duration?

9. Ordered: Novolin R 10 units and Novolin N 40 units subcutaneous every AM ½ hr before meals. How many total units will you give? What is the duration?

10. Ordered: 15 units of Novolog at 0830 before breakfast. Available: Novolog (aspart). How many units will you administer? When will it peak?

IV Insulin

During acute phases of illness, regular insulin is given by the IV route to ensure a controlled supply of medication that will vary depending on laboratory monitoring. A piggyback infusion is always administered with an IV-controlled infusion device. Discard the first 2 to 3 mL of combined infusion through IV tubing to prevent the insulin from binding to the tubing.

CLINICAL ALERT!
Only **clear regular** insulin can be used intravenously. Discard if cloudy (Figure 9–13).

FIGURE 9-13 **A,** Regular and Humalog (lispro), Novolog (aspart), and Apidra (glulisine) should always look clear. **B,** Insulin at the bottom of the bottle; do not use if insulin stays on the bottom of the bottle after gentle rolling. **C,** Clumps of insulin; do not use if there are clumps of insulin in the liquid or on the bottom of the vial. **D,** Bottle appears frosted; do not use if particles of insulin are on the bottom or sides of the bottle and give it a frosty appearance. (Copyright Eli Lilly and Company. All rights reserved. Used with permission.)

WORKSHEET 9D | IV Insulin Calculations

Answers on page 347

Answer questions 1 through 3 using Figure 9–14.

BG (mg/dL)	Std. Infusion Rate (units/hour)	☐ Stress Infusion Rate (units/hour)	☐ Customized (units/hour)
<80	0.2	0.2	_____
80-100	0.5	1.0	_____
101-140	1.0	2.0	_____
141-180	1.5	3.0	_____
181-220	2.0	4.0	_____
221-260	2.5	5.0	_____
261-300	3.0	6.0	_____
301-340	4.0	8.0	_____
>340	5.0	10.0	_____

FIGURE 9-14 Standard insulin infusion chart. (Modified from Scottsdale Healthcare, Scottsdale, Ariz.)

RULE Begin the problem with the known amount of medication in the total solution.

The pharmacy standard insulin drip: 100 units Human Regular in 100 mL of NS.

Example Ordered: Regular human insulin 5 units per hr IV drip. Pharmacy has delivered 100 mL 0.9% NS with 100 units of regular human insulin.
- How many mL per hr will infuse 5 units per hr?
- For how many hours will the IV infuse?

Step 1 KNOW   WANT TO KNOW   FRACTION CROSS PRODUCT

100 units : 100 mL = 5 units : x mL

$100x = 100 \times 5 = 500$

$100x = 500$

$x = 5$ mL per hr = 5 units of insulin

PROOF

$100 \times 5 = 500$

$100 \times 5 = 500$

Step 2 KNOW   WANT TO KNOW   FRACTION CROSS PRODUCT

5 mL : 1 hr = 100 mL : x hr

$5x = 100$

$x = 20$ hr

PROOF

$20 \times 5 = 100$

$1 \times 100 = 100$

1. The patient's BG level is 310 mg per dL at 0820 hr.
   a. At what rate will you set the IV infusion device?
   b. At 0920 hr the BG level is 270 mg per dL. What will be the rate for the IV infusion device?

2. The patient's blood glucose level is 235 mg per dL at 0400 hr.
   a. At what rate will you set the infusion rate?
   b. In 1 hour, the BG level is 270 mg per dL. What will be the new IV rate?
   c. At 0600 hr the physician called and inquired about the BG level. He asked how many units of insulin the patient had received since the IV was started. What will you tell the physician?

3. Your patient is receiving insulin IV. The standard rate of 100 units in 100 mL of NS is sent from the pharmacy. The BG q1h is as follows: 350 mg per dL, 330, 270, 210, 190, 165, 145, 120 mg per dL. How many total units has the patient received?

4. The pharmacy has sent 50 mL of NS with 100 units of insulin. The order is for 5 units per hr until the BG level is stable at 130 mg per dL.
   a. At how many mL per hr will you set the IV infusion device?
   b. It took 16 hours for the BG level to stabilize at 130 mg per dL. How many total units of insulin did the patient receive during the 16 hours?

5. Ordered: 100 units Human Regular insulin in 50 mL of NS to be infused at 3 mL per hr until the blood glucose level is stable at 120 mg per dL.
   a. How many units per hr will be delivered?
   b. If it took 8 hours for the blood glucose level to stabilize at 120 mg per dL, how many total units of insulin did the patient receive?

For Problems 6 through 10, calculate the following:
- **mL per hr necessary to infuse the ordered amount via an infusion device**
- **length of time the IV is to infuse**

6. Ordered: Humulin R IV at 10 units per hr. Available: 150 mL of 0.9% NS with 100 units Humulin (lispro) R insulin.

7. Ordered: Humulin R in 50 mL to infuse at 8 units per hr. Available: 50 mL 0.9% NS with 50 units Humulin R insulin.

8. Ordered: Humulin R in 50 mL to infuse at 12 units per hr. Available: 50 mL 0.9% NS with 75 units Humulin R insulin.

9. Ordered: 120 units Humulin R insulin IV at 10 units per hr. Available: 100 mL of NS 0.9% with 120 units Humulin R insulin.

10. Ordered: 150 units Humulin R insulin IV at 12 units per hr. Available: 150 mL of NS 0.9% with 150 units Humulin R insulin.

Frequent Blood Glucose Monitoring/Insulin Drip Record

Normal Blood Glucose M 75-110 mg/dL F 65-105 mg/dL

DATE 12/5/16

Time	Glucose (mg/dL)	Intervention Insulin (units/h) or other	Ketones S/M/L/Neg	Initial
00				
01				
02				
03		IV Insulin Drip Started		
04 15	350	5.0		JB
05 15	303	4.0		JB
06 15	310	4.0		JB
07 15	270	3.0		JB
08 15	180	1.5		JB
09 15	165	1.5		JB
10 15	150	1.5		JB
11				
12 15	140	1.0		JB
13 15	130	1.0		JB
14				
15 15	135	1.0		JB
16				
17 15	140	1.0		JB
18		Converted to Subcutaneous Insulin		
19				
20				
21				
22				
23				
Insulin Total Daily Dose (TDD)				

Initial	Signature
JB	J Booth

DATE

Time	Glucose (mg/dL)	Intervention Insulin (units/h) or other	Ketones S/M/L/Neg	Initial
00				
01				
02				
03				
04				
05				
06				
07				
08				
09				
10				
11				
12				
13				
14				
15				
16				
17				
18				
19				
20				
21				
22				
23				
Insulin Total Daily Dose (TDD)				

Initial	Signature

DATE

Time	Glucose (mg/dL)	Intervention Insulin (units/h) or other	Ketones S/M/L/Neg	Initial
00				
01				
02				
03				
04				
05				
06				
07				
08				
09				
10				
11				
12				
13				
14				
15				
16				
17				
18				
19				
20				
21				
22				
23				
Insulin Total Daily Dose (TDD)				

Initial	Signature

Original in Medical Chart   Copy to Pharmacy

Diabetes flow sheet. Note: IV insulin should always be used with an infusion device, never via gravity feed. (Modified from Scottsdale Healthcare, Scottsdale, Ariz.)

Oral Diabetes Medications

Oral diabetes medications (ODMs) are used to treat type 2 DM. They are taken alone or in combination with insulin. Blood glucose levels determine the strength of oral medication needed. ODMs are *not* insulin. Many ODMs are combinations of two types of drugs. Examples include: Prandimet, Janumet, and Xigduo XR. Other type 2 ODMs have a specific action, as listed in the table below.

Class	Brand Name	Generic Name	Action
Biguanides	Glucophage, Glucophage XR	metformin	Decreases amount of glucose made by the liver.
Meglitinides	Prandin, Starlix	repaglinide nateglitinide	Stimulates the pancreas to produce a quick burst of insulin, plus it decreases glucose production in the liver.
	Prandimet	metformin and repaglinide	
Sulfonylurea	Diabeta	glyburide	Stimulates pancreas to increase insulin production. These are sometimes used in conjunction with insulin injections.
	Amaryl	glimepiride	
	Glucotrol	glipizide	
Alpha-glucosidase inhibitors	Precose	acarbose	Slows the absorption of starches
	Glyset	miglitol	
DPP-4 inhibitors	Nestina	alogliptin	Stimulates insulin production when blood sugar rises. Boosts incretin gut hormone to help lower blood glucose.
	Onglyza	sazagliptin	
	Tradjenta	linagliptin	
	Januvia	sitagliptin	
	Janumet	sitagliptin and metformin	
SGLT 2 inhibitors	Jardiance	empagliflozin	Causes excess blood glucose to be excreted in urine. Stops glucose from getting reabsorbed by the kidneys.
	Invokana	canagliflozin	
	Farxiga	dapagliflozin	
	Farxiga and Glucophage	dapagliflozin and metformin	
Thiazolidinedones	Actos	pioglitazone	Makes body tissue more sensitive to insulin
	Avandia	rosiglitazone	

Oral Antidiabetic Drug Labels

Example The following are some examples of prescribers' orders for oral antidiabetics, along with the drug labels:

GLUCOPHAGE® (metformin hydrochloride tablets) 500 mg — 500 Tablets — NDC 0087-6060-10

Each tablet contains 500 mg of metformin hydrochloride. See enclosed package insert for dosage information. Caution: Federal law prohibits dispensing without prescription. Store between 15°–30° C (59°–86° F). Dispense in light resistant container. Glucophage is a registered trademark of LIPHA s.a. Licensed to Bristol-Myers Squibb Company. Distributed by Bristol-Myers Squibb Company, Princeton, NJ 08543 USA. 606010DRL-2 34-007102-01

Glucophage 500 mg PO tid with meals.

CHAPTER 9 Insulin Administration and Type 2 Diabetes Medications

Glucotrol XL 2.5 mg daily with breakfast.

Prandin 1 mg PO tid 30 minutes ac.

Insulin Infusion Devices

Nurses must understand how to care for patients who are admitted with insulin pumps. It is the nurse's responsibility to ascertain the patient's knowledge of pump management. Patients must be able to manage their diabetes, monitor their blood glucose level four times a day, calculate carbohydrate intake (grams), and determine when a bolus dose is needed. Many times the patient is admitted because of a lack of knowledge or lack of compliance with the regimen. Most hospitals do not keep a supply of insulin pumps or batteries for the pump; therefore, determine if the patient has made arrangements for these supplies.

An insulin pump is a battery-powered pump that delivers a continuous subcutaneous insulin infusion (CSII) (Figure 9-15). The pump is attached to an infusion set (Figure 9-16) that has a very fine-gauge cannula inserted subcutaneously in the abdomen and is attached to the insulin reservoir via tubing. The reservoir can hold either 150 units, or, more commonly, 300 units of U-100 rapid-acting insulin. Insulin pumps generally take only rapid or short-acting insulin. Ketoacidosis can develop quickly if the insulin is interrupted. Because of this significant risk, *the device must not be stopped or disconnected without supplemental insulin coverage.* If the insulin pump has to be disconnected for computerized tomography scans and magnetic resonance imaging tests, the blood sugar level should be checked before disconnecting and after reconnecting the pump. An insulin IV may be needed during the tests.

FIGURE 9-15 Paradigm Link blood glucose monitor and Paradigm 515 pump. (From Medtronic, Minneapolis, Minn.)

FIGURE 9-16 Quick-set infusion sets. (From Medtronic Diabetes, Northridge, Calif.)

When using insulin pumps, the blood glucose should be checked before meals and at bedtime. A continuous glucose monitoring (CGM) system device is a device worn by the patient to transmit glucose levels to the insulin pump. It is programmed to take blood glucose levels every 5 minutes. The blood glucose value is sent to the insulin pump, where the number is displayed.

Sensor glucose (SG) readings are taken from interstitial fluids. Fingersticks taken with the glucometer are taken from blood vessels. Therefore, the blood glucose (BG) level and the sensor level values are expected to be different. A big difference between the SG and the BG will most likely be after eating or exercising.

The patient will program the pump according to the basal rate set by the health care provider and the patient. If the basal rate is set correctly, the blood glucose should not fluctuate between meals. Basal rates are specific to each patient. They are set in units per hr. See Table 9-3, Basal Rates, Insulin Units Based on Required CHO Intake and Weight.

Insulin Dosage Based on Carbohydrate Intake

Because blood glucose levels fluctuate during the day (Figure 9-17), insulin doses should also fluctuate rather than being a constant dose every day. To keep the blood glucose level as close to the desired range as possible, carbohydrate intake must be calculated for each meal based on current blood glucose levels. This technique produces a more constant glucose level, which will help to minimize the detrimental effects of wide variations in blood glucose levels during the day. However, blood glucose levels must be measured before each meal and at bedtime. Usually, an insulin pump is used. If the carbohydrate ratio is high, the insulin pump can provide a bolus dose.

The health care provider will set a daily dose of long-acting insulin. For example, Lantus is used to cover blood glucose levels outside of meal times and is set for individualized parameters for each patient, depending on metabolic needs, such as exercise. The best type of diabetes management for some diabetics is the carbohydrate ratio technique, which is the closest way of replacing insulin made by the pancreas. A high level of compliance is needed for successful management. Rapid-acting insulin is used in the carbohydrate intake-to-weight ratio.

Week Starting / /	Sunday		Monday		Tuesday		Wednesday		Thursday		Friday		Saturday	
	Before	After	Before	After	Before	After	Before	After	Before	After	Before	After	Before	After
Breakfast	220	245												
Lunch	180	200												
Dinner	235	250												
Bed time	210													

Week Starting / /	Sunday		Monday		Tuesday		Wednesday		Thursday		Friday		Saturday	
	Before	After	Before	After	Before	After	Before	After	Before	After	Before	After	Before	After
Breakfast														
Lunch														
Dinner														
Bed time														

FIGURE 9-17 Preprandial and postprandial blood glucose level (BGL) Tracker

remember Blood glucose levels should be checked before meals and after meals for optimal diabetes control (see Figure 9-17).

Example Based on blood glucose level (BGL) and carbohydrate (CHO) intake.
- Desired blood glucose level is 130 mg per dL
- Order: Give 1 unit of insulin for every 15 mg per dL above 130 mg. Give 1 unit of insulin for every 10 g of CHO consumed.

Lunch	CHO
• ¾ cup of potato salad	21 g
• 2 slices of whole wheat bread	42 g
• 2 slices of Swiss cheese	2 g
• 2 slices of ham	2 g
• Mustard	1 g
• 1 12-oz. can of Pepsi	42 g
• Total	110 g CHO

Step 1 Desired BGL is 130 mg per dL. The BGL before lunch was 145 mg per dL. The difference between 130 and 145 is 15. The order states to give 1 unit of insulin for each 15 mg per dL above the desired 130 mg per dL. Therefore, 1 unit of insulin is required to treat the blood glucose level.

R & P Formula

15 mg : 1 unit = 15 mg : x units
15x = 15
x = 1 unit

Fraction Cross Product

$$\frac{15 \text{ mg}}{1 \text{ unit}} \times \frac{15 \text{ mg}}{x \text{ unit}}$$

Easy Method

Divide the BGL difference by the order.
15 divided by 15 = 1 unit

Step 2 Total CHO for lunch is 110 g
Order: give 1 unit of insulin for each 10 g of CHO consumed.

R & P Formula

10 g : 1 unit = 110 g : x units
10x = 110
x = 11 units
Round to nearest whole number.

Fraction Cross Product

$$\frac{10}{1} \times \frac{110}{x}$$

Easy Method

Divide the total grams of CHO by the order.
110 divided by 10 = 11 units

Give: 1 unit because the blood glucose level is above 15 g and give 11 units for the amount of CHO consumed. Give a total of 12 units of insulin.

Answers on page 348

WORKSHEET 9E: Insulin Dosage Based on CHO Intake

Use the following order to answer questions 1, 2, and 3. Round answers to the nearest whole number. Calculate the total number of insulin units required on the basis of the BGL and the CHO intake.

Ordered: BGL of 130 mg per dL is desired for this patient. Give 1 unit of insulin for each 10 mg above 130 mg. Give 1 unit of insulin for every 8 g of CHO consumed.

1. Breakfast   BGL is 150 mg per dL
   - ¾ cup Total cereal   CHO = 23 g
   - 8 oz. low-carb milk   3 g
   - ½ cup blueberries   1 g
   - 1 slice wheat toast   21 g
   - 1 pat butter   0 g
   - 1 cup black coffee   0 g
   - Total units _____

2. Lunch   BGL is 135 mg per dL
   - 8 oz. yogurt   CHO = 25 g
   - ⅓ cup dried cranberries   33 g
   - 2 apple slices   1 g
   - 5 grapes   1 g
   - 5 saltines   11 g
   - Plain iced tea   0 g
   - Total units _____

3. Dinner   BGL is 145 mg per dL
   - 1 pork chop   CHO = 0 g
   - ¾ cup mashed potatoes   34 g
   - ¾ cup broccoli   0 g
   - 8 oz. plain iced tea   0 g
   - Total units _____
   - Bedtime snack   BGL is 145 mg per dL
   - ¾ cup low-fat ice cream   CHO = 15 g
   - Total units _____

Use the following order to calculate the total insulin units in questions 4 and 5.

Ordered: The desired BGL is 140 mg per dL. Give 1 unit of insulin for every 10 mg above 140 mg per dL. Give 1 unit of insulin for every 10 g of CHO consumed.

4. Breakfast   BGL is 135 mg per dL
   - 2 eggs   CHO = 1 g
   - 2 slices wheat toast   42 g
   - 2 slices bacon   0 g
   - 2 cups black coffee   0 g
   - Total units _____

5. Lunch   BGL is 160 mg per dL
   - 4 oz. hamburger patty   CHO = 0 g
   - 1 hamburger bun   28 g
   - ½ cup cole slaw   20 g
   - 1 small serving fries   45 g
   - Total units _____

SAMPLE

Logbook Based on CHO Intake, BG and Insulin

Name: *John Doe* Start Date: 3-15-16 End Date:

Date	RC	24	1	2	3	4	5	6	7	8	9	10	11	12	13	14	15	16	17	18	19	20	21	22	23
						A.M. (Night/Morning)											P.M. (Afternoon/Evening)									
Mon	Blood Glucose									240					250				245				245		
	Carbs									150					130				140				15		
	Insulin Bolus									2					2				3				2		
	Total Daily Dose:												**Basal Dose:**												
Tues	Blood Glucose																								
	Carbs																								
	Insulin Bolus																								
	Total Daily Dose:												**Basal Dose:**												
Wed	Blood Glucose																								
	Carbs																								
	Insulin Bolus																								
	Total Daily Dose:												**Basal Dose:**												
Thurs	Blood Glucose																								
	Carbs																								
	Insulin Bolus																								
	Total Daily Dose:												**Basal Dose:**												
Fri	Blood Glucose																								
	Carbs																								
	Insulin Bolus																								
	Total Daily Dose:												**Basal Dose:**												
Sat	Blood Glucose																								
	Carbs																								
	Insulin Bolus																								
	Total Daily Dose:												**Basal Dose:**												
Sun	Blood Glucose																								
	Carbs																								
	Insulin Bolus																								
	Total Daily Dose:												**Basal Dose:**												
Ave	Blood Glucose																								
	Carbs																								
	Insulin Bolus																								
	Total Daily Dose:												**Basal Dose:**												

FIGURE 9-18 Logbook based on CHO intake, BG and Insulin

WORKSHEET 9F | Insulin Dosage Based on Blood Glucose and CHO Intake

Answers on page 349

Calculate the insulin requirements in questions 1, 2, and 3. The BGL readings and CHO requirements are based on the following orders. **Mark each syringe** with the total dose required.

Ordered: Give 1 unit of insulin for every 20 mg BGL above 160 mg per dL. Give 1 unit of insulin for every 15 g of CHO consumed.

1. BGL is 190 mg per dL; 98 g of CHO were consumed.
   How many total units of insulin are required?

2. BGL is 180 mg per dL; 40 g of CHO were consumed.
   How many total units of insulin are required?

3. BGL is 210 mg per dL; 118 g of CHO were consumed.
   How many total units of insulin are required?

Calculate the total insulin requirements in questions 4 through 7. The BGL reading and CHO requirements are based on the following orders. Mark each syringe with the total dose required.

Ordered: Give 1 unit of insulin for every 30 mg BGL above 150 mg per dL. Give 1 unit of insulin for every 10 g of CHO consumed.

4. BGL is 240 mg per dL; 58 g of CHO were consumed. How many total units of insulin are required?

338 Drug Calculations: *Ratio and Proportion Problems for Clinical Practice*

5. BGL is 180 mg per dL; 120 g of CHO were consumed. How many total units of insulin are required?

6. BGL is 260 mg per dL; 58 g of CHO were consumed. How many total units of insulin are required?

7. BGL is 160 mg per dL; 28 g of CHO were consumed. How many total units of insulin are required?

Sliding-Scale Calculations

Insulin administered according to a sliding scale is predicated on the blood glucose reading, the type of diabetes, insulin resistance, weight, age, renal status, and activity level. Blood glucose levels determine how much insulin to give. Blood glucose readings may be taken several times a day to determine daily insulin requirements. Sliding scales can vary greatly because they are individualized. Evidence-based computerized medical records information systems used in place of individualized sliding scales result in better glycemic control. The study was completed by the Department of Medicine, University of Washington, Seattle, WA, USA.

Example Ordered: Regular insulin q6h to follow the sliding scale.

Blood Sugar (mg per dL)	Low-Dose Scale
<70	Initiate Hypoglycemia Protocol
70-130	0 units
131-180	2 units
181-240	4 units
241-300	6 units
301-350	8 units
351-400	10 units
>400	12 units and call physician

Repeat blood glucose measurement 4 hr after it peaks.

At 1700 hr, the patient's blood glucose level was 168 mg per dL. How much regular insulin should be given? Shade the amount in the syringe.

Estimating Insulin-to-Carbohydrate Ratio

This formula is based on estimates of insulin needs according to CHO intake and weight. It is a simple formula that gives estimates for categories of weight based on Table 9-3. Also given is the kilogram ratio for the same number of pounds.

Example Breakfast = 44 CHO. The patient's weight is 165 lb. Refer to Table 9-3. The ratio is 1 unit of insulin to 11 g of CHO consumed.

R & P Method

1 unit : 11 CHO = x units : 44 CHO
$11x = 44$
$x = 4$ units of R insulin

Fraction Cross Product

$$\frac{1}{11} \times \frac{x}{44}$$

Total grams of CHO (Divided by) unit-to-CHO Ratio = Insulin Needs

44 (divided by) 11 = 4 units

Basal Rates

Table 9-3 Insulin Units Required Based on CHO Intake and Weight

Weight in Pounds	Weight in Kg	Unit: grams of CHO
100-109	45.5-49.5	1:16
110-129	50-58.6	1:15
130-139	59-63.2	1:14
140-149	63.6-67.7	1:13
150-159	68.2-72.3	1:12
160-169	72.7-76.8	1:11
170-179	77.3-81.4	1:10
180-189	81.8-85.9	1:9
190-199	86.4-90	1:8
200-239	90.9-108.6	1:7
240+	109.1+	1:6

Answers on page 350

WORKSHEET 9G: Insulin Dosage Based on CHO Intake and Weight

Calculate the insulin requirements for the following CHO intake related to the patient's weight. Refer to Table 9–3. Use either method shown in the example.

1. The patient ate 26 g CHO for breakfast. She weighs 142 lb. How many units of R are required?

2. The patient weighs 83 kg and ate 80 g CHO for lunch. How many units of R are required?

3. The patient ate 18 g CHO for lunch. She weighs 108 lb. How many units of R are required?

4. The patient consumed 90 g CHO for dinner and weighs 240 lb. How many units of R are required?

5. The patient weighs 162 lb. The total CHO intake during a 24-hour period was 160 g. How many units of R has the patient received in 24 hours?

6. The patient weighs 100 kg. The patient's total CHO intake during 24 hours was 145 g. How many units of R did she receive?

7. The physician calls at 1500 hours and wants to know how many total units of R his patient has received for the day. You calculate the following: breakfast included 45 g CHO, and he ate half of the CHO plus three quarters of his lunch, which had 72 g CHO. The patient weighs 190 lb. How many total units of R has the patient received?

8. You estimate that the patient ate half of his carbohydrates for lunch. The total CHO on his lunch menu was 50 g. His weight is 81 kg. How many units of R should he receive?

9. The patient weighs 70 kg. He has consumed 44 g CHO for breakfast, 72 g CHO for lunch, and 48 g CHO for dinner. His bedtime snack had 15 g CHO. What is the total amount of CHO the patient has consumed? What is the total amount of R he requires for the day?

10. Breakfast included 38 g CHO. The patient ate half of the CHO on the tray. Lunch included 50 g of CHO, and she ate one quarter of the CHO on the tray. Dinner included 48 g CHO, and she ate one third of the CHO. She weighs 112 lb. What is the total amount of CHO the patient has consumed? What is the total amount of R she requires for the three meals?

Answers on page 351

WORKSHEET 9H | Multiple-Choice Practice

Calculate units per hr, mL per hr, and hours to infuse.

1. The IV is infusing at 10 mL per hr. You have NS 250 mL with 100 units of R insulin. How many units per hr of insulin is the patient receiving?
   a. 8 units	b. 2 units	c. 10 units	d. 4 units

2. Using the units per hr in question 1, calculate how many hours it will take to infuse the 100 units of insulin.
   a. 50 hr	b. 25 hr	c. 15 hr	d. 5 hr

3. Ordered: 15 units of Lantus (glargine) subcutaneous. What is the length of effectiveness of the insulin?
   a. 12 hr	b. 4 hr	c. 36 hr	d. 24 hr

4. Ordered: 10 units of R insulin per hr IVPB. Available: 500 mL NS with 100 units of R insulin. At what rate will you set the IV infusion device?
   a. 50 mL per hr	b. 25 mL per hr	c. 100 mL per hr	d. 5 mL per hr

5. Ordered: 30 units of R insulin to be infused over 12 hr. Available: 50 mL NS with 30 units of insulin. How many units per hr will be infused?
   a. 1.5 units	b. 2.5 units	c. 5 units	d. 4 units

   At how many mL per hr will you set the infusion device?
   a. 4 mL per hr	b. 12 mL per hr	c. 41 mL per hr	d. 8 mL per hr

6. The type of insulin that is used for infusions is
   a. Humulin N	b. Levemir	c. Humulin R	d. Lantus

7. You have 100 mL of NS with 100 units of R insulin as an IVPB. The patient's BG level at 0600 is 300 mg per dL. Using the Standard Infusion Insulin Chart (see Figure 9–15), at what rate per hour will you start the IV?
   a. 5 mL per hr   b. 4 mL per hr   c. 3 mL per hr   d. 2.5 mL per hr

8. Ordered: Humulin N 20 units subcutaneous at 0730. When will it peak?
   a. 4-5 hr   b. 4-10 hr   c. 1-3 hr   d. 3-4 hr

9. Lantus (glargine) is the preferred insulin because it:
   a. peaks in 15 minutes   b. has a duration of 16 hr
   c. is absorbed quickly   d. is peakless

10. Lantus (glargine) is usually given subcutaneously:
    a. at breakfast   b. at bedtime   c. at midday   d. anytime

Critical Thinking Exercises

Critical Thinking Exercises provide math and medication-related patient safety issues for student discussion. Answers are not provided.
Analyze the following scenario.

1. Mr. Johnson's blood glucose level was 350 mg per dL. The orders on his chart read: Give 10 units of Humalog stat and check the BMBG in 1 hour. The nurse gave the insulin at 1400 hr. After the change of shift, at 1430 hr, Mr. Johnson was incoherent. On checking the Diabetes Flow Sheet the nurse found that Mr. Johnson had been given 1 mL (100 units) of Humalog.

   Ordered:

   Given:

   Error(s):

   ### Discussion

   What would be your immediate action?

   How did this error occur?

   How could this error have been prevented?

   Do you think the nurse should have known the safe dosage range?

   What were the potential injuries to the patient?

   How can a safety issue like this be reconciled?

2. Mrs. B. was admitted to the surgical unit through the emergency department with a diagnosis of diabetic ulceration on right ankle. She has used an insulin pump for over 1 year and said it works well for her as she is able to be more ambulatory and free from giving herself multiple daily injections. At the time of admission, she did not have any diabetic supplies to care for the insulin pump. At 1100 hr, she asked the nurse to fill the reservoir on her insulin pump. The nurse checked the order, which read: Fill reservoir with 3 mL of U-100 insulin PRN. After filling the reservoir, the nurse then inserted the reservoir into Mrs. B.'s infusion device. After the change of shift at 1600 hr, the evening nurse noticed that Mrs. B. looked flushed. Her skin was warm and dry, and her reflexes were slow. The nurse took her vitals and found: BP 90/75, respirations 14, pulse 60 and weak. The nurse detected a fruity odor to her breath. The reservoir on the insulin device showed 2.5 mL left. The nurse then tested Mrs. B.'s blood glucose and found it to be 400 mg per dL.

Discussion:
What would be your immediate action?
What error occurred?
Was the order specific?
Should the nurse have known the type of insulin to put in the reservoir?
How can this type of error be remediated to ensure patient safety?

3. After shoulder replacement surgery, Mr. H., who is a type 1 diabetic, returned to the surgical unit in your care. He has an IV with 100 units of insulin in 100 mL of 0.9% normal saline infusing at 4 units per hr and heparin IV infusing with 1000 units of heparin in 250 mL infusing at 10 mL per hr. The PACU nurse transferred the MAR and stated that Mr. H. had been given a 5000-unit bolus dose of heparin and 10 mg morphine 10 minutes ago. When taking his vitals, the assigned nurse noticed Mr. H.'s blood glucose level had escalated to 300 mg per dL, probably due to the stress of surgery. When the nurse contacted the physician by phone, the physician ordered a bolus of 20 units of insulin and then a recheck of the blood glucose level in 1 hour. The nurse wrote the order and had it checked by the supervisor, who initialed it as being a correct order. The assigned nurse proceeded to give the 20 units into the IV port as a bolus dose.

After 1 hour, the nurse checked the blood glucose level and found it to be 380 mg per dL. The nurse contacted the supervisor and the physician. The two nurses analyzed the situation and realized that the assigned nurse had given a bolus dose of 20 units of heparin in place of the insulin.
What would be your first action?
Insulin is a high-alert drug; therefore, what preventative measures should have been followed?
What are the potential serious consequences for the patient?

CHAPTER 9 Final

1. Ordered: Humalog insulin 15 units stat. Available: Humalog insulin.
   a. How many units will you give? 15

   b. Which syringe will give a precise measurement? Shade in correct amount.

2. The blood glucose level is 280. How many units of Regular insulin will you give subcutaneously? Use the sliding scale on page 339. 6 units

3. Ordered: Novolin R 16 units with Novolin N insulin 30 units at 0700. Shade in the amount of regular insulin. Shade in the amount of N insulin and label.

   clear — cloudy

   Novolin N   Novolin R

4. Ordered: Humalog 18 units before breakfast at 0930.
   a. How many units will you give? 18 units

   b. Which syringe is easier to read? → more distinction between units

344   Drug Calculations: Ratio and Proportion Problems for Clinical Practice

5. Ordered: Glucophage 850 mg tab and Novolin N 15 units before breakfast. How many total units will you give? Shade in the correct amount.

6. Ordered: 10 units per hr Novolin R insulin IV. Available: 500 mL 0.9% saline with 250 units Novolin R regular insulin.
   a. How many mL per hr will deliver 10 units per hr? ⟨20 mL/hr⟩
   b. How many hours will the IV infuse? ⟨25 hours⟩

$$\frac{250 \text{ units}}{500 \text{ mL}} = \frac{1 \text{ unit}}{2 \text{ mL}} \times \frac{1 \text{ hr}}{10 \text{ units}}$$

7. Ordered: 6 units per hr Novolin R IV. Available: 100 units Humulin R insulin in 250 mL of 0.9% saline.
   a. How many mL per hr will infuse 6 units of insulin? ⟨15 mL/hr⟩
   b. How many hours will the IV infuse? ⟨16.7 hours⟩

$$\frac{2 \text{ units}}{5 \text{ mL}} \times \frac{1 \text{ hr}}{6 \text{ units}}$$

8. Ordered: 8 units per hr Novolin R IV. Available: 250 mL NS with 100 units insulin.
   a. How many mL per hr will infuse 8 units of insulin? ⟨20 mL/hr⟩
   b. How many hours will the IV infuse? ⟨12.5 hours⟩

$$\frac{5 \text{ mL}}{2 \text{ units}} \cdot \frac{8 \text{ units}}{1 \text{ hr}} = \frac{40}{2} \quad \boxed{20 \text{ mL/hr}}$$

9. Ordered: 7 units per hr Novolin R IV. Available: 200 mL NS with 100 units Novolin R.
   a. How many mL per hr will infuse 7 units per hr?
   b. How many hours will the IV infuse? ⟨14.3 hours⟩

$$\frac{2 \text{ mL}}{1 \text{ unit}} \cdot \frac{7 \text{ units}}{\text{hr}} \quad \boxed{14 \text{ mL/hr}}$$

10. Ordered: Humulin R 9 units per hr IV. Available: 500 mL NS IV solution with 100 units Humulin R.
   a. How many mL per hr will infuse 9 units per hr?
   b. For how many hours will the IV infuse? ⟨11.1 hours⟩

$$\frac{9 \text{ units}}{1 \text{ hr}} \cdot \frac{5 \text{ mL}}{1 \text{ unit}} = \boxed{45 \text{ mL/hr}}$$

evolve Refer to the Advanced Calculations section of Drug Calculations, version 5 on Evolve for additional practice problems.

Answer Key

9 Insulin Administration and Type 2 Diabetes Medications

WORKSHEET 9A (page 316)

1. 27 units
2. 68 units
3. 16 units
4. 44 units
5. 32 units
6. 78 units
7. 42 units
8. 39 units
9. 23 units
10. 18 units

WORKSHEET 9B (page 319)

1. b
2. b
3. a
4. a
5. a

WORKSHEET 9C (page 324)

1. Total units: 68
   a is correct
   b insulins are reversed—drawn up incorrectly.
2. Total units: 39
   a is correct
3. Total units: 23
   a is correct
4. Total units: 38
   b is correct
5. Total units: 48
   b is correct
6. 42 units
   Peak: 2 to 4 hr for R
   Duration: 1 to 18 hr for N
7. 10 units
   Onset: 10 to 15 min
8. 44 units
   Peak: 2-10 hr
   Duration: 10 to 18 hr

346

9. 50 units
Duration: 10 to 18 hr

10. 15 units
Peak: 30-90 minutes

WORKSHEET 9D (page 328)

1. a. 4 units per hr
   b. 3 units per hr

2. a. KNOW WANT TO KNOW
100 units : 100 mL = 2.5 units : x mL
100x = 100 × 2.5 = 250
x = 2.5 mL/hr $\dfrac{100}{100} \times \dfrac{2.5}{x}$
PROOF
100 × 2.5 = 250
100 × 2.5 = 250
   b. Change IV rate to 3 mL/hr
   c. 5.5 units

3. 19 total units
Do not give insulin when BG is 120 mg per dL

4. a. KNOW WANT TO KNOW
50 mL : 100 units = x mL : 5 units
100x = 50 × 5 = 250
x = 2.5 mL/hr $\dfrac{50}{100} \times \dfrac{x}{5}$
PROOF
100 × 2.5 = 250
50 × 5 = 250
   b. 5 units per hour × 16 hours = 80 units of insulin

5. a. KNOW WANT TO KNOW
100 units : 50 mL = x units : 3 mL
50x = 100 × 3 = 300
x = 6 units/hr $\dfrac{100}{50} \times \dfrac{x}{3}$
PROOF
100 × 3 = 300
50 × 6 = 300
   b. 8 hr × 6 units per hr = 48 units

6. KNOW WANT TO KNOW
100 units : 150 mL = 10 units : x mL
100x = 150 × 10 = 1500
100x = 1500 $\dfrac{100}{150} \times \dfrac{10}{x}$
x = 15 mL/hr = 10 units insulin
PROOF
100 × 15 = 1500
150 × 10 = 1500
KNOW WANT TO KNOW
15 mL : 1 hr = 150 mL : x hr
15x = 150 $\dfrac{15}{1} \times \dfrac{150}{x}$
x = 10 hr to infuse 100 units insulin
PROOF
15 × 10 = 150
1 × 150 = 150

7. KNOW WANT TO KNOW
50 mL : 50 units = x mL : 8 units
50x = 50 × 8 = 400
50x = 400
 x = 8 mL/hr = 8 units of insulin

$\dfrac{50}{50} \times \dfrac{x}{8}$

PROOF
50 × 8 = 400
50 × 8 = 400

KNOW WANT TO KNOW
8 mL : 1 hr = 50 mL : x hr
8x = 50
 x = 6.25 hr to infuse 50 units insulin or 6 hr 15 min

$\dfrac{8}{1} \times \dfrac{50}{x}$

PROOF
8 × 6.25 = 50
1 × 50 = 50

8. KNOW WANT TO KNOW
50 mL : 75 units = x mL : 12 units
75x = 50 × 15 = 750
75x = 600
 x = 8 mL/hr = 12 units

$\dfrac{50}{75} \times \dfrac{x}{12}$

PROOF
50 × 15 = 750
75 × 10 = 750

KNOW WANT TO KNOW
10 mL : 1 hr = 50 mL : x hr
10x = 50
 x = 5 hours to infuse

$\dfrac{10}{1} \times \dfrac{50}{x}$

PROOF
1 × 50 = 50
10 × 5 = 50

9. KNOW WANT TO KNOW
100 mL : 120 units = x mL : 10 units
120x = 100 × 10 = 1000
120x = 1000
 x = 8.33 mL/hr to deliver 10 units of insulin

$\dfrac{100}{120} \times \dfrac{x}{10}$

PROOF
120 × 8.33 = 999.6
100 × 10 = 1000

KNOW WANT TO KNOW
8 mL : 1 hr = 100 mL : x hr
8x = 1 × 100 = 100
8x = 100
 x = 12.5 hr to infuse 120 units of regular insulin

$\dfrac{8}{1} \times \dfrac{100}{x}$

PROOF
8 × 12.5 = 100
1 × 100 = 100

10. KNOW WANT TO KNOW
150 mL : 150 units = x mL : 12 units
150x = 150 × 12
150x = 1800
 x = 12 mL/hr to deliver 12 units of insulin

$\dfrac{150}{150} \times \dfrac{x}{12}$

PROOF
150 × 12 = 1800
12 × 150 = 1800

KNOW WANT TO KNOW
12 mL : 1 hr = 150 mL : x hr
12x = 150
 x = 12.5 hr to infuse 150 units of regular insulin, or 12 hr 30 min

$\dfrac{12}{1} \times \dfrac{150}{x}$

12 × 12.5 = 150
1 × 150 = 150

WORKSHEET 9E (page 336)

1. BGL difference is 20 divided by 10 = 2 units of R
 CHO is 48 g divided by 8 = 6 units R
 Total units = 8

2. BGL difference is 5 divided by 10 = 0.5 = 1 unit R (rounded to nearest whole number)
 CHO is 71 g divided by 8 = 8.87 = 9 units R
 Total units = 10

3. BGL difference is 15 divided by 10 = 1.5 = 2 units R
 CHO is 34 g divided by 8 = 4.25 = 4 units R
 Total units = 6

 Snack: BGL difference is 15 divided by 10 = 1.5 = 2 units R
 CHO is 15 g divided by 8 = 1.87 = 2 units R
 Total insulin for the day = 28 units

348 Answer Key

4. BGL difference is −5 = 0 units R
CHO is 43 g divided by 10 = 4.3 = 4 units R
Total units = 4

5. BGL difference is 20 divided by 10 = 2 units
CHO is 93 g divided by 10 = 9.3 = 9 units R
Total units = 11

WORKSHEET 9F (page 338)

1. BGL difference is 30 divided by 20 = 1.5 = 2 units R
CHO is 98 g divided by 15 = 6.5 = 7 units R
Total = 9 units R

2. BGL difference is 20 divided by 20 = 1 = 1 unit R
CHO is 40 g divided by 15 = 2.6 = 3 units R
Total = 4 units R

3. BGL difference is 50 divided by 20 = 2.5 = 3 units R
CHO is 118 g divided by 15 = 7.8 = 8 units R
Total = 11 units R

4. BGL difference is 90 divided by 30 = 3 units R
CHO is 58 g divided by 10 = 5.8 = 6 units R
Total = 9 units R

5. BGL difference is 30 divided by 30 = 1 unit R
CHO is 120 g divided by 10 = 12 units R
Total = 13 units R

6. BGL difference is 110 divided by 30 = 3.6 = 4 units R
CHO is 58 g divided by 10 = 5.8 = 6 units R
Total = 10 units R

7. BGL difference is 10 divided by 30 = 0.3 = 0 units R
CHO is 28 g divided by 10 = 2.8 = 3 units R
Total = 3 units R

8. BGL difference is 10 divided by 20 = 0.5 = 1 unit R
CHO is 45 g divided by 8 = 5.6 = 6 units R
Total = 7 units R

9. BGL difference is 30 divided by 20 = 1.5 = 2 units R
CHO is 80 g divided by 8 = 10 units R
Total = 12 units R

10. BGL difference is −10 = 0 units R
CHO is 85 g divided by 8 = 10.6 = 11 units R
Total = 11 units R

WORKSHEET 9G (page 340)

1. $\dfrac{\text{total g}}{\text{units}} = \dfrac{26}{13} = 2$ units R

2. $\dfrac{\text{total g}}{\text{units}} = \dfrac{80}{9} = 8.8 = 9$ units R

3. $\dfrac{\text{total g}}{\text{units}} = \dfrac{18}{16} = 1.1 = 1$ unit R

4. $\dfrac{\text{total g}}{\text{units}} = \dfrac{90}{6} = 15$ units R

5. $\dfrac{\text{total g}}{\text{units}} = \dfrac{160}{11} = 14.5$ units = 15 units R for 24 hr

6. $\dfrac{\text{total g}}{\text{units}} = \dfrac{145}{7} = 20.7 = 21$ units R for 24 hr

7. $\dfrac{1}{2}$ of 45 = 22.5 + $\dfrac{3}{4}$ of 75 = 56.25 = 78.75; 78.75 ÷ 8 = 9.8 = 10 units R

8. 50 g divided by 2 = $\dfrac{25 \text{ g}}{10}$ = 2.5 = 3 units R

9. Total amount of CHO = 179 g

   $\frac{179}{12}$ = 14.9 = 15 units for the day

10. $\frac{1}{2}$ of 38 = 19 g; $\frac{1}{4}$ of 50 = 12.5 g; $\frac{1}{3}$ of 48 = 16 g

    Total CHO grams = 47.5 = 3 units total for the 3 meals

WORKSHEET 9H (page 341)

1. d. 4 units
KNOW   WANT TO KNOW
250 mL : 100 units = 10 mL : x units
250x = 100 × 10 = 1000
    x = 4 units/hr $\frac{250}{100} \times \frac{10}{x}$
PROOF
250 × 4 = 1000
100 × 10 = 1000

2. b. 25 hr
KNOW   WANT TO KNOW
4 units : 1 hr = 100 units : x hr
4x = 100
    x = 25 hr $\frac{4}{1} \times \frac{100}{x}$
PROOF
1 × 100 = 100
4 × 25 = 100

3. d. 24 hr

4. a. 50 mL/hr
KNOW   WANT TO KNOW
500 mL : 100 units = x mL : 10 units
100x = 500 × 10 = 5000
    x = 50 mL/hr $\frac{500}{100} \times \frac{x}{10}$
PROOF
100 × 50 = 5000
500 × 10 = 5000

5. b. 2.5 units/hr
KNOW   WANT TO KNOW
30 units : 12 hr = x units : 1 hr
12x = 30
    x = 2.5 units/hr $\frac{30}{12} \times \frac{x}{1}$
PROOF
30 × 1 = 30
12 × 2.5 = 30

a. 4 mL/hr
50 mL : 12 hr = x mL : 1 hr
12x = 50
    x = 4.16 = 4 mL/hr $\frac{50}{12} \times \frac{x}{1}$
PROOF
50 × 1 = 50
12 × 4.16 = 4.9

6. c. Humulin R

7. c. 3 mL/hr
KNOW   WANT TO KNOW
100 units : 100 mL = 3 units : x mL
100x = 100 × 3 = 300
    x = 3 mL/hr $\frac{100}{100} \times \frac{3}{x}$
PROOF
100 × 3 = 300
100 × 3 = 300

8. b. 4 to 10 hr

9. d. is peakless

10. b. at bedtime

CHAPTER 9 FINAL: INSULIN ADMINISTRATION AND TYPE 2 DIABETES MEDICATIONS (page 344)

1. 15 units
   b

2. Sliding scale
   Give 6 units.

3. 16 units Humulin R
   30 units Humulin N
   Total amount is 46 units.

4. 18 units Humalog
   b is easier to read

5. 15 units Novolin N

6. 20 mL per hr = 10 units
   25 hr to infuse. An IV solution can hang for only 24 hr (CDC guidelines).

7. 15 mL per hr to infuse 6 units insulin
   16.6 hr to infuse = 16 hr 36 min

8. 20 mL per hr to infuse 8 units insulin
   12.5 hr to infuse = 12 hr 30 min

9. 14 mL per hr to infuse 7 units insulin
   14.28 hr to infuse = 14 hr 17 min

10. 45 mL per hr to infuse 9 units insulin
    11.1 hr to infuse = 11 hr 6 min

Parenteral Nutrition

Objectives
- Calculate grams of protein, dextrose, and lipids per order.
- Calculate the percentage of protein, dextrose, and lipids per infusion.
- Discuss the reasons different concentrations of additives are used in peripheral and central lines.
- Calculate the kilocalories for protein, dextrose, and lipids per infusion.
- Calculate the total kilocalories per infusion.
- Compare the ordered amount of parenteral nutrition with the infusion label.
- Analyze medication errors using critical thinking.

Introduction The IV requirements for patients who are unable to ingest food and fluid are calculated on a daily basis. Concentrations of nutrients are calculated to show the differing strengths and percentages of additives for peripheral and central lines. The percentage of additives is calculated to ensure that the electrolyte and mineral requirements are being met. Standard orders for peripheral and central lines are compared. The importance of parenteral orders and of verification of the labels on the bag is stressed.

Vocabulary **AA:** Amino acids or protein.

CHO: Dextrose or sugar.

CPN: Nutrition delivered by central (venous) parenteral infusion.

Diabetes Mellitus (DM): A chronic metabolic disorder resulting in hyperglycemia caused by inadequate production of insulin by the islets of Langerhans in the pancreas.

Diabetic Ketoacidosis (DKA): A complication of diabetes diagnosed by elevated blood glucose (above 250 mg per dL), elevated ketones in the blood and urine and a blood pH below 7.3; this condition is an emergency because death may result.

Glucagon: A hormone produced by the beta cells of the islets of Langerhans in the pancreas that increases the blood glucose level by stimulating the liver to convert stored glycogen to glucose. Used to reverse hypoglycemia and insulin shock by opposing the action of insulin.

Home Parenteral Nutrition (HPN): Peripheral or central nutrition administered in the home.

Hyperglycemia: Blood glucose level above the basic normal values of 80 to 120 mg per dL.

Hypoglycemia: Blood glucose level below 70 mg per dL.

Insulin Shock: Blood sugar level below 60 mg per dL (hypoglycemia) caused by too much insulin in the blood. Treated by giving glucose orally or intravenously, depending on the patient's condition.

Kcal: A unit of energy; 1 kcal = 1000 small calories = 1 calorie USA.

Liposyn: A prepared intravenous fat emulsion.

PICC: Peripherally inserted central (venous) catheter.

PPN: Nutrition delivered by peripheral (venous) parenteral infusion.

TPN: Total parenteral nutrition; the venous administration of dextrose, amino acids, lipids, electrolytes, and vitamins.

Type 1 DM: failure of the pancreas to produce insulin.

Type 2 DM: Inadequate insulin secretion or insulin resistance due to decrease sensitivity of muscle cells to uptake insulin.

Total Parenteral Nutrition

Nutritional support of the sick patient in the hospital as well as in the home has become increasingly important. More people are being treated with total parenteral nutrition (TPN) in the home, and it is the nurse's responsibility to teach the patient and the family to care for the catheter insertion site and the infusion pump, and to educate them about possible side effects of the infusion. Survival of the patient with a gastrointestinal problem has been made possible by advances in the field of parenteral nutrition.

TPN permits the venous administration of dextrose, amino acids, lipids, electrolytes, and vitamins to sustain life when the gastrointestinal system must be bypassed or during serious illness or injury (e.g., burns). A TPN bag is shown in Figure 10-1.

FIGURE 10-1 TPN bag. The content label will be put on the bag by the pharmacist.

CLINICAL ALERT!

Medication incompatibility can occur when IV drugs are delivered along with TPN administration. A pharmacist with special training in intravenous TPN should be consulted to determine compatibility. A dedicated PICC line, Groshong catheter, Hickman/Broviac port should be established.

A, Hickman catheter. **B,** Broviac catheter. **C,** Groshong catheter. (From Clayton BD, Willihnganz MJ: *Basic pharmacology for nurses,* ed. 16, St. Louis, 2013, Elsevier.)

A routine maintenance IV solution of 1000 mL with 5% dextrose delivered over an 8-hour period provides approximately 200 calories derived from dextrose. If a patient is restricted from ingesting anything by mouth (NPO, npo) and receives 3 liters of D5W a day, the 600 total calories received would not be enough to promote or maintain health for a sustained period. In contrast, TPN may deliver as much as 1 calorie per mL, depending on the concentration of nutrients.

TPN administered via a central vein such as the subclavian or internal jugular is known as *central parenteral nutrition (CPN)*. Peripheral administration, known as *peripheral parenteral nutrition (PPN)*, is delivered via peripheral veins. The choice depends on the patient, vein condition, and how long the patient will need the therapy. The larger central veins are selected for longer-term therapy and higher concentration of nutrients. The contents of TPN are customized according to the patient's condition and need, the venous route, relevant laboratory values, and the patient's weight. Orders for the contents may be changed daily. TPN formulas are specific to the patient and are determined by the individual's energy, protein, fluid, and caloric requirements. Special formulas are created for patients with diabetes, renal or hepatic problems, bowel obstruction, or pancreatitis. This list is not all inclusive.

PPN is used for nutritional therapy lasting 2 weeks or less. A PPN solution must be kept at the following concentration levels to prevent vein irritation: amino acids, 5.5%; dextrose, 10%; lipids, 10%. CPN permits higher levels of concentration because it is infused into larger veins. CPN solutions are hypertonic and have higher osmolarity. CPN is used when nutritional therapy is needed for more than 2 weeks. CPN concentrations usually are as follows: amino acids, 8.5%; dextrose, 20% to 70%; lipids, 20%. Dextrose administered with amino acids spares the protein for tissue repair. Parenteral nutrition must always be administered by an infusion pump—**never** by gravity.

A three-in-one solution, or total nutrition admixture, combines lipids, amino acids, and dextrose. The solution is white because of the lipids, which make precipitation difficult to observe. The three-in-one solution is used for both hospital and home therapy. When lipids are administered with dextrose and amino acids, the osmolarity of the solution will improve the tolerance for peripheral venous administration. Lipids are isotonic because of added glycerol and can therefore be administered either peripherally or centrally. Lipids can also be administered separately (Figure 10-2). Lipids help control hyperglycemia, which is a complication of parenteral nutrition. After 12 hours, lipids may become unstable. If a fat embolus could be a problem, monitor the patient closely. Amino acids, vitamins, and other life-supporting additives are easily denigrated when exposed to sunlight. Home therapy TPN is usually run for 12 hours to give the patient some infusion-free time.

FIGURE 10-2 A, Liposyn II (fat emulsion) 20% for parenteral nutrition. Notice the opaque contents contrasted with the parenteral infusion without lipids (fat emulsion). **B,** Fat emulsion (lipid) order. (**A,** From Abbott Laboratories, Abbott Park, Ill.)

Types of IV Lines

There are many types of IV tubing used for temporary and long-term access to veins and arteries (Figure 10-3).
- **Peripheral** A peripheral line is usually used for fluid replacement and temporary intermittent medication administration. The IV line is inserted in the hand, arm, or possibly leg if the hand or arm cannot be accessed. Foot and scalp sites are used for infants.
- **Peripherally inserted central catheter (PICC)** A PICC line (Figure 10-4) is longer than a central catheterline (approximately 22 inches in length). The insertion point is usually the vein in the antecubital region of the arm, where the line is then advanced into the superior vena cava. It is inserted by a PICC-certified RN or physician. Only solutions with an osmolarity of less than 10% should be administered via peripheral lines.

FIGURE 10-3 Central venous access sites. **A,** Subclavian catheter. **B,** Peripherally inserted central catheter (PICC). **C,** Femoral catheter. **D.** Hickman catheter. **E,** Subclavian catheter with implantable vascular access port. **F,** Implantable vascular access port. (**F,** from Perry AG, Potter PA: *Clinical nursing skills and techniques,* ed. 6, St. Louis, 2006, Mosby.)

A Subclavian Catheter Site
B Peripherally Inserted Central Catheter (PICC)
C Femoral Catheter Site
D Hickman Catheter Site
E Subclavian Catheter with Implantable Vascular Access Port
F Implantable Vascular Access Port

FIGURE 10-4 Peripherally inserted central catheter (PICC). The double-lumen catheter is used to draw blood samples. (From Perry AG, Potter PA: *Clinical nursing skills and techniques,* ed. 7, St. Louis, 2010, Mosby.)

CHAPTER 10   Parenteral Nutrition   357

- **Central line** A central line (Figure 10-5) is inserted directly into the jugular or subclavian vein and then into the superior vena cava. This type of line is for therapy requiring a longer period of time or when a peripheral line is not possible. The femoral vein may also be used as a central line site.

FIGURE 10-5 Central line with a mediport. (From Perry AG, Potter PA: *Clinical nursing skills and techniques,* ed. 7, St. Louis, 2010, Mosby.)

CLINICAL ALERT!
Only solutions with an osmolarity of less than 10% should be administered via peripheral lines.

Table 10-1 is a guide that can be used to maintain patency by flushing intermittent-access locks. Always refer to manufacturer's insert or hospital protocol for type of solution, volume, and frequency.

Table 10-1 Intermittent Flushing Ranges

Catheter	Flush Solution	Volume
Peripheral	Normal saline	1-3 mL
Peripherally inserted central catheter (PICC)	Normal saline	3-5 mL
Central venous	Heparinized saline	5-10 mL of saline followed with 3 mL heparin 1:100 units per mL

CLINICAL RELEVANCE
When flushing peripheral IV lines, prefilled sterile normal saline should be used. The syringe should be twice the volume of the solution. Smaller syringes may create greater pressure within the IV line, causing damage to the vein.

Automatic dose calculators (Figure 10-6) or electronic infusion devices (EIDs) are programmed by the patient's caregiver to deliver lipids and parenteral nutrition at the accurate mL per hour ordered. Gravity infusion tubing should ***never*** be used because the rate could fluctuate and harm the patient.

FIGURE 10-6 Automatic dose calculation device showing lipid infusing. (From Perry AG, Potter PA, Ostendorf WR: *Clinical nursing skills and techniques,* ed. 8, St. Louis, 2014, Mosby.)

A tunneled catheter is surgically inserted into a vein in the neck or chest and passes under the skin (Figure 10-7). This type of catheter allows freedom of movement for the patient during long-term parenteral nutrition.

FIGURE 10-7 Tunneled catheter used for central parenteral nutrition given at home. (From Perry AG, Potter PA: *Clinical nursing skills and techniques,* ed. 8, St. Louis, 2013, Mosby.)

Validation of TPN Label With the Physician's Order

Validate the contents listed on the TPN bag label (Figure 10-8) with the physician's order (Figure 10-9).

The 341 mL of qsad (quantity sufficient additive) sterile water includes the volume for the additives of calcium gluconate, magnesium sulfate, potassium phosphate, sodium chloride, and multivitamins. In this order, the pharmacist included all of the additives except for the 10 units of insulin, which the nurse will add immediately before administering the bag of TPN.

```
                TPN Bag label
          HOME INFUSION PHARMACY

RX#37856

AMINO*ACIDS 10%=425ML DEXTROSE*70%=357ML
STER*WATER=341ML LIPIDS*20%=125ML
MVI=10ML/DAY *ADDITIVES PER LITER*
SOD*CHLOR=35mEq POT*PHOS=15mM CALCIUM=5mEq
MAGNESIUM=5mEq

QTY#       TPN 40-51GM PROTEIN+LIPIDS
INFUSE NIGHTLY 8PM TO 8AM THRU IV PICC LINE
VIA SIGMA PUMP. *****ADD 10 UNITS
HUMULIN-R TO EACH BAG JUST PRIOR TO
INFUSION***** **NOTE:CONTAINS TPN
SOLN+LIPIDS:RATE ADJUSTED** SETTINGS:
RATE=104ML/HR VOLUME=1248ML
          *** REFRIGERATE ***

EXPIRATION DATE:01/06/17
```

FIGURE 10-8 TPN bag label. It is the nurse's responsibility to check the label on the TPN bag with the physician's order. Quantities of nutrients and additives are calculated based on 1 liter. The total volume (TV) is calculated by adding the amount over 1 liter as a decimal (e.g., 1248 mL = 1.248 L).

CLINICAL ALERT!

It is the nurse's responsibility to check the physician's order to determine if the pharmacy has filled the order according to the directions. Compare the order shown in Figure 10-9 with the label shown in Figure 10-8.

Example Refer to Figure 10-9, a sample physician's order form.

Calculate grams, percentage of concentration, and kilocalories per bag of TPN.

TPN ORDER SHEET

HOME HEALTH
DATE
PATIENT
ADDRESS

TPN FORMULA:

AMINO ACIDS: ☐ 5.5% ☐ 8.5% ☑ 10%	425 mL
☐ WITH STANDARD ELECTROLYTES	
DEXTROSE: ☐ 10% ☐ 20% ☐ 40% ☐ 50% ☑ 70% (check one)	357 mL
LIPIDS: ☐ 10% ☑ 20% FOR ALL-IN-ONE FORMULA	125 mL

FINAL VOLUME qsad STERILE WATER FOR INJECTION *400 mL*	1248 mL

Calcium Gluconate	0.465 mEq/mL	5 mEq
Magnesium Sulfate	4 mEq/mL	5 mEq
Potassium Acetate	2 mEq/mL	___ mEq
Potassium Chloride	2 mEq/mL	___ mEq
Potassium Phosphate	3 mM/mL	15 mM
Sodium Acetate	2 mEq/mL	___ mEq
Sodium Chloride	4 mEq/mL	35 mEq
Sodium Phosphate	3 mM/mL	___ mM
TRACE ELEMENTS CONCENTRATE	☐ 4 ☐ 5 ☐ 6	___ mL

Patient Additives:
- ☐ MVC 9 + 3 10 mL Daily
- ☐ HUMULIN-R __10__ units DAILY
- ☐ FOLIC ACID _____ mg _____ times weekly
- ☐ VITAMIN K _____ mg _____ times weekly
- ☐ OTHER: *MVI 10 mL/daily*
- ☐ OTHER: _____

Directions:

INFUSE: ☐ DAILY
☐ _____ TIMES WEEKLY

OTHER DIRECTIONS:
_____
_____
_____
_____

Rate:
- ☐ CYCLIC INFUSION: OVER ____ HOURS (TAPER UP AND DOWN)
- ☐ CONTINUOUS INFUSION: AT ____ mL PER HOUR
- ☑ STANDARD RATE: AT __104__ mL PER HOUR FOR __12__ HOURS

LAB ORDERS:

☐ STANDARD LAB ORDERS
SMAC-20, CO2, Mg+2 TWICE WEEKLY
CBC WITH AUTO DIFF WEEKLY
UNTIL STABLE, THEN:
SMAC-20, CO2, Mg+2 WEEKLY
CBC WITH AUTO DIFF MONTHLY

☐ OTHER: _____

VALIDATION:

_____
DOCTOR'S SIGNATURE

Print Name: _____
Office Address: _____
Phone: _____

WHITE: Home Health CANARY: Physician

FIGURE 10-9 Sample physician's order for Worksheet 10A.

Total Grams per Bag

Formula: % × mL = g/L

Step 1
Amino acids (AA) 10% in 425 mL
0.10 × 425 = 42.5 g/L

Formula g/L × TV*/L = g/bag

Step 2
42.5 g/L × 1.248 TV/L = 53 g/bag
There are 53 g of AA in 1248 mL of TPN

Shortcut method: % × mL = g/L × TV/L = g/bag
AA 10% in 425 mL
0.10 × 425 = 42.5 g/L × 1.248 TV/L = 53 g of AA in the bag

Shortcut method: % × mL = g/L × TV/L = g/bag

Dextrose 70% in 357 mL
0.70 × 357 = 250 g/L × 1.248 TV/L = 312 g of dextrose per bag

Shortcut method: % × mL = g/L × TV/L = g/bag

Lipids 20% in 125 mL

Step 1   **Step 2**
0.20 × 125 = 25 g/L × TV/L 1.248 ml = 31.2 g/bag
There are 31.2 g of lipids in 1248 mL per bag

Percentage of Amino Acids, Dextrose, and Lipids per Bag

Formula: $\dfrac{g/bag}{TV} = \%/bag$

AA $\dfrac{53}{1248} = 0.042 = 4.2\%$ of bag is AA (PRO)

Dextrose $\dfrac{312}{1248} = 0.250 = 25\%$ of bag is dextrose (CHO)

Lipids $\dfrac{31.2}{1248} = 0.0250 = 2.5\%$ of bag is lipids (FAT)

Percentage of Additives

Formula: **Step 1**   mEq/L × TV/L = mEq/bag
                     Step 2   mEq/bag ÷ TV = % in bag
Shortcut method: mEq/L × TV/L ÷ TV = % in bag
Calcium gluconate   5 mEq × 1.248 TV = 6.24 mEq/bag
                                  6.24 ÷ 1248 TV = 6.24 mEq in bag
Magnesium sulfate   5 mEq × 1.248 TV = 6.24 ÷ 1248 = 0.5% in bag
Potassium phosphate   15 mEq × 1.248 TV = 18.72 ÷ 1248 = 1.5% in bag
Sodium chloride   35 mEq × 1.248 TV = 43.68 ÷ 1248 = 3.5% in bag

A milliequivalent (mEq) is a measurement of weight that represents 1000th of a gram.

mL per Hour to Set the Pump

$\dfrac{TV}{Total\ Time\ (hr)} = mL\ per\ hr$ $\dfrac{1248}{12} = 104\ mL\ per\ hr$

TV, Total volume.

Kilocalories (kcal) per Bag

Formula: kcal/g × g/bag = kcal/bag
1 g CHO = 4 kcal   312 g × 4 kcal = 1248 kcal of CHO
1 g PRO = 4 kcal   53 g × 4 kcal = 212 of PRO
1 g FAT = 9 kcal   31.2 g × 9 kcal = __281__ kcal of FAT
                    Total kcal =   1741 per bag of TPN

CLINICAL ALERT!
Begin TPN at a slow rate of 40 to 60 mL per hour and gradually increase by 25 mL per hour every 6 hours to the ordered rate, according to hospital protocol. Maintain a steady rate of infusion (within 10% of the ordered dose) to reduce the chance of a sudden onset of hyperglycemia. TPN should never be abruptly stopped because this may precipitate sudden, severe hypoglycemia.

CLINICAL RELEVANCE
- Patients receiving TPN must be monitored for hyperglycemia and serum potassium level as well as for all electrolytes.
- The TPN and lipid administration set should be changed every 24 hours. When administering lipids only, change tubing every 12 hours.
- The fat emulsions filter should be a 1.2-micron size.
- The TPN and lipid solutions should be refrigerated at 39° F or 4° C until time of administration.
- TPN solutions should be filtered with a 0.22-micron filter.
- It is not recommended to administer other medications via the Y port line or piggyback before consulting with the pharmacist for compatibility. There can be many metabolic complications as the result of the type of additives in the TPN solution.

CLINICAL ALERT!
The admixture of fat emulsions with the dextrose and amino acids may produce bacterial growth. Discard the solution after 24 hours.

Answers on page 374

WORKSHEET 10A | Central Parenteral Nutrition Calculations

Use Figure 10-10 to answer the following questions.

1. What are the total grams per bag of:
   a. Amino acids (AA)
   b. Dextrose
   c. Lipids

2. What are the percentages of concentration per bag of:
   a. AA
   b. Dextrose
   c. Lipids

3. How many kilocalories are there per bag of:
   a. CHO
   b. PRO
   c. FAT
   d. What is the total number of kilocalories per bag?

4. For how many mL per hour will you set the infusion device?

5. 1500 mL of D50W provides how many grams of dextrose?

A sample MAR for parenteral nutrition is shown in Figure 10-11.

TPN ORDER SHEET

HOME HEALTH
DATE _____

PATIENT _____ ADDRESS _____

TPN FORMULA:

AMINO ACIDS: ☐ 5.5% ☐ 8.5% ☑ 10% ☐ WITH STANDARD ELECTROLYTES		**425** mL
DEXTROSE: ☐ 10% ☐ 20% ☐ 40% ☐ 50% ☑ 70% (check one)		**357** mL
LIPIDS: ☐ 10% ☑ 20% FOR ALL-IN-ONE FORMULA		**125** mL

FINAL VOLUME		
qsad STERILE WATER FOR INJECTION **400 mL**		**1307** mL

Calcium Gluconate	0.465 mEq/mL	**5** mEq
Magnesium Sulfate	4 mEq/mL	**5** mEq
Potassium Acetate	2 mEq/mL	___ mEq
Potassium Chloride	2 mEq/mL	___ mEq
Potassium Phosphate	3 mM/mL	**22** mM
Sodium Acetate	2 mEq/mL	___ mEq
Sodium Chloride	4 mEq/mL	**35** mEq
Sodium Phosphate	3 mM/mL	___ mM
TRACE ELEMENTS CONCENTRATE	☐ 4 ☐ 5 ☐ 6	___ mL

Patient Additives:

☐ MVC 9 + 3 10 mL Daily

☐ HUMULIN-R **10** units DAILY

☐ FOLIC ACID _____ mg
    _____ times weekly

☐ VITAMIN K _____ mg
    _____ times weekly

☐ OTHER: **MVI 12 10 mL/daily**

☐ OTHER: _____

Directions:

INFUSE: ☑ DAILY
    ☐ ____ TIMES WEEKLY

OTHER DIRECTIONS:

_____

_____

_____

_____

Rate:
☐ CYCLIC INFUSION:
   OVER ____ HOURS
   (TAPER UP AND DOWN)
☐ CONTINUOUS INFUSION:
   AT ____ mL PER HOUR
☑ STANDARD RATE:
   AT **110** mL PER HOUR
   FOR **12** HOURS

LAB ORDERS:

☐ STANDARD LAB ORDERS
SMAC-20, CO2, Mg+2 TWICE WEEKLY
CBC WITH AUTO DIFF WEEKLY
UNTIL STABLE, THEN:
SMAC-20, CO2, Mg+2 WEEKLY
CBC WITH AUTO DIFF MONTHLY

☐ OTHER: _____

VALIDATION:

_____

DOCTOR'S SIGNATURE

Print Name: _____

Office Address: _____

_____

Phone: _____

WHITE: Home Health   CANARY: Physician

FIGURE 10-10 Sample physician's order form for TPN example calculation in Figure 10-8.

			MR#:		M	MEDICATION
Acct:			Age:		A	ADMINISTRATION
Admitted:			HT:		R	RECORD
Att Phys:			WT:			
Diagnosis:					Page: 3	
Allergies:					From: 10/10/15 0730	
					Thru: 10/11/15 0730	

Start Date/Time	Stop Date/Time	RN/ LPN	Medication		0731-1530	1531-2330	2331-0730
10/10/15 1800	10/11/15 1759		PICC Line Flush FLush Q12H IV Flush PICC Q 12 HRS with NS 10 ML when PICC line used for TPN	(1 Inject) #022		1800	0600
10/10/15 1800	10/11/15 1759		Amino Acid 8.5% 600 ML Dextrose 50% 600 ML Sodium Chloride CO 58 MEQ Potassium Acetate 12 MEQ Magnesium Sulfate 6 MEQ	(600 ML) (600 ML) (14.5 ML) (6 ML) (1.5 ML)		1800	
			Calcium Gluconate 6 MEQ Infuvite Multivitamin 10 ML Trace Elements 1 ML Sodium Phosphate 26 MEQ Insulin Humulin Regu 21 units	(12.84 ML) (10 ML) (1 ML) (6.5 ML) (0.21 ML)			
			50 ML/HR Q24H IV Central	#047			
			Store in Refrigerator				

The preprinted MAR from the pharmacy shows the contents of the TPN, the time it is to be started, and the times and amount of NS to be used to flush the central and PICC lines. The nurse will initial next to the preprinted time as well as initial and sign the bottom of the MAR. The MAR is for 24 hours only.

Order Date	RN INIT.	Date/Time To Be Given	One Time Orders and Pre-Operatives Medication-Dose-Route	Actual Time Given	Site Codes		Dose Omission Code	
					Arm	LA RA	A = pt absent	
					Deltoid	LD RD	H = hold	
					Ventrogluteal	LVG RVG	M = med absent	
					Gluteal	LG RG	N = NPO	
					Abdomen	LUQ RUQ	O = other	
					Abdomen	LLQ RLQ	R = refused	
							U = unable to tolerate	
					INIT	Signature	INIT	Signature

CHART

60321 (8/98)A

FIGURE 10-11 Sample medication administration record.

Answers on page 374

WORKSHEET 10B: Peripheral Parenteral Nutrition Calculations

Use Figure 10-12 to answer the following questions.

1. What are the total grams per bag of:
   a. Amino acids (AA)
   b. Dextrose
   c. Lipids

2. What are the percentages of concentration per bag of:
   a. AA
   b. Dextrose
   c. Lipids

3. How many kilocalories are there per bag of:
   a. PRO
   b. CHO
   c. FAT
   d. What is the total number of kilocalories per bag?

4. For how many mL per hour will you set the infusion device?

5. How many kilocalories are in 750 g of dextrose?

TPN ORDER SHEET

HOME HEALTH DATE _____

PATIENT _____ ADDRESS _____

TPN FORMULA:

AMINO ACIDS: ☐ 5.5% ☑ 8.5% ☐ 10% ☐ WITH STANDARD ELECTROLYTES	**500** mL
DEXTROSE: ☐ 10% ☐ 20% ☐ 40% ☑ 50% ☐ 70% (check one)	**500** mL
LIPIDS: ☑ 10% ☐ 20% FOR ALL-IN-ONE FORMULA	**250** mL

FINAL VOLUME qsad STERILE WATER FOR INJECTION	**1500** mL

Calcium Gluconate	0.465 mEq/mL	**5** mEq
Magnesium Sulfate	4 mEq/mL	**15** mEq
Potassium Acetate	2 mEq/mL	**8.3** mEq
Potassium Chloride	2 mEq/mL	mEq
Potassium Phosphate	3 mM/mL	**35** mM
Sodium Acetate	2 mEq/mL	mEq
Sodium Chloride	4 mEq/mL	**35** mEq
Sodium Phosphate	3 mM/mL	mM
TRACE ELEMENTS CONCENTRATE	☐ 4 ☐ 5 ☐ 6	mL

Patient Additives:

☐ MVC 9 + 3 10 ml Daily

☐ HUMULIN-R __**10**__ units DAILY

☐ FOLIC ACID _____ mg _____ times weekly

☐ VITAMIN K _____ mg _____ times weekly

☑ OTHER: *MVI 12 1.5mL/daily*

☐ OTHER: _____

Directions:

INFUSE: ☑ DAILY

☐ ____ TIMES WEEKLY

OTHER DIRECTIONS:
_____
_____
_____
_____

Rate:
☐ CYCLIC INFUSION: OVER __**12**__ HOURS (TAPER UP AND DOWN)
☐ CONTINUOUS INFUSION: AT ____ mL PER HOUR
☑ STANDARD RATE: AT ____ mL PER HOUR FOR __**12**__ HOURS

LAB ORDERS:

☑ STANDARD LAB ORDERS
SMAC-20, CO2, Mg+2 TWICE WEEKLY
CBC WITH AUTO DIFF WEEKLY
UNTIL STABLE, THEN:
SMAC-20, CO2, Mg+2 WEEKLY
CBC WITH AUTO DIFF MONTHLY

☐ OTHER: _____

VALIDATION:

_____
DOCTOR'S SIGNATURE

Print Name: _____

Office Address: _____

Phone: _____

WHITE: Home Health CANARY: Physician

FIGURE 10-12 Sample physician's order for Worksheet 10B.

Answers on page 375

WORKSHEET 10C | Central Parenteral Nutrition Calculations

Use Figure 10-13 to answer the following questions. Use the formulas on pages 362 and 363.

1. Total grams per bag:
   a. How many total grams of amino acids (AA) are there per bag?
   b. How many total grams of dextrose are there per bag?

2. Percentages of concentration per bag:
   a. What is the percentage of amino acids per bag?
   b. What is the percentage of dextrose per bag?

3. Kilocalories per bag:
   a. AA
   b. CHO
   c. Total number of kilocalories

4. How many hours will it take for the contents of the parenteral nutrition bag to be infused?

5. 8.5% AA in 1000 mL provides how many grams of AA?

Amino Acid 10%	(900 ML)
Dextrose 70%	(430 ML)
Sterile Water For Injection	(70 ML)
Sodium Chloride Conc 140 MEQ	(35 ML)
Potassium Phosphate 41 MEQ	(9.318 ML)
Potassium Chloride 43 MEQ	(21.5 ML)
Magnesium Sulfate 7 MEQ	(1.75 ML)
Calcium Gluconate 7 MEQ	(14.98 ML)
Insulin Humulin Regular 20 units	(0.2 ML)
Infuvite Multivitamin A 10 ML	(10 ML)

Total: 1492.748

** Continued **

DO NOT START AFTER 24 HOURS

Rate: 55 mL/hr   Freq: Q24H
Modified Central TPN
Hang Date/Time: 1800 11/19/15
Expir:
Init: DF
Refrigerate
Prep. By: /_____

DO NOT START AFTER 24 HOURS

FIGURE 10-13 Sample CPN label for Worksheet 10C.

Answers on page 375

WORKSHEET 10D | Peripheral Parenteral Nutrition Calculations

Use Figure 10-14 to answer the following questions. Use the formulas on pages 362 and 363.

1. Total grams per bag:
   a. Amino acids (AA)
   b. Dextrose

2. Percentages of concentration per bag:
   a. Amino acids
   b. Dextrose

3. Kilocalories per bag:
   a. AA
   b. CHO
   c. Total number of kilocalories
   d. What is the total number of kilocalories per bag?

4. How many hours will it take for the contents to be infused?

5. 20% of lipids in 500 mL provides how many kilocalories?

```
Amino Acid 8% (Hepatic)            (600 ML)
Dextrose 20%                       (600 ML)
Sodium Chloride Conc 42 MEQ        (10.5 ML)
Potassium Phosphate 26 MEQ         (5.909 ML)
Potassium Acetate 10 MEQ           (5 ML)
Calcium Gluconate 6 MEQ            (12.84 ML)
Magnesium Sulfate 6 MEQ            (1.5 ML)
Infuvite Multivitamin A 10 ML      (10 ML)
Insulin Humulin Regular 24 units   (0.24 ML)

                        Total: 1245.989

** Continued **

         DO NOT START AFTER 24 HOURS

Rate: 50 mL/hr    Freq: Q24H
Peripheral
Hang Date/Time: 1800 11/19/15
Expir:
Init: MM

Prep. By:  /_____

         DO NOT START AFTER 24 HOURS
```

FIGURE 10-14 Sample PCN label for Worksheet 10D.

Answers on page 376

WORKSHEET 10E | Multiple-Choice Practice

1. Have: A three-in-one TPN solution with 20% lipids in 175 mL. The total volume (TV) is 1200 mL. How many grams of lipids are in the solution?
   a. 42 g per bag   **b.** 48 g per bag   **c.** 52 g per bag   **d.** 36 g per bag

2. What is the percentage of concentration of grams per bag for lipids in question 1?
   a. 2.7%   **b.** 3.5%   **c.** 5.6%   **d.** 7%

3. Have: Potassium acetate 12 mEq/L. The TV is 1385 mL. What is the percentage of potassium acetate in the bag?
   a. 2.2%   **b.** 3.6%   **c.** 1.2%   **d.** 2.6%

4. The TV of the parenteral nutrition (PN) solution is 1275 mL. The infusion rate is 110 mL per hour. The infusion is started at 1800 hr. What time will it be completed?
   a. 0659 hr   **b.** 0459 hr   **c.** 0535 hr   **d.** 0345 hr

5. Have: CPN solution with 8.5% AA in 375 mL. The TV is 1500 mL. How many grams of protein are in the solution?
   a. 50 g per bag   **b.** 77.7 g per bag   **c.** 62 g per bag   **d.** 47.8 g per bag

6. What is the percentage of concentration of grams per bag of the AA in question 5?
   a. 4.6%   **b.** 3%   **c.** 8.2%   **d.** 4.7%

7. Have: Calcium gluconate additive of 6 mEq/L. The TV of the TPN is 1350 mL. What is the percentage of calcium gluconate in the bag?
   a. 0.3%   **b.** 1%   **c.** 0.4%   **d.** 0.6%

8. Have: Magnesium sulfate additive 10 mEq/L. The TV is 1258 mL. What is the percentage of magnesium sulfate in the bag?
   a. 1%   **b.** 10.2%   **c.** 1.8%   **d.** 11%

9. Have: CPN solution with 40% dextrose in 400 mL. The TV is 1450 mL. How many grams of dextrose are in the bag?
   a. 232 g per bag   **b.** 130 g per bag   **c.** 160 g per bag   **d.** 260 g per bag

10. What is the percentage of concentration per bag for dextrose in question 9?

Critical Thinking Exercises

Critical Thinking Exercises provide math and medication-related patient safety issues for student discussion. Answers are not provied.

Analyze the following scenarios.

1. Your patient, Mary Braun, is receiving peripheral parenteral nutrition (PPN). On assessment, she complains that the IV site burns. When the site is checked, the solution is infusing well at the correct rate. The label on the solution is 8.5% amino acids and 70% dextrose.

   Error(s):

   Causes of error(s):

   Nursing interventions:

   Preventive measures:

   Discussion

   What will be your first action?

   Why are the percentages of amino acids and dextrose important to know?

   What is the percentage difference for PPN and CPN infusion?

   How can this situation be reconciled to reduce potential risks?

2. Mrs. S. had been hospitalized for 5 days for ulcerative colitis that was not responding to the treatment. During this time she was receiving a TPN solution with 8.5% amino acids and 40% dextrose with multivitamins 1.5 mL daily. She was then scheduled for a total colectomy. After the surgery, Mrs. S. was returned to the surgical unit. The postoperative orders were PCA 1.5 mg morphine every 6 minutes, Ambien 10 mg prn for sleep, and continue daily TPN with Aminosyn II 15%, dextrose 40%, multivitamins 10 mL, and 10 units of Humulin R added to the bag. After 3 days, Mrs. S. complained of nausea and her skin appeared flushed.

   What would be your first reaction to her signs and symptoms?

   What medication is she receiving that might cause an adverse reaction?

   What are the side effects of Aminosyn?

   If this is an adverse reaction, do you think the benefit of the medication outweighs the reaction?

   How can you make Mrs. S. more comfortable to alleviate the signs and symptoms?

3. A 1500-mL TPN infusion of 5% amino acids, 40% dextrose, and 10% lipids is ordered to be infused in 12 hours. The infusion was started at 1430 hr. At 630 hr, the nurse checked the infusion and found that it still had 300 mL in the bag. She checked the infusion pump, which was set at 100 mL per hour.

Ordered:

Error:

Discussion:

What would be your first action?

Why do you think the infusion time of 12 hours is important?

How was the patient's safety jeopardized?

At what rate should the TPN be infusing?

You are the person who found the error. Will you make out the incident report?

How would an error like this be reconciled in the future?

CHAPTER 10 Final

Calculate and solve the following problems using a calculator, moving decimals, reducing ratios, and labeling your answers. Prove your work.*

1. Why is a 50% dextrose solution infused via a central line?

2. What is the major difference between a PPN line and a CPN line?
   Peripheral   central

3. A three-in-one TPN solution has lipids 20% in 110 mL. The total volume is 1145 mL.
   a. How many grams of lipids will the patient receive?
   b. How many kilocalories of fat will the patient receive?

4. The TPN order reads: Dextrose 40% in 400 mL. The TV is 1325 mL.
   a. How many grams of dextrose will the patient receive?
   b. How many kilocalories of carbohydrate will the patient receive?

5. A TPN order reads: Amino acids 8.5% in 550 mL. The TV of the TPN infusion is 1430 mL.
   a. How many grams of AA will the patient receive through the central line?
   b. How many kilocalories of protein will the patient receive?

6. A TPN order reads dextrose 10% in 475 mL.
   a. How many grams of dextrose will be infused?
      The total volume is 1550 mL in the peripheral line.
   b. How many kilocalories of dextrose will the patient receive?

7. A TPN solution has 48 g of protein, 255 g of carbohydrate, and 38.6 g of fat. How many total kilocalories will the patient receive?

8. A PPN order reads: Amino acids 5% in 350 mL. The TV is 1280 mL.
   a. How many grams of AA will the patient receive?
   b. How many kilocalories of protein will the patient receive?

9. The TPN of 1420 mL is to start at 1800 hr. The rate is 108 mL per hour. What time will the infusion be completed?   13.15 hours   0709

10. A TPN of 1320 mL is infusing at 120 mL per hour. How many hours will it take to infuse?
    11 hours

evolve Refer to the Advanced Calculations section of Drug Calculations Companion, version 5 on Evolve for additional practice problems.

---

*It may be acceptable to withdraw small amounts of large-volume IV solutions equal to the number of milliliters of drug to be added so as to simplify calculations and flow rates. Follow your hospital's policy.

Answer Key

10 Parenteral Nutrition

WORKSHEET 10A (page 363)

1. Total grams per bag:
   % × mL = g/L   g/L × TV/L = g/bag
   a. AA 0.055 × 400 = 22 g/L   22 × 1.350 = 29.7 g/bag
   b. Dextrose 0.10 × 350 = 35 g/L   35 × 1.350 = 47.25 g/bag
   c. Lipids 0.10 × 200 = 20 g/L   20 × 1.350 = 27 g/bag

2. Percentage of concentration:
   g/bag ÷ TV = % of concentration
   a. AA 29.7 g ÷ 1350 = 2.2%
   b. Dextrose 47.25 ÷ 1350 = 3.5%
   c. Lipids 27 ÷ 1350 = 2%

3. kcal per bag:
   a. CHO 47.25 × 4 = 189   PRO = 4 kcal/g
   b. PRO 29.7 × 4 = 118.8   CHO = 4 kcal/g
   c. FAT 27 × 9 = 243   FAT = 9 kcal/g
   d. Total kcal 550.8

4. mL/hr to set infusion device
   $$\frac{TV}{TT} = mL/hr$$ $$\frac{1350}{12} = 112.5 = 113 \text{ mL/hr}$$

   Percentage is based on 100
5. 0.50 × 1500 = 750 g CHO

WORKSHEET 10B (page 366)

1. Total grams per bag:
   % × mL = g/L   g/L × TV/L = g/bag
   a. 0.085 × 500 = 42.5 g/L AA   42.5 × 1.5 = 63.75 g/bag
   b. 0.50 × 500 = 250 g/L DEX   250 × 1.5 = 375 g/bag
   c. 0.10 × 250 = 25 g/L LIP   25 × 1.5 = 37.5 g/bag

2. Percentage of concentration
   g/bag ÷ TV = % of concentration
   a. 63.75 ÷ 1500 = 4.25% AA
   b. 375 ÷ 1500 = 25% DEX
   c. 37.5 ÷ 1500 = 2.5% LIP

3. kcal per bag
   a. 63.75 × 4 = 255 kcal PRO   CHO = 4 kcal/g
   b. 375 × 4 = 1500 kcal CHO   PRO = 4 kcal/g
   c. 37.5 × 9 = 337.5 kcal FAT   FAT = 9 kcal/g
   d. Total kcal = 2092.5

4. mL/hr to set infusion device

$$\frac{TV}{TT} = mL/hr$$

$$\frac{1500}{12} = 125 \text{ mL/hr}$$

5. 750 g × 4 = 3000 kcal CHO

WORKSHEET 10C (page 368)

1. Total grams per bag
Formula: % × mL = g/L
Shortcut method: % × mL = g/L × TV/L = g/bag
AA 0.10 × 900 = 90 × 1.492 = 134.28 g/bag
Dex 0.70 × 430 = 301 × 1.492 = 449 g/bag

Formula: g/L × TV/L = g/bag

Percentage of concentrate per bag

2. Formula: $\frac{g/bag}{TV} = \%/bag$

AA $\frac{134.28}{1492.74} = 0.0899 = 9\%$

Dex $\frac{449}{1492.74} = 0.30 = 30\%$

3. Total kcal per bag
  a. Protein 134.28 g × 4 = 537 kcal
  b. Carbohydrate 449 g × 4 = 1796 kcal
  c. Total kcal = 2333

4. KNOW   WANT TO KNOW
55 mL : 1 hr = 1492 mL : x hr
55x = 1 × 1492 = 1492
  x = 27.127 = 27 hr
27 hr 8 min
PROOF
55 mL × 27.127 = 1491.9 = 1492
1 × 1492 = 1492

5. 1000 × 0.085 = 85 g of AA

WORKSHEET 10D (page 369)

1. Total grams per bag
Formulas: % × mL = g/L
g/L × TV/L = g/bag
Shortcut method: % × mL = g/L × TV/L = g/bag
AA 0.08 × 600 = 48 × 1.246 = 59.8 = 60 g/bag
Dex 0.20 × 600 = 120 × 1.246 = 149.5 = 150 g/bag

Percentage of concentrate per bag

2. Formula: $\frac{g/bag}{TV} = \%/bag$

AA $\frac{60}{1246} = 0.048 = 4.8\%/bag$

Dex $\frac{150}{1246} = 0.120 = 12\%/bag$

3. Formula: 1 g of protein = 4 kcal; 1 g of dextrose = 4 kcal; 1 g of fat = 9 kcal
   a. AA 60 × 4 = 240 kcal
   b. CHO 150 × 4 = 600 kcal
   c. Total kcal = 840

4. KNOW   WANT TO KNOW
   50 mL : 1 hr = 1246 mL : x hr
   50x = 1 × 1246 = 1246
      x = 24.92   Convert .92 into minutes: 0.92 × 60 = 55 min
      x = 24 hr 55 min
   PROOF
   1 × 1246 = 1246
   50 × 24.92 = 1246

5. 500 mL × 0.20 = 100 g × 9 = 900 kcal

WORKSHEET 10E (page 370)

1. a. 0.20 × 175 = 35 × 1.200 = 42 g lipids/bag

2. b. $\frac{42}{1200}$ = 0.035 = 3.5% conc. of lipids

3. c. 12 × 1.385 = 16.62 ÷ 1385 = 0.012 = 1.2% potassium

4. c. KNOW   WANT TO KNOW   FRACTION CROSS PRODUCT
   110 mL : 1 hr = 1275 mL : x hr   OR $\frac{110 \text{ mL}}{1 \text{ hr}} = \frac{1275 \text{ mL}}{x \text{ hr}}$
   110x = 1275   110x = 1275
      x = 11.59 hr = 11 hr 35 min   x = 11.59 = 11 hr 35 min
   PROOF
   1 × 1275 = 1275
   110 × 11.59 = 1275
   IV started at 1800 hours plus 11 hr 35 min = 0535 hr

5. d. 0.085 × 375 = 31.8 × 1.500 = 47.8 g/bag of AA

6. b. $\frac{47.8}{1500}$ = 0.03 = 3% conc. of AA

7. d. 6 × 1.350 = 8.1 ÷ 1350 = 0.006 = 0.6% calcium gluconate

8. a. 10 × 1.258 = 12.5 ÷ 1258 = 0.01 = 1% magnesium sulfate

9. a. 0.40 × 400 = 160 × 1.450 = 232 g/bag of dextrose

10. b. $\frac{232}{1450}$ = 0.16 = 16% conc. of dextrose

CHAPTER 10 FINAL: PARENTERAL NUTRITION (page 373)

1. 50% dextrose has a high osmolarity that would be harmful to smaller veins.

2. The size and location of the veins. Central lines can tolerate higher percentages of dextrose and amino acids.

3. a. 25 g/bag of lipids
   b. 225 kcal of fat

4. a. 212 g/bag of dextrose
   b. 848 kcal of dextrose

5. a. 66.85 g/bag of AA
   b. 267.4 kcal of PRO

6. a. 73.62 g/bag of dextrose
   b. 294.5 kcal of CHO

7. 1559 total kcal

8. a. 22.4 g/bag of AA
   b. 89.6 kcal of PRO

9. At 0709 hr the infusion will be completed

10. 11 hr to infuse

Anticoagulants

Objectives
- Compare the actions of oral, subcutaneous, and intravenous anticoagulants.
- Measure a dose in a tuberculin syringe.
- Measure subcutaneous heparin using various concentrations.
- Titrate intravenous heparin for bolus dose, units per kg, units per hr, and mL per hr.
- Calculate the length of time to infuse.
- Analyze medication errors using critical thinking.

Introduction

Anticoagulant medications are administered subcutaneously, intravenously, or orally. They are all high-alert medications capable of doing great harm if a dose is measured incorrectly and administered. Anticoagulant drugs are designed to inhibit the coagulation cascade to decrease the chance for the formation of thrombi. The purpose is to extend the clotting time of blood to prevent venous or arterial thrombosis, which could result in an embolus causing pulmonary or cerebral damage.

Vocabulary

Activated Partial Thromboplastin Time (aPTT): A shortened form of the prothrombin time (PT) test used to monitor heparin therapy. Normal control time is 30 to 40 seconds. This is not a standardized test like the INR, therefore results may vary depending on the agents used.

Anticoagulant: A drug that prevents or delays blood coagulation.

Anti-Xa Assay: A test to measure heparin and low molecular weight heparin (LMWH) levels and to monitor anticoagulant therapy effectiveness. Dosages are titrated to maintain anticoagulant effectiveness.

Deep Vein Thrombosis (DVT): Complication of immobilization, orthopedic surgery, or any type of surgery.

Embolus: A blood clot that travels from its original location, usually in the leg.

Heparin: Heparin sodium or heparin calcium (unfractionated) is a parenteral drug that has a faster effect than oral warfarin or other oral medications. It is administered subcutaneously or intravenously. Heparin is usually administered in a hospital setting because the partial thromboplastin time must be monitored every 4 to 6 hours. Heparin inhibits coagulation by forming antithrombin, thereby preventing the conversion of prothrombin to thrombin. It is used as an anticoagulant in the prevention and treatment of thrombosis and embolism.

Heparin Lock (Heplock): A port on the IV to administer medications.

Heparin (Heplock) Flush: Can be a saline flush or a heparin flush of 10 to 100 units per mL to prevent the IV catheter from clotting.

International Normalized Ratio (INR): A rating scale used by laboratories around the world that standardizes the prothrombin time (PT) result. The INR was introduced by the World Health Organization (WHO) in 1983. Normal blood has an INR of 1. Therapeutic target range for blood of anticoagulated patients is 2.0 to 3.0.

Heparin-Induced Thrombocytopenia (HIT): A low platelet count as a result of the administration of various forms of the anticoagulant heparin. HIT predisposes the patient to thrombosis.

Heparin-Induced Thrombocytopenia and Thrombosis (HITT): A low platelet count with the formation of a thrombus. Several drugs are available that will not reduce the platelet count any further. The new drugs are lepirudin and argatroban.

Low Molecular Weight Heparin: The most bioavailable fractionized product of heparin. It has a more precise anticoagulant effect than unfractionated heparin. It is used to treat DVT, pulmonary embolus, and coronary episodes.

Petechiae: Small, purplish hemorrhagic spots on the skin that appear in patients with platelet deficiencies.

Platelet Count: The number of platelets, or thrombocytes, in blood is normally 150,000 to 400,000 per mcL. A count of less than 200,000 platelets contributes to a risk for bleeding. Platelets release factors that initiate the first stages of clotting.

Protamine Sulfate: An antidote to reverse the effects of heparin and heparinoids.

Prothrombin Time (PT or Pro Time): No longer used for monitoring warfarin therapy. It is not as reliable as the standardized INR to monitor anticoagulated blood values.

Pulmonary Embolus (PE): A blood clot usually from a DVT that has traveled from its original source and obstructs a pulmonary artery in the lungs. This is an extreme emergency.

Thrombocytopenia: An abnormal decrease in the number of platelets. Watch for signs of hemorrhage.

Thrombolytic Agent: An intravenous drug that lyses or dissolves clots to reverse a cerebral vascular accident (CVA) or a pulmonary embolus.

Vitamin K: An antidote to reverse the effects of warfarin (Coumadin).

Injectable Anticoagulants

Heparin sodium injection, USP, is a fast-acting drug used to interrupt the clotting process. It affects the ability of the blood to coagulate, thereby preventing clots from forming. It is used to treat deep vein thrombosis (DVT) and pulmonary embolism (PE); during cardiac surgery; during hemodialysis, myocardial infarction (MI), and disseminated intravascular coagulation (DIC); and prophylactically for immobilized patients. It may be given in therapeutic doses or in small, diluted doses to maintain the patency of IV or intraarterial (IA) lines.

Because it is inactive orally, heparin sodium is administered intravenously or subcutaneously. If administered intramuscularly, the drug produces a high level of pain and may cause hematomas. The orders for heparin are highly individualized and are based on the weight of the patient and coagulation values. Heparin comes in various strengths, including 1000, 5000, 10,000, 20,000, and 50,000 units per mL. Heparin also comes in 10 and 100 units per mL for IV patency flushes. The vial must be checked carefully before administration. Heparin is fast acting.

Low molecular weight heparins (LMWH) are fractionalized heparin. They have replaced unfractionated heparin (UFH) to prevent and treat venous thrombosis, unstable angina, and pulmonary embolus. They are safer than UFH and just as effective. Once-daily subcutaneous dosing and a lower incidence of heparin-induced thrombocytopenia (HIT) and osteopenia make LMWH the choice drug. Natural or unfractionated heparin is less predictable than LMWH.

Differences between injectable (UFH) and LMWH (fractionated) include the following:
- The unfractionated weight of a heparin molecule is about 15 kDa.
- The fractionated weight of an LMWH molecule is about 4.5 kDa.

- Less frequent subcutaneous dosing is required for LMWH than UFH for postoperative prophylaxis of venous thromboembolism.
- With LMWH there is no need to monitor aPTT coagulation, which is necessary with UFH.
- Possibly a lower risk for bleeding.
- Lower risk of osteoporosis in long-term use.
- Less chance of heparin-induced thrombocytopenia.
- The anticoagulant effects of heparin are reversible with protamine sulfate.
- Protamine sulfate is less effective on LMWH.
- LMWH can inactivate factor Xa, activating (AT) antithrombin.
- UFH is unable to inactivate factor Xa, which can produce thrombocytopenia and osteoporosis.

The LMWH subcutaneous injectable drugs are Lovenox (enoparin), Arixtra (fondaparinux), Fragmin (dalteparin), and Innohep (tinzaparin). Figure 11-1 shows anticoagulant injection sites. Figure 11-2 demonstrates how subcutaneous heparin injections are documented.

FIGURE 11-1 Subcutaneous injection sites. The abdominal sites are better for absorption of injectable anticoagulant.

MEDICATION ADMINISTRATION RECORD (MAR)

ADM. DX :
DIET :
HT :
WT :
ALLERGIES:

Start Date/Time	Stop Date/Time	RN/LPN	Medication	0731-1530	1531-2330	2331-0730
12/13/15		NB	Heparin sodium 5,000 units subcut	0800 RLQ		
		NB	Heparin sodium 5,000 units subcut	1400 LLQ		
		KR	Heparin sodium 5,000 units subcut		2000 RLQ	

Order Date	RN INIT.	Date/Time To Be Given	One Time Orders and Pre-Operatives Medication-Dose-Route	Actual Time Given

Site Codes

Arm	LA	RA
Deltoid	LD	RD
Ventrogluteal	LVG	RVG
Gluteal	LG	RG
Abdomen	LUQ	RUQ
Abdomen	LLQ	RLQ

Dose Omission Code

A = pt absent
H = hold
M = med absent
N = NPO
O = other
R = refused
U = unable to tolerate

INIT	Signature	INIT	Signature
NB	Nancy Berg RN		
KR	Kay Rae RN		

FIGURE 11-2 Sample MAR. (Modified from Scottsdale Healthcare, Scottsdale, Ariz.)

Check laboratory values for clotting times before administering heparin. Heparin therapy must not be interrupted and is incompatible with other medications.

Heparin has a half-life of 1 to 6 hours. To maintain a therapeutic level in the blood, heparin is usually given as a continuous IV drip during hospitalization. The heparin level is titrated on the basis of partial thromboplastin time (PTT) levels, which are taken every 6 hours to correlate with the half-life of heparin. Heparin can be counteracted with protamine sulfate.

► CLINICAL ALERT!

Heparin is a high-alert medication that carries a risk of causing serious injury if the wrong dosage is administered. Anticoagulant dosages require two licensed nurses to verify the ordered dosage for accuracy.

Lovenox (enoxaparin) and Fragmin (dalteparin), Arixtra (fondaparinux), and Innohep (tinzaparin) are low molecular weight (LWMH) anticoagulants. They are prescribed for the prevention and treatment of DVT and PE and also after knee and hip surgery. LMWHs have a longer half-life than heparin. Because of their low level of activity in the blood, there is a reduced need for PTT tests. These four drugs have more predictable peaks and durations of action. The preferred sites for LMWH anticoagulants are the anterolateral abdominal wall.

► CLINICAL ALERT!

Lovenox, Fragmin, Arixtra, and Innohep should never be given intramuscularly because they may cause large hematomas.

Example Ordered: Lovenox 30 mg subcutaneous q12h after hip replacement. The pharmacy has sent 40 mg per 0.4 mL in a prefilled syringe. How many milliliters will be administered? How many milliliters will be discarded?

LOVENOX®
(enoxaparin sodium) Injection
40 mg/0.4 mL Syringe
LOT 506572A
RHÔNE-POULENC RORER PHARMACEUTICALS INC.
COLLEGEVILLE, PA 19426
Made in France   L-5560A

HAVE | WANT TO HAVE | FRACTION CROSS PRODUCT

40 mg : 0.4 mL = 30 mg : x mL

$$\frac{40}{0.4} = \frac{30}{x \text{ mL}}$$

$40x = 0.4 \times 30 = 12$ $40x = 30 \times 0.4 = 12$
$40x = 12$ $x = 0.3$ mL
$x = 0.3$ mL

PROOF $40 \times 0.3 = 12$
$0.4 \times 30 = 12$

0.1 mL will be discarded.

Arixtra (fondaparinux sodium) is a nonheparin (fractionated) anticoagulant made by chemical synthesis and not from animal origin (Figure 11-3). It is a specific inhibitor of the activated factor X (Xa).

Arixtra is used for prophylaxis of venous thromboembolism (VTE), such as deep vein thrombosis (DVT), which may lead to pulmonary embolism (PE) in patients undergoing hip fracture surgery, knee replacement or hip replacement surgery, and for those at risk for thromboembolitic complications from abdominal surgery.

Warfarin can be administered in conjunction with Arixtra for the treatment of acute DVT when initiated while the patient is hospitalized.

FIGURE 11-3 Arixtra single-dose syringes.

> ### CLINICAL ALERT!
> Arixtra is NOT intended for intramuscular use. It CANNOT be used interchangeably with heparin or other low molecular weight (LMW) heparinoids such as Lovenox (enoxaparin) and Fragmin (dalteparin).
>
> There is a risk of hemorrhage for patients with impaired renal function and for those who are at increased risk of hemorrhage from thrombocytopenia. If the platelet count falls below 100,000/mm^3, discontinue Arixtra. This is known as heparin-induced thrombocytopenia (HIT) (see Vocabulary).

Subcutaneous Heparin Injections

Example Ordered: Heparin 3500 units subcutaneous q6h. Available: Vial containing 5000 units per mL. How many milliliters will the patient receive? Shade in the dose on the tuberculin syringe.

KNOW	WANT TO KNOW	FRACTION CROSS PRODUCT
5000 units : 1 mL = 3500 units : x mL		$\dfrac{5000}{1} = \dfrac{3500}{x \text{ mL}}$
$5000x = 3500$		$50x = 35$
$x = 0.7$ mL		$x = 0.7$ mL

PROOF $5000 \times 0.7 = 3500$
$1 \times 3500 = 3500$

CHAPTER 11 Anticoagulants

Example Ordered: Fragmin 8000 international units subcutaneous q6h. How many milliliters will you give? Shade in the dose on the syringe.

KNOW WANT TO KNOW
10,000 international units : 1 mL = 8000 international units : x mL

FRACTION CROSS PRODUCT

$10x = 1 \times 8 = 8$

$\dfrac{10,000}{1 \text{ mL}} = \dfrac{8000}{x \text{ mL}}$

$x = 0.8$ mL

$10x = 1 \times 8 = 8$

$x = 0.8$ mL

PROOF $1 \times 8000 = 8000$
$10,000 \times 0.8 = 8000$

10,000 international units/mL
9.5 mL multidose vial
NDC 0013-2436-06

The product, as depicted in this label, is no longer available. This image was authorized for use by Pfizer Inc. for educational purposes only.

CLINICAL ALERT!

Do not substitute insulin syringes for tuberculin syringes. Insulin syringes are calibrated in 100 units per mL and tuberculin syringes are calibrated in tenths per mL.

CLINICAL RELEVANCE

Do not massage the injection site because this increases the incidence of bleeding and hematoma development.

The U.S. Pharmacopeia (USP) and the Institute for Safe Medication Practices (ISMP) require that manufacturers of heparin sodium injection and heparin lock flush solutions clearly state the total strength per volume per vial as well as the unit strength per milliliter for the heparin sodium injection. Hospitals may have both types of labels available as they transition to all new labels. Compare the old label and the new label (see Worksheet 11A, question 1).

Answers on page 405

WORKSHEET 11A | Subcutaneous Injections

Multidose vials are available in 10, 100, 1000, 5000, 10,000, 20,000, and 50,000 units per mL. Read the labels carefully. Answer the following questions and show your proofs (carry out to nearest hundredth). Shade in doses on syringes.

1. Ordered: Heparin 6000 units subcutaneous.
   Available: Heparin 10,000 units/mL. How many milliliters will the patient receive?

2. Ordered: Lovenox 35 mg subcut daily following hip replacement surgery. How many milliliters will the patient receive?

CHAPTER 11 Anticoagulants

3. Ordered: Heparin 15,000 units subcutaneous q8h. Available: Heparin 20,000 units/mL. How many milliliters will the patient receive?

4. Ordered: Fragmin 7500 units subcutaneous q6h. Available: Fragmin 10,000 international units/mL. How many milliliters will the patient receive?

10,000 international units/mL
9.5 mL multidose vial
NDC 0013-2436-06

The product, as depicted in this label, is no longer available. This image was authorized for use by Pfizer Inc. for educational purposes only.

5. Ordered: Heparin 17,000 units subcutaneous stat dose. Available: Heparin 10,000 units/mL and 20,000 units/mL. Which strength will you choose? How many milliliters will the patient receive?

> **CLINICAL ALERT!**
> The subcutaneous dosage of heparin should not exceed 1 mL.

6. Ordered: Heparin 750 units subcutaneous q4h. Available: Heparin 1000 units/mL. How many milliliters will the patient receive?

7. Ordered: Heparin 800 units subcutaneous q8hr. Available: Heparin 1000 units/mL in a multidose vial. How many milliliters will the patient receive?

CLINICAL ALERT!
Check your patient's chart for allergies. Heparin is made from pork and beef.

8. Ordered: Heparin 3000 units subcutaneous q8h. Available: Heparin 5000 units/mL in a multidose vial. How many milliliters will the patient receive?

IV Flushes

9. Ordered: Heparin flush 5 units after each medication administration to prevent clot formation in the heparin lock. Available: Heparin 10 units/mL. How many units of medication are in the vial? How many milliliters will the patient receive?

```
NDC 63323-557-01     505701
HEPARIN
LOCK FLUSH
SOLUTION, USP
10 USP Units/mL
(Derived from Porcine
Intestinal Mucosa)
Preservative Free    Rx only
1 mL Single Dose Vial
```

Follow hospital protocol for saline and heparin flushes after medication administration.

CLINICAL RELEVANCE
Heparin resistance has been documented in elderly patients; therefore large doses may be ordered.

CLINICAL ALERT!
Symptoms of overdose are nosebleed, bleeding gums, tarry stools, petechiae, and easy bruising. An electric razor should be used for shaving.

10. Ordered: Heparin flush 50 units q12h for IV site patency. Available: Heparin 100 units/mL. How many milliliters will the patient receive?

IV Flushes

Peripheral lines are gently flushed with 2 to 3 mL of normal saline.

Heparin locks provide patients with mobility while they are receiving IV medications. Heparin flushes are used to prevent clot formation in the central line. Central lines are used for access to large veins. Hyperosmolarity solutions can be used without causing vein damage. Heparin flushes for central lines come in prefilled 12-mL syringes with 5 mL of 10 units per mL of heparin. Heparin flushes are also available in prefilled 12-mL syringes with 10 mL of 100 units per mL of heparin. Multiple-dose vials of various strengths are also available.

⊖ CLINICAL ALERT!

Heparin IV flushes are available in many different strengths and multiple-dose vials. READ LABELS CAREFULLY. Hospital protocol will specify the strength and the amount to administer.

Polypharmacy

Many people who take prescription drugs also take over-the-counter (OTC) medication. Researchers from the University of Chicago found that about 91% of older adults use at least one medication, and nearly 30% have at least five prescriptions. The study also indicated that many of these older people are taking anticoagulants or antiplatelet agents, which puts them at high risk for adverse drug reactions. It is imperative that all OTC and prescription drugs be charted and the physician notified.

IV Heparin

When intermittent or continuous IV therapy is used, blood should be drawn for a PTT and a hematocrit level to determine the course of therapy. Therapeutic anticoagulant dosage is regulated according to the results of the PTT and the patient's weight.

Pharmacies are standardizing IV heparin preparations in concentrations of 25,000 units/500 mL and 25,000 units/250 mL. Dispensing charts indicating mL/hr and units/hr are available for each concentration. This will reduce overdosing and underdosing. Protamine sulfate is the antagonist for heparin. It is the nurse's responsibility to have protamine sulfate available.

The usual dosage for protamine sulfate is 1 mg for every 100 IU of active heparin, not to exceed 50 mg, given slowly over a 10-minute interval. This is used to reverse large doses of heparin administered IV during surgery, especially heart surgery. Monitor aPTT 5 to 15 minutes after the dose is administered, then again in 2 to 8 hours.

CLINICAL RELEVANCE

Patients receiving IV heparin may experience a complex of symptoms (systemic reaction) when the infusion is started. The symptoms include fever, chills, high blood pressure, fast heart rate, shortness of breath, and chest pain. This happens in about 25% of people who have HIT. Others may develop a skin rash consisting of red spots.

Answers on page 407

WORKSHEET 11B — IV Heparin Calculations: mL per hr

Answer the following questions and show your proofs (carry out to the nearest hundredth). The heparin will be administered with an infusion device.

Example Ordered: Heparin 1400 units per hr IV. Available: 500 mL of NS with 25,000 units of heparin sodium.
  a. How many mL per hr will deliver 1400 units per hr?
  b. How many hours will it take to infuse?

KNOW

500 mL : 25,000 units = x mL : 1400 units

250x = 500 × 14 = 7000
250x = 7000 units
  x = 28/mL per hr. Set infusion pump to deliver 28 mL per hr.

FRACTION CROSS PRODUCT

$$\frac{500}{25000 \text{ units}} \times \frac{x \text{ mL}}{1400 \text{ units}}$$

250x = 5 × 1400 = 7000
x = 28 mL

PROOF 500 × 1400 = 7000
250 × 28 = 7000

KNOW

28 mL : 1 hr = 500 mL : x hr

28x = 1 × 500 = 500
28x = 500
  x = 17.85 hr
60 × 0.85 = 51. The IV will take 17 hr 51 minutes to infuse.

FRACTION CROSS PRODUCT

$$\frac{28 \text{ mL}}{1 \text{ hr}} \times \frac{500 \text{ mL}}{x \text{ hr}}$$

28x = 500
x = 17.85

PROOF 500 × 1 = 500
28 × 17.85 = 499.8 = 500

1. Ordered: Heparin 2500 units per hr IV. Available: 50,000 units per 1000 mL 0.9% NS.
   a. How many mL per hr will deliver 2500 units per hr?
   b. How many hours will it take to infuse?

2. Ordered: Heparin 10,000 units in 15 hr. Pharmacy has sent 1000 mL NS with 10,000 units of heparin. The infusion was started at 0830.
   a. How many units per hr will the patient receive?
   b. How many mL per hr will be infused?
   c. The 0700 hr shift reports that 300 mL have been infused. When will the infusion finish? How many hours remain for the infusion?

CHAPTER 11 Anticoagulants

3. Ordered: Heparin 1500 units per hr IV. Pharmacy has sent 1 L 0.9% saline with 20,000 units of heparin.
   a. How many mL per hr will deliver 1500 units?
   b. How many hours will it take to infuse this bag?

4. Ordered: Heparin sodium 20,000 units IV in 12 hr. Pharmacy has sent 1000 mL of 0.9% normal saline with 20,000 units heparin sodium.
   a. At how many mL per hr should the IV infuse?
   b. How many units per hr will infuse?
   c. The shift report states that 250 mL have been infused. How many hours remain for the infusion?

5. Ordered: Heparin 1200 units per hr. Available: 500 mL NS with 10,000 units of heparin.
   a. How many mL per hr will infuse 1200 units per hr?
   b. How many hours will it take to infuse this bag?

6. Ordered: Heparin sodium 1000 units/hr IV. Available: 1 L of 0.9% saline with 20,000 units of heparin.
   a. How many mL per hr will deliver 1000 units?
   b. How many hours will it take to infuse the bag?

7. Ordered: Heparin 1000 units per hr. Your patient is on fluid restrictions. The pharmacy has sent 20,000 units per 250 mL of NS.
   a. How many mL per hr will deliver 1000 units per hr?
   b. How many hours will it take to infuse?

8. Ordered: Heparin 1300 units per hr IV. Available: 500 mL with 25,000 units of heparin sodium.
   a. How many mL per hr will deliver 1300 units per hr?
   b. How long will it take to infuse?

9. Ordered: Heparin 1800 units per hr IV. Your patient is on fluid restrictions; therefore the pharmacy has sent a concentrated solution of 25,000 units per 250 mL of NS.
   a. How many mL per hr will deliver 1800 units per hr?
   b. How many hours will it take to infuse?

10. Ordered: Heparin 1500 units per hr IV. Available: 25,000 units per 500 mL.
    a. How many mL per hr will deliver 1500 units per hr?
    b. How many hours will it take to infuse?

WORKSHEET 11C — IV Heparin Calculations Titrated to Kilograms

All intravenous anticoagulants are based on the PTT results. Loading (bolus) doses are individualized and are titrated to weight in kilograms. Hospital protocol is usually standardized for each institution. It is important that the nurses know what the protocol standards are and where they are located. Protocols and literature may vary, but the loading doses are usually between 70 and 100 units per kg. Infusion rates for heparin sodium also vary but are usually between 15 and 25 units per kg per hr.

Example Ordered: IV heparin loading dose to infuse at 15 units per kg per hr. The patient weighs 190 lb.
Available: 20,000 units of heparin sodium in 1000 mL of D5W.
At what rate will you set the IV infusion pump?

Change 190 lb to kg.   190 divided by 2.2 = 86.36 = 86 kg.
Multiply units per hr by the patient's weight in kg.   15 × 86 = 1290 units per hr.

Ratio and Proportion Method

KNOW   WANT TO KNOW   FRACTION CROSS PRODUCT

15 units : 1 kg = x units : 86 kg $\frac{15 \text{ units}}{1 \text{ kg}} \times \frac{x \text{ units}}{86 \text{ kg}}$

x = 15 × 86 = 1290   x = 15 × 86 = 1290
x = 1290 units per hr   x = 1290 units per hr

PROOF 15 × 86 = 1290
1 × 1290 = 1290

KNOW   WANT TO KNOW   FRACTION CROSS PRODUCT

20,000 units : 1000 mL = 1290 units : x mL $\frac{20 \text{ units}}{1 \text{ mL}} \times \frac{1290 \text{ units}}{x \text{ mL}}$

20x = 1 × 1290 = 1290   20x = 1290
20x = 1290   x = 64.5 = 65

PROOF 1 × 1290 = 1290
20 × 64.5 = 1290

x = 64.5 mL per hr = 65 mL per hr. Set infusion pump to deliver 65 mL per hr.

Directions: Follow the above example to calculate the loading dose, units per hr, and mL per hr.

1. Ordered: Heparin sodium 90 units per kg. Infuse at 25 units per kg per hr. Available: 1000 mL 0.45% NS with 25,000 units of heparin. The patient weighs 210 lb.
   a. How many units is the loading dose?
   b. How many units per hr will the patient receive?
   c. At what rate will you set the mL per hr?

2. Ordered: 80 units per kg of heparin as a loading dose. Set infusion rate to deliver 1500 units per hr. Available: 1000 mL NS with 30,000 units of heparin. The patient weighs 160 lb.
   a. Calculate the loading dose.
   b. Calculate the mL per hr.

> **CLINICAL ALERT!**
> Always have protamine sulfate available as an antidote for heparin.

3. Ordered: Heparin sodium 70 units per kg bolus loading dose. Infusion rate to run at 20 units per kg per hr. Available: 1000 mL D5W with 25,000 units of heparin. The patient weighs 176 lb.
   a. Calculate the loading dose.
   b. Calculate the units per hr based on weight.
   c. Calculate the mL per hr.

4. Ordered: Loading dose of 75 units per kg; then infuse at 20 units per kg per hr. Available: 1000 mL 0.9% NS with 50,000 units of heparin. The patient weighs 300 lb.
   a. Calculate the loading dose.
   b. How many units per hr will the patient receive?
   c. At what rate will you set the infusion device?

5. Ordered: A bolus dose of heparin at 70 units per kg. Run the infusion at 18 units per kg per hr. Available: 1000 mL D5W with 30,000 units of heparin. The patient weighs 194 lb.
   a. How many units will you give as the bolus dose?
   b. How many units per hr will infuse?
   c. At what rate will you set the infusion device?

6. Ordered: Loading dose of 65 units per kg. Set the infusion to run at 15 units per kg per hr. Available: 500 mL 0.45% NS with 30,000 units of heparin. The patient weighs 145 lb.
   a. How many units is the loading dose?
   b. How many units per hr will infuse?
   c. At what rate will you set the infusion device?

7. Ordered: Bolus dose of heparin at 80 units per kg. Titrate infusion to run at 1000 units per hr. Available: 1000 mL D5W with 25,000 units of heparin. The patient weighs 120 kg.
   a. Calculate the number of units for the loading dose.
   b. Calculate mL per hr to infuse 1000 units per hr.

8. Ordered: Loading dose of heparin 75 units per kg. Infuse at 17 units per kg per hr. Available: 1000 mL D5W with 20,000 units of heparin. The patient weighs 185 lb.
   a. How many units is the loading dose?
   b. How many units per hr will the patient receive?
   c. At what rate will you set the infusion device?

9. Ordered: A loading dose of heparin at 95 units per kg. Pharmacy has sent 1000 mL 0.9% NS with 20,000 units of heparin. Run the infusion at 20 units per kg per hr. The patient weighs 136 kg.
   a. How many units is the loading dose?
   b. How many units per hr will infuse?
   c. At what rate will you set the infusion device?

10. Ordered: Heparin 100 units/kg bolus dose. Infuse at 18 units per kg per hr. Available: 1000 mL 0.45% NS with 35,000 units of heparin. The patient weighs 108 kg.
    a. How many units is the loading dose?
    b. How many units per hr will infuse?
    c. At what rate will you set the infusion device?

WORKSHEET 11D: Dosing Guidelines

The sequence of IV administration usually follows a process of bolus or loading dose, the titrated dose, and a rebolus rate adjusted to the aPTT result.

Directions:

Use the Dosing Guidelines for (DVT-PE) Treatment Chart (Table 11-1) to calculate the units per hour for the IV rate for a patient who weighs 70 kg. The standard infusion bag holds 25,000 units per 250 mL (100 units per mL).

Table 11-1 Dosing Guidelines for (DVT-PE) Treatment Chart

(Based on Raschke[1] nomogram)
Obtain baseline aPTT, prothrombin time (PT), CBC, platelet count.
Check for contraindications to heparin therapy.

Patient name:	Location:
Height: 70 inches **Weight:** 70 kg	**Dosing weight:** 70 kg

Standard infusion bag concentration: 25,000 units per 250 mL (100 units per mL).
Also, all infusion rates below are rounded to the nearest **100** units.

Initial bolus dose (80 units per kg): 5600 units
Initial infusion rate (18 units per kg per hr): 1300 units per hr (13 mL per hr)

aPTT (seconds)*	Dose Change (units per kg per hr)	Additional Action	Next aPTT
<35 (1.2 × mean normal)	Increase by 4 units per kg per hr (300 units) or 3 mL per hr	Rebolus with 80 units per kg (5600 units)	6 hours
35 to 45 (1.2 to 1.5 × mean normal)	Increase by 2 units per kg per hr (100 units) or 1 mL per hr	Rebolus with 40 units per kg (2800 units)	6 hours
46 to 70 (1.5 to 2.3 × mean normal)	No change		6 hours†
71 to 90 (2.3 to 3.0 × mean normal)	Decrease by 2 units per kg per hr (100 units) or 1 mL per hr		6 hours
>90 (>3 × mean normal)	Decrease by 3 units per kg per hr (200 units) or 2 mL per hr	Stop infusion 1 hour	6 hours

*The therapeutic range in seconds should correspond to a plasma heparin level of 0.2 to 0.4 IU per mL by protamine sulfate or 0.3 to 0.6 IU per mL by amidolytic assay.
†Repeat aPTT every 6 hours during the first 24 hours; thereafter, monitor aPTT once every morning, unless it is outside the therapeutic range.

1. Calculate the initial bolus dose of 80 units per kg for the patient who weighs 70 kg.

2. Calculate the units per hour.

3. Calculate the infusion rate.

The 6-hour aPTT is 30. Rebolus with 80 units per kg (5600 units) and increase the rate by 4 units per kg.

4. a. Calculate the increased units per hour.
   b. What is the new units-per-hour rate?

5. Calculate the new infusion rate.

The 6-hour aPTT is 40. Increase the IV rate by 2 units per kg per hour. Rebolus with 40 units per kg.

6. Calculate the bolus dose.

7. a. Calculate the increased units per hour.
   b. What is the new units-per-hour rate?

8. Calculate the new infusion rate.

The 6-hour aPTT is 55 = no change
The 6-hour aPTT is 85 = decrease the rate by 2 units per kg per hour.

9. a. Calculate the decreased units per hour.
   b. What is the new units-per-hour rate?

10. Calculate the new infusion rate.

The 6-hour aPTT is 95 = decrease the rate by 3 units per kg per hour.

11. a. Calculate the decreased units per hour.
    b. What is the new units-per-hour rate?

12. Calculate the new infusion rate.

13. What will be your next action?

Oral Anticoagulants

Warfarin (Coumadin) (Figure 11-4) is used as prophylaxis after an episode of thrombolytic complications and for atrial fibrillation to prevent blood coagulation. The drug inhibits the activity of vitamin K, which is required for the activation of clotting factors. Patients receiving heparin therapy are converted to an oral anticoagulant in the hospital while still receiving heparin injections. The level of warfarin in the blood is monitored by the laboratory value of the international normalized ratio (INR). The INR is a standardized measurement of the prothrombin time (PTT). The INR should be maintained at 2 to 3 for best results, depending on the illness being treated. Dosing for all anticoagulants is individualized. The antidote for warfarin is vitamin K (Figure 11-5), plasma, or whole blood.

FIGURE 11-4 Coumadin tablets come in a variety of dosages. (From *Mosby's Drug Consult 2007*, St Louis, 2007, Mosby.)

FIGURE 11-5 Vitamin K may be given as an antidote for warfarin.

CLINICAL RELEVANCE

When discharging a patient who will be going home on Coumadin (warfarin), it is extremely important that the patient is knowledgeable about medications that can potentiate the anticoagulation effect of Coumadin. A list of these medications is available from the pharmacist. Also, there are medications that can inhibit the effect of the Coumadin and over-the-counter medications that can increase the effects of the anticoagulant. Foods high in vitamin K should be avoided until the INR level has been stabilized. Compliance to daily dosage and diet restrictions is essential.

Because of the potential harmful effects of anticoagulants, these medications deserve special protocols for use and compliance with the blood-testing regimen. The importance must be stressed that all PT/INR tests be taken at the scheduled times. Signs and symptoms of bleeding or clotting must be reported immediately.

Oral anticoagulant warfarin (Coumadin) has been used to treat atrial fibrillation (AF) for many years. People with defibrillation have had to rely on warfarin to control their blood clotting cascade. The major drawback with warfarin use is the weekly or monthly blood testing to monitor the INR. A strict diet is necessary, and some medications may interfere with the anticoagulant property of warfarin. The effects of warfarin can be counteracted with vitamin K.

The new class of oral medications called *target-specific oral anticoagulants* (TSOACs) act rapidly and do not require monitoring because their actions are predictable. No special diet is required; however, compliance to take the medication as ordered is essential because they have a shorter half-life than warfarin. Missing a dose could cause problems. The downside of the newer drugs is that there is no medication to counteract or reverse the anticlotting effect (Table 11-2).

CLINICAL RELEVANCE

It is important for the nurse to be familiar with the hospital's preferred clotting factor protocols to treat bleeding associated with TSOACs.

Table 11-2 Warfarin Oral Anticoagulant vs. New Oral Anticoagulants (TSOACs)

Drug Name (Brand Name)	Pros	Cons
Warfarin (Coumadin)	Predictable benefits and risks Take once daily Can be reversed rapidly with vitamin K	Weekly or monthly blood test to monitor prothrombin time (PT) and INR
Dabigatran (Pradaxa)	No blood monitoring required Lower risk of stroke or brain bleeding than warfarin	Take twice daily, making missed doses more likely More likely than warfarin to cause stomach upset
Rivaroxaban (Xarelto)	Take once daily Lower rates of brain bleeding than warfarin	Slightly higher risk of gastrointestinal bleeding than with apixaban or warfarin
Apixaban (Eliquis)	Lower risk of brain bleeding than with warfarin Major bleeding rate lower than with warfarin Lower rate of upset stomach than with dabigatran	Take twice daily Missed doses can become a problem

Patients taking Coumadin are at increased risk for medication interactions. The patient must always report to the health care provider all medications, including over-the-counter medications being taken.

Clopidogrel (Plavix) is an antiplatelet agent that blocks the formation of blood clots by preventing the clumping of platelets. Plavix is used for the prevention of heart attacks, unstable angina, recent stroke, or peripheral vascular disease. As with warfarin, there are many drug interactions associated with the efficacy of this drug. Atorvastatin (Lipitor) may potentiate the action of Plavix. A proton pump inhibitor (PPI) may subject the patient to another heart attack. The only PPI found to be safe for patients taking Plavix is pantoprazole (Protonix).

Missed doses: Warfarin and Plavix are usually taken once a day. If a dose is missed at the patient's usual dosing time, he or she should take it as soon as possible afterward. If it is missed closer to the 24-hour period, then the patient should resume his or her regular dose the next day. DO NOT DOUBLE THE DOSE.

Acetylsalicylic acid (aspirin) is also an antiplatelet agent that prevents the formation of blood clots. Sometimes a low dose of aspirin is prescribed for concurrent use along with warfarin, as these two drugs work in different ways. Warfarin prevents clotting of blood, and aspirin prevents clumping of platelets that can form blood clots.

⊙ CLINICAL ALERT!

There are many over-the-counter and prescribed medications that can adversely affect the efficacy of warfarin (Coumadin) and clopidogrel (Plavix). A list of medications and foods that interact with Coumadin and Plavix must be discussed with the patient before discharge. It is essential that the patient understand the necessity of compliance.

WORKSHEET 11E — Multiple-Choice Practice

Answers on page 413

1. Ordered: Administer a bolus of heparin sodium IV. The hospital protocol is 80 units per kg. The patient weighs 160 lb. How many units will you give?
   a. 5840 units
   b. 6620 units
   c. 4320 units
   d. 2420 units

2. Ordered: IV heparin to infuse at 18 units per kg per hr. Available: 1000 mL D5W with 20,000 units heparin. The patient weighs 175 lb. How many units per hr will the patient receive?
   a. 1220 units per hr
   b. 880 units per hr
   c. 1280 units per hr
   d. 1440 units per hr

   At what rate will you set the infusion device?
   a. 110 mL per hr
   b. 85 mL per hr
   c. 68 mL per hr
   d. 72 mL per hr

3. Ordered: Fragmin subcutaneous q12h titrated to kg. Titrate Fragmin to 120 international units per kg subcutaneous. The patient weighs 132 lb. How many kilograms does the patient weigh?
   a. 50 kg
   b. 120 kg
   c. 60 kg
   d. 45 kg

   How many international units of Fragmin will you prepare?
   a. 7000 international units
   b. 5000 international units
   c. 83,000 international units
   d. 7200 international units

4. Refer to question 3. How many milliliters of Fragmin will you give? Available: 10,000 IU per mL multidose vial.
   a. 0.7 mL
   b. 0.5 mL
   c. 1 mL
   d. 1.2 mL

5. Ordered: Fragmin subcutaneous. Titrate to 120 international units per kg q12h for 3-5 days. The patient weighs 185 lb. How many international units of Fragmin will you administer for each dose?
   a. 5800 international units
   b. 1800 international units
   c. 10,080 international units
   d. 6400 international units

6. Refer to question 5. Available: 25,000 IU per mL multidose vial of Fragmin. How many milliliters of Fragmin will you give?
   a. 2.2 mL
   b. 0.4 mL
   c. 4.4 mL
   d. 0.2 mL

7. Ordered: Heparin drip at 40 units per kg. Available: 25,000 units of heparin in 1000 mL of D5W. The patient weighs 75 kg. At what rate will you set the infusion device?
   a. 100 mL per hr
   b. 120 mL per hr
   c. 75 mL per hr
   d. 82 mL per hr

8. Ordered: Heparin IV drip at 500 units/hr. Available: 500 mL 0.9% NS with 10,000 units of heparin. At what hourly rate will you set the infusion?
   a. 50 mL per hr
   b. 75 mL per hr
   c. 100 mL per hr
   d. 25 mL per hr

9. Ordered: Fragmin subcutaneous titrated to 120 international units per kg q12h for 3-8 days. Begin treatment at 0800 hr. The patient weighs 220 lb. How many kg does the patient weigh?

   a. 100 kg　　b. 120 kg　　c. 110 kg　　d. 60 kg

   How many international units of Fragmin will the patient receive per dose?
   a. 10,000 international units
   b. 15,000 international units
   c. 8000 international units
   d. 12,000 international units

10. Refer to question 9. Available: Fragmin 10,000 international units per mL and Fragmin 25,000 international units per mL multidose vials. Which multidose vial will you use? How many mL will you give?

    a. 1 mL　　b. 0.75 mL　　c. 0.48 mL　　d. 0.66 mL

Critical Thinking Exercises

Critical Thinking Exercises provide math and medication-related patient safety issues for student discussion. Answers are not provided.

Analyze the following scenarios.

1. Mrs. Smith, a 76-year-old woman, was recuperating after abdominal surgery. The physician wrote the following order: *2000 units heparin subcut stat*. The nurse administered a 1-mL dose taken from a multidose vial labeled 20,000 units/mL. Later that day, the physician reduced the heparin order. He wrote: *Reduce heparin to 1000 units q8h*. While the nurse is preparing the 1000-unit dose from the multidose vial of 20,000 units/mL, she realizes the error when the first dose of heparin was administered.

   Order:

   Given:

   Error(s):

   Potential injuries:

   Preventive measures:

   Discussion
   What factors contributed to the error?
   How many units of heparin did Mrs. Smith receive for the first dose?
   How was the patient's safety jeopardized?
   What medication should always be on hand when a patient is receiving heparin?
   What safety measures should have been implemented?
   How can this type of error be reconciled?

2. Mr. G., an 80-year-old man, was admitted with a diagnosis of pulmonary embolism. He was given a bolus dose of 80 units of heparin and then was started on an IV drip of 25,000 units of heparin in 500 mL of D5W for 3 days. He has an order to start Coumadin 10 mg daily 72 hours before being discharged. Mr. G.'s discharge orders are for Coumadin (warfarin) 10 mg daily and blood tests for INR status once a week for the first 2 weeks. What precautions will Mr. G. need to be aware of while taking Coumadin?

Discussion:
What types of food might interfere with the desired effects of Coumadin?
What safety precautions should Mr. G. be aware of concerning possible bleeding?
What are some of the OTC medications that could enhance the effect of Coumadin?
What is the need for INR blood tests every week for the first 2 or 3 weeks?
How do you think that noncompliance with diet, medications, lifestyle, and blood testing could interfere with the patient's safety?

3. A 68-year-old woman who had a hip replacement just returned to the general surgery floor. The woman is a type 1 diabetic. The physician wrote a new order that read: *Start IV drip with 500 units of insulin in 1 liter of NS. Infuse over 24 hr. Heparin 250 units subcut q6h.* The nurse charted on the MAR: 500 units of heparin subcut. 250 units of insulin R added to the liter of NS. The nurse on the next shift noticed that the wrong medication and the wrong amount of heparin and insulin were charted for the IV and the subcut injection.

Order:

Given:

Discussion:
What factors contributed to the error?
What measures could be implemented for patient safety?
Why is it important to have another licensed nurse check the order?
What hospital protocols should be addressed to remediate these types of errors?
Do you think that the first nurse was aware of the error?

CHAPTER 11 Final

1. Ordered: Heparin 3000 units subcutaneous for prophylaxis of cerebral thrombosis. Available: 5000 units/mL. How many milliliters will the patient receive?

   $\dfrac{5000 \text{ units}}{1 \text{ mL}} \times \dfrac{1 \text{ dose}}{3000 \text{ units}}$ = **0.6 mL/dose**

2. Ordered: Heparin 2500 units q4h subcutaneous to prevent thrombi from recurring. Available: 10,000 units/mL vial. How many milliliters will the patient receive?

   $\dfrac{2500 \text{ units}}{\text{dose}} \times \dfrac{1 \text{ mL}}{10,000 \text{ units}}$ = **0.25 mL/dose**

3. Ordered: Heparin 2000 units q4h subcutaneous for venous stasis. Available: 5000 units/mL and 10,000 units/mL. Which vial will you choose? If a tuberculin syringe is used, how many milliliters will the patient receive?

   $\dfrac{2000 \text{ units}}{1 \text{ dose}} \times \dfrac{1 \text{ mL}}{\text{units}}$

   5,000 units/mL: **0.4 mL/dose**

   10,000 units/mL: **0.2 mL/dose**

4. Ordered: Heparin 7000 units subcutaneous q8h before initiating a heparin infusion for a venous thromboembolism. Available: 5000, 10,000, and 20,000 units per mL. Which one will you choose? How many milliliters will the patient receive?

$\dfrac{7000 \text{ units}}{1 \text{ dose}} \times \dfrac{1 \text{ mL}}{\square \text{ units}}$

[Label: HEPARIN Sodium Injection, USP 5,000 USP units per mL, 1 mL Vial]

1.4 mL/dose

[Label: HEPARIN Sodium Injection, USP 10,000 USP units per mL, 1 mL Vial]

0.7 mL/dose

[Label: HEPARIN Sodium Injection, USP 20,000 USP units per mL, 1 mL Multi-Dose Vial]

0.35 mL/dose

5. Ordered: Heparin 650 units subcutaneous every 4 hours as a prophylaxis for immobility. Available: Heparin 1000 units per mL. How many milliliters will the patient receive?

[Label: HEPARIN Sodium Injection, USP 1,000 USP units per mL, 1 mL Vial]

$\dfrac{650 \text{ units}}{1 \text{ dose}} \times \dfrac{1 \text{ mL}}{1000 \text{ units}}$

0.65 mL/dose

6. Ordered: 700 units per hr IV to infuse. Available: 20,000 units per 500 mL. How many mL per hr will provide 700 units per hr? For how many hours will the IV infuse? 28.6 hours (24 hours) regulated by CDC

$\dfrac{700 \text{ units}}{\text{hour}} \times \dfrac{500 \text{ mL}}{20000 \text{ units}}$ 17.5 mL/hr

7. Ordered: 1500 units per hr IV for hyperlipidemia. Available: 25,000 units per 500 mL. How many mL per hr will provide 1500 units per hr? For how many hours will the IV infuse?

$\dfrac{1500 \text{ units}}{1 \text{ hour}} \times \dfrac{500 \text{ mL}}{25,000 \text{ units}}$ 30 mL/hr   16 hrs 40 min

8. Ordered: Heparin 35,000 units IV in 24 hr for atrial fibrillation. Available: 1000 mL 0.9% NS with 35,000 units of heparin sodium. How many mL per hr will the patient receive? How many units per hr will the patient receive?

$$\frac{35000 \text{ units}}{24 \text{ hrs}} \times \frac{1000 \text{ mL}}{35000 \text{ units}}$$

41.7 mL/hr
1458 units/hr

9. Ordered: Heparin 2000 units per hr IV for pulmonary emboli. Available: Heparin 20,000 units in 1000 mL 0.9% NS. How many mL per hr will be delivered via the infusion device? For how long will the IV infuse?

$$\frac{2000 \text{ units}}{1 \text{ hr}} \times \frac{1000 \text{ mL}}{20000 \text{ units}}$$

100 mL/hr
10 hours

10. Ordered: Heparin 25,000 units IV in 24 hr for peripheral arterial embolization. Available: 1000 mL with 25,000 units of heparin sodium. How many mL per hr will give 25,000 units in 24 hr? How many units per hr will infuse?

$$\frac{25,000 \text{ units}}{24 \text{ hours}} \times \frac{1000 \text{ mL}}{25,000 \text{ units}}$$

41.7 mL/hr
1042 units/hr

evolve — Refer to the Advanced Calculations section of Drug Calculations Companion, version 5 on Evolve for additional practice problems.

Answer Key

11 Anticoagulants

WORKSHEET 11A (page 385)

1. KNOW   WANT TO KNOW   FRACTION CROSS PRODUCT

10,000 units : 1 mL = 6000 units : x mL $\dfrac{10{,}000}{10x} = \dfrac{6000}{x\ mL}$

10x = 6   10x = 6
 x = 0.6 mL   x = 0.6 mL

PROOF
1 × 6000 = 6000
10,000 × 0.6 = 6000

2. KNOW   WANT TO KNOW   FRACTION CROSS PRODUCT

40 mg : 0.4 mL = 35 mg $\dfrac{40\ mg}{0.4} = \dfrac{35\ mg}{x\ mL}$

40x = 0.4 × 35 = 14   40x = 0.4 × 35 = 14
 x = 0.35   x = 0.35

PROOF
40 × 0.35 = 14
0.4 × 35 = 14

3. KNOW   WANT TO KNOW   FRACTION CROSS PRODUCT

20,000 units : 1 mL = 15,000 units : x mL $\dfrac{20{,}000}{1} = \dfrac{15000}{x\ mL}$

20x = 15   20x = 15
 x = 0.75 mL   x = 0.75 mL

PROOF
1 × 15,000 = 15,000
20,000 × 0.75 = 15,000

4. KNOW   WANT TO KNOW

10,000 international units : 1 mL = 7500 international units : x mL
100x = 75
   x = 0.75 mL Fragmin

PROOF
1 × 75 = 75
100 × 0.75 = 75

405

5. KNOW   WANT TO KNOW   FRACTION CROSS PRODUCT

20,000 units : 1 mL = 17,000 units : x mL } use the 20,000 units per mL strength $\dfrac{20{,}000}{1} = \dfrac{17{,}000}{x \text{ mL}}$

20x = 17
   x = 0.85 mL
PROOF
1 × 17 = 17
20 × 0.85 = 17

6. KNOW   WANT TO KNOW
1000 units : 1 mL = 750 units : x mL
100x = 75
   x = 0.75 mL
PROOF
1000 × 0.75 = 750
1 × 750 = 750

7. KNOW   WANT TO KNOW
1000 units : 1 mL = 800 units : x mL
10x = 8
   x = 0.8 mL
PROOF
10 × 0.8 = 8
1 × 8 = 8

8. KNOW   WANT TO KNOW
5000 units : 1 mL = 3000 units : x mL
5x = 3
   x = 0.6 mL
PROOF
1 × 3 = 3
5 × 0.6 = 3

9. KNOW   WANT TO KNOW
100 units : 1 mL = 50 units : x mL
10x = 5
   x = 0.5 mL
PROOF
1 × 5 = 5
10 × 0.5 = 5

10. KNOW   WANT TO KNOW
100 units : 1 mL = 50 units : x mL
10x = 5
   x = 0.5 mL
PROOF
1 × 5 = 5
10 × 0.5 = 5

WORKSHEET 11B (page 391)

1. a. KNOW   WANT TO KNOW
50,000 units : 1000 mL = 2500 units : x mL
500x = 25 × 1000 = 25,000
5x = 250
x = 50 mL per hr
PROOF
500 × 50 = 25,000
1000 × 25 = 25,000

b. KNOW   WANT TO KNOW
50 mL : 1 hr = 1000 mL : x hr
50x = 1000
x = 20 hr
PROOF
50 × 20 = 1000
1 × 1000 = 1000

2. a. KNOW   WANT TO KNOW
10,000 units : 15 hr = x units : 1 hr
15x = 10,000
x = 666.6 units per hr = 667 units per hr
PROOF
15 × 666.6 = 9999
10,000 × 1 = 10,000

b. $\dfrac{1000}{15}$ = 66.6 or 67 mL per hr

c. KNOW   WANT TO KNOW
67 mL : 1 hr = 700 mL : x hr
67x = 700
x = 10.45 hr or 10 hr 27 min remaining
The IV will be infused at 1727 hours.
PROOF
1 × 700 = 700
67 × 10.45 = 700

3. a. KNOW   WANT TO KNOW
20,000 units : 1000 mL = 1500 units : x mL
200x = 15,000
x = 75 mL per hr = 1500 units heparin
PROOF
200 × 75 = 15,000
1000 × 15 = 15,000

b. KNOW   WANT TO KNOW
75 mL : 1 hr = 1000 mL : x hr
75x = 1000
x = 13.33 hr or 13 hr, 20 min
PROOF
1 × 1000 = 1000
75 × 13.33 = 999.75

4. a. $\dfrac{1000}{12}$ = 83.3 or 83 mL per hr

b. KNOW   WANT TO KNOW
20,000 units : 12 hr = x units : 1 hr
12x = 20,000
x = 1666.6 units per hr = 1667 units per hr
PROOF
20,000 × 1 = 20,000
12 × 1666 = 19,992

c. KNOW   WANT TO KNOW
83 mL : 1 hr = 750 mL : x hr
83x = 750
x = 9 hr remaining
PROOF
1 × 750 = 750
83 × 9 = 747

5. a. KNOW   WANT TO KNOW
10,000 units : 500 mL = 1200 units : x mL
100x = 6000
x = 60 mL per hr
PROOF
500 × 12 = 6000
100 × 60 = 6000

b. KNOW   WANT TO KNOW
60 mL : 1 hr = 500 mL : x hr
60x = 500
x = 8.33 hr or 8 hr 20 min
PROOF
60 × 8.33 = 499.8
1 × 500 = 500

6. a. KNOW   WANT TO KNOW
20,000 units : 1000 mL = 1000 units : x mL
20x = 1000
x = 50 mL per hr = 1000 units heparin
PROOF
20 × 50 = 1000
1000 × 1 = 1000

b. KNOW   WANT TO KNOW
50 mL : 1 hr = 1000 mL : x hr
50x = 1000
x = 20 hr
PROOF
1 × 1000 = 1000
50 × 20 = 1000

7. a. KNOW   WANT TO KNOW
20,000 units : 250 mL = 1000 units : x mL
$20x = 250$
$x = 12.5$ mL per hr or 13 mL per hr
PROOF
$20 \times 12.5 = 250$
$250 \times 1 = 250$

b. KNOW   WANT TO KNOW
13 mL : 1 hr = 250 mL : x hr
$13x = 250$
$x = 19.23$ hr or 19 hr 14 min
PROOF
$1 \times 250 = 250$
$13 \times 19.23 = 249.9$

8. a. KNOW   WANT TO KNOW
25,000 units : 500 mL = 1300 units : x mL
$250x = 6500$
$x = 26$ mL per hr
PROOF
$26 \times 250 = 6500$
$500 \times 13 = 6500$

b. KNOW   WANT TO KNOW
26 mL : 1 hr = 500 mL : x hr
$26x = 500$
$x = 19.23$ hr or 19 hr 14 min
PROOF
$1 \times 500 = 500$
$26 \times 19.23 = 499.98$

9. a. KNOW   WANT TO KNOW
25,000 units : 250 mL = 1800 units : x mL
$250x = 250 \times 18 = 4500$
$250x = 4500$
$x = 18$ mL per hr
PROOF
$250 \times 18 = 4500$
$250 \times 18 = 4500$

b. KNOW   WANT TO KNOW
18 mL : 1 hr = 250 mL : x hr
$18x = 250$
$x = 13.88$ hr or 13 hr 53 min
PROOF
$1 \times 250 = 250$
$18 \times 13.8 = 248.4$

10. a. KNOW   WANT TO KNOW
25,000 units : 500 mL = 1500 units : x mL
$250x = 500 \times 15 = 7500$
$25x = 750$
$x = 30$ mL per hr
PROOF
$250 \times 30 = 7500$
$500 \times 15 = 7500$

b. KNOW   WANT TO KNOW
30 mL : 1 hr = 500 mL : x hr
$30x = 500$
$3x = 50$
$x = 16.66 = 16$ hr 40 min
PROOF
$1 \times 500 = 500$
$30 \times 16.66 = 499.8$

WORKSHEET 11C (page 393)

1. lb to kg = 210 lb divided by 2.2 = 95.5 = 96 kg
   a. KNOW   WANT TO KNOW
   90 units : 1 kg = x units : 96 kg
   $x = 90 \times 96 = 8640$
   $x = 8640$ units loading dose
   PROOF
   $1 \times 8640 = 8640$
   $90 \times 96 = 8640$
   b. KNOW   WANT TO KNOW
   25 units : 1 kg/hr = x units : 96 kg/hr
   $x = 25 \times 96 = 2400$
   $x = 2400$ units per hr
   PROOF
   $25 \times 96 = 2400$
   $1 \times 2400 = 2400$
   c. KNOW   WANT TO KNOW
   1000 mL : 25,000 units = x mL : 2400 units
   $250x = 1000 \times 2400 = 2400$
   $25x = 2400 = 96$
   $x = 96$ mL per hr
   PROOF
   $96 \times 25 = 2400$
   $1 \times 2400 = 2400$

2. lb to kg = 160 lb divided by 2.2 kg = 72.7 = 73 kg
   a. KNOW   WANT TO KNOW
   80 units : 1 kg = x units : 73 kg
   $x = 80 \times 73 = 5840$
   $x = 5840$ units loading dose
   PROOF
   $1 \times 5840 = 5840$
   $73 \times 80 = 5840$
   b. KNOW   WANT TO KNOW
   1000 mL : 30,000 units = x mL : 1500 units
   $300x = 1000 \times 15 = 15{,}000$
   $3x = 150$
   $x = 50$ mL per hr
   PROOF
   $50 \times 300 = 15{,}000$
   $15 \times 1000 = 15{,}000$

3. lb to kg = 176 ÷ 2.2 = 80 kg
   a. KNOW   WANT TO KNOW
   70 units : 1 kg = x units : 80 kg
   $x = 70 \times 80 = 5600$ units loading dose
   PROOF
   $1 \times 5600 = 5600$
   $70 \times 80 = 5600$
   b. KNOW   WANT TO KNOW
   20 units : 1 kg per hr = x units : 80 kg per hr
   $x = 20 \times 80 = 1600$
   $x = 1600$ units per hr
   PROOF
   $1 \times 1600 = 1600$
   $20 \times 80 = 1600$
   c. KNOW   WANT TO KNOW
   1000 mL : 25,000 units = x mL : 1600 units
   $250x = 1000 \times 16 = 16{,}000$
   $x = 64$ mL/hr
   PROOF
   $64 \times 250 = 16{,}000$
   $16 \times 1000 = 16{,}000$

4. lb to kg = 300 lb divided by 2.2 = 136.3 = 136 kg
   a. KNOW   WANT TO KNOW
   75 units : 1 kg = x units : 136 kg
   $x = 75 \times 136 = 10{,}200$
   $x = 10{,}200$ units bolus dose
   PROOF
   $1 \times 110{,}200 = 10{,}200$
   $75 \times 136 = 10{,}200$
   b. KNOW   WANT TO KNOW
   20 units : 1 kg = x units : 136 kg
   $x = 20 \times 136 = 2720$
   $x = 2720$ units per hr
   PROOF
   $1 \times 2720 = 2720$
   $20 \times 136 = 2720$
   c. KNOW   WANT TO KNOW
   1000 mL : 50,000 units = x mL : 2720 units
   $50x = 1 \times 2720 = 2720$
   $50x = 2720$
   $x = 54.4 = 54$ mL per hr
   PROOF
   $1 \times 2720 = 2720$
   $54.4 \times 50 = 2720$

5. lb to kg = 194 divided by 2.2 = 88 kg
   a. KNOW　　　　　WANT TO KNOW
      70 units : 1 kg = x units : 88 kg
      x = 70 × 88 = 6160
      x = 6160 units bolus dose
      PROOF
      1 × 6160 = 6160
      70 × 88 = 6160
   b. KNOW　　　　　WANT TO KNOW
      18 units : 1 kg = x units : 88 kg
      x = 18 × 88 = 1584
      x = 1584 units per hr
      PROOF
      1 × 1584 = 1584
      18 × 88 = 1584
   c. KNOW　　　　　WANT TO KNOW
      1000 mL : 30,000 units = x mL : 1584 units
      30x = 1584 × 1 = 1584
      30x = 1584
      　x = 52.8 = 53 mL per hr
      PROOF
      30 × 52.8 = 1584
      1 × 1584 = 1584

7. a. KNOW　　　　　WANT TO KNOW
      80 units : 1 kg = x units : 120 kg
      x = 80 × 120 = 9600
      x = 9600 units bolus dose
      PROOF
      1 × 9600 = 9600
      80 × 120 = 9600
   b. KNOW　　　　　WANT TO KNOW
      1000 mL : 25,000 units = x mL : 1000 units
      25x = 1000
      　x = 40 mL per hr
      PROOF
      25 × 40 = 1000
      1 × 1000 = 1000

6. lb to kg = 145 divided by 2.2 = 65.9 = 66 kg
   a. KNOW　　　　　WANT TO KNOW
      65 units : 1 kg = x units : 66 kg
      x = 65 × 66 = 4290
      x = 4290 units bolus dose
      PROOF
      1 × 4290 = 4290
      65 × 66 = 4290
   b. KNOW　　　　　WANT TO KNOW
      15 units : 1 kg per hr = x units : 66 kg per hr
      x = 15 × 66 = 990 units
      x = 990 units per hr
      PROOF
      1 × 990 = 990
      15 × 66 = 990
   c. KNOW　　　　　WANT TO KNOW
      500 mL : 30,000 units = x mL : 990 units
      30x = 5 × 990 = 4950
      30x = 495
      　x = 16.5 = 17 mL per hr
      PROOF
      990 × 500 = 495,000
      30,000 × 16.5 = 495,000

8. lb to kg = 185 divided by 2.2 = 84.09 = 84 kg
   a. KNOW　　　　　WANT TO KNOW
      75 units : 1 kg = x units : 84 kg
      x = 75 × 84 = 6300
      x = 6300 units bolus dose
      PROOF
      1 × 6300 = 6300
      75 × 84 = 6300
   b. KNOW　　　　　WANT TO KNOW
      17 units : 1 kg per hr = x units : 84 kg per hr
      x = 17 × 84 = 1428
      x = 1428 units per hr
      PROOF
      1 × 1428 = 1428
      17 × 84 = 1428
   c. KNOW　　　　　WANT TO KNOW
      1000 mL : 20,000 units = x mL : 1428 units
      20x = 1 × 1428 = 1428
      20x = 1428
      　x = 71.4 = 71 mL per hr
      PROOF
      1 × 1428 = 1428
      20 × 71.4 = 1428

9. **a.** KNOW   WANT TO KNOW
   95 units : 1 kg = x units : 136 kg
   $x = 95 \times 136 = 12{,}920$
   $x = 12{,}920$ units loading dose
   PROOF
   $1 \times 12{,}920 = 12{,}920$
   $95 \times 136 = 12{,}920$

   b. KNOW   WANT TO KNOW
   20 units : 1 kg per hr = x units : 136 kg per hr
   $x = 20 \times 136 = 2720$
   $x = 2720$ units per hr
   PROOF
   $1 \times 2720 = 2720$
   $20 \times 136 = 2720$

   c. KNOW   WANT TO KNOW
   1000 mL : 20,000 units = x mL : 2720 units
   $20x = 1 \times 2720 = 2720$
   $20x = 2720$
      $x = 136$ mL per hr
   PROOF
   $2000 \times 136 = 272{,}000$
   $1000 \times 272 = 272{,}000$

10. **a.** KNOW   WANT TO KNOW
    1000 units : 1 kg = x units : 108 kg
    $x = 1000 \times 108 = 108{,}000$
    $x = 108{,}000$ units loading dose
    PROOF
    $1 \times 108{,}000 = 108{,}000$
    $1000 \times 108 = 108{,}000$

    b. KNOW   WANT TO KNOW
    18 units : 1 kg = x units : 108 kg
    $x = 18 \times 108 = 1944$
    $x = 1944$ units per hr
    PROOF
    $1 \times 1944 = 1944$
    $18 \times 108 = 1944$

    c. KNOW   WANT TO KNOW
    1000 mL : 35,000 units = x mL : 1944 units
    $35x = 1944$
       $x = 55.54 = 56$ mL per hr
    PROOF
    $35 \times 55.54 = 1943.9$
    $1944 \times 1 = 1944$

WORKSHEET 11D (page 395)

1. Give initial bolus dose = 80 units/kg
   KNOW   WANT TO KNOW
   80 units : 1 kg = x units : 70 kg
   $x = 70 \times 80 = 5600$
   $x = 5600$ units initial bolus dose

   PROOF
   $80 \times 70 = 5600$
   $1 \times 5600 = 5600$

2. Initial infusion rate: 18 units per kg per hr
   KNOW   WANT TO KNOW
   18 units : 1 kg per hr = x units : 70 kg
   $x = 70 \times 18 = 1260$
   $x = 1260$ units per hr. Round off units to nearest whole number = 1300 units per hr

   PROOF
   $18 \times 70 = 1260$
   $1 \times 1260 = 1260$

3. KNOW   WANT TO KNOW
   250 mL : 25,000 units = x mL : 1300 units
   $250x = 250 \times 13 = 3250$
      $x = 13$ mL per hr

   PROOF
   $250 \times 1300 = 325{,}000$
   $13 \times 25000 = 325{,}000$

   After 6 hours the aPTT is 30. Rebolus with 80 units/kg (5600 units). Increase the rate by 4 units per kg per hr.

4. **a.** KNOW   WANT TO KNOW
   4 units : 1 kg = x units : 70 kg
   $x = 4 \times 70 = 280$ units round to 300 units

   PROOF
   $4 \times 70 = 280$
   $1 \times 280 = 280$

   b. 1300 units/hr increased by 300 units = 1600 units/hr

5. Reset infusion rate to:
   KNOW   WANT TO KNOW
   250 mL : 25,000 units = x mL : 1600 units
   $25{,}000x = 250 \times 1600 = 400{,}000$
   $25x = 400$
      $x = 16$ mL per hr is the new rate for the infusion

   PROOF
   $250 \times 1600 = 400{,}000$
   $16 \times 25{,}000 = 400{,}000$

   After 6 hours the aPTT is 40. Increase IV rate by 2 units per kg per hr. Rebolus with 40 units per kg.

6. KNOW   WANT TO KNOW   **PROOF**

    40 units : 1 kg = x units : 70 kg   40 × 70 = 2800

    x = 40 × 70 = 2800   1 × 2800 = 2800

    x = 2800 units bolus dose

7. KNOW   WANT TO KNOW   **PROOF**

  a. 2 units : 1 kg = x units : 70 kg   2 × 70 = 140

      x = 2 × 70 = 140   1 × 140 = 140

      x = 140 units per hr rounded to 100 units

  b. 1600 units per hr increased by 100 units = 1700 units per hr

    Reset infusion rate to:

8. KNOW   WANT TO KNOW   **PROOF**

    250 mL : 25,000 units = x mL : 1700 units   250 × 1700 = 425,000

    250x = 250 × 17 = 4250   17 × 25,000 = 425,000

       x = 17 mL per hr is the new rate for the infusion

    6-hour aPTT is 55 = no change in the rate.

    6-hour aPTT is 85. Decrease rate by 2 units per kg per hr.

9. KNOW   WANT TO KNOW   **PROOF**

  a. 2 units : 1 kg = x units : 70 kg   2 × 70 = 140

      x = 2 × 70 = 140   1 × 140 = 140

      x = 140 rounded to 100 units per hr decrease

  b. 1700 units/hr decreased by 100 units/hr = 1600 units per hr new rate

    Reset infusion rate to:

10. KNOW   WANT TO KNOW   **PROOF**

    250 mL : 25,000 units = x mL : 1600 units   250 × 1600 = 400,000

    250 = 250 × 1600 = 4,000   16 × 25,000 = 400,000

    25x = 400

      x = 16 mL per hr new rate to set the IV pump

    6-hr aPTT is 95. Decrease rate by 3 units per kg per hr.

11. KNOW   WANT TO KNOW   **PROOF**

  a. 3 units : 1 kg = x units : 70 kg   3 × 70 = 210

      x = 3 × 70 = 210   1 × 210 = 210

      x = 210 units = 200 units/hr decrease

  b 1600 units per hr decreased by 200 units per hr = 1400 units per hr new rate

    Reset infusion rate to:

12. KNOW   WANT TO KNOW   **PROOF**

    250 mL : 25,000 units = x mL : 1400 units   250 × 1400 = 350,000

    250x = 250 × 14 = 3500   25,000 × 14 = 350,000

    250x = 3500

      x = 14 mL per hr new IV rate.

13. Stop infusion for 1 hour before resuming IV rate. Next aPTT in 6 hours.

WORKSHEET 11E (page 399)

1. a. KNOW   WANT TO KNOW
80 units : 1 kg = x units : 73 kg
$x = 80 \times 73 = 5840$
$x = 5840$ units of heparin
PROOF
$1 \times 5840 = 5840$
$80 \times 73 = 5840$

2. d. KNOW   WANT TO KNOW
18 units : 1 kg = x units : 80 kg
$x = 18 \times 80 = 1440$
$x = 1440$ units/hr
PROOF
$1 \times 1440 = 1440$
$18 \times 80 = 1440$

   d. KNOW   WANT TO KNOW
1000 mL : 20,000 units = x mL : 1440 units
$20{,}000x = 1000 \times 1440 = 1{,}440{,}000$
       $x = 72$ mL per hr
PROOF
$1000 \times 1440 = 1{,}440{,}000$
$72 \times 20{,}000 = 1{,}440{,}000$

3. c. KNOW   WANT TO KNOW
1 kg : 2.2 lb = x kg : 132 lb
$2.2x = 132$
  $x = 60$ kg
PROOF
$1 \times 132 = 132$
$2.2 \times 60 = 132$

   d. KNOW   WANT TO KNOW
120 international units : 1 kg =
          x international units : 60 kg
$x = 60 \times 120$
$x = 7200$ international units q12h
PROOF
$1 \times 7200 = 7200$
$60 \times 120 = 7200$

4. a. KNOW   WANT TO KNOW
10,000 international units : 1 mL =
       7200 international units : x mL
$10{,}000x = 7200$
     $x = 0.72 = 0.7$ mL
PROOF
$7200 \times 1 = 7200$
$10{,}000 \times 0.72 = 7200$

5. c. KNOW   WANT TO KNOW
120 international units : 1 kg =
          x international units : 84 kg
$x = 120 \times 84 = 10{,}080$
$x = 10{,}080$ international units of Fragmin
PROOF
$120 \times 84 = 10{,}080$
$1 \times 10{,}080 = 10{,}080$

6. b. KNOW   WANT TO KNOW
25,000 international units : 1 mL =
          10,080 : x mL
$25{,}000x = 10{,}080$
     $x = 0.4$ mL
PROOF
$1 \times 10{,}080 = 10{,}080$ (units can be rounded up or down)
$0.4 \times 25{,}000 = 10{,}000$

7. b. KNOW   WANT TO KNOW
1000 mL : 25,000 units = x mL : 3000 units
$25{,}000x = 3{,}000{,}000$
    $25x = 3000 = 120$ mL per hr
PROOF
$25 \times 120 = 3000$
$1000 \times 3 = 3000$

8. d. KNOW   WANT TO KNOW
10,000 units : 500 mL = 500 units : x mL
$10{,}000x = 250{,}000$
     $x = 25$ mL per hr
PROOF
$25 \times 10{,}000 = 250{,}000$
$500 \times 500 = 250{,}000$

Answer Key

9. a. 220 divided by 2.2 = 100 kg

    d. KNOW   WANT TO KNOW

       120 international units : 1 kg =

                      x international units : 100 kg

       $x = 120 \times 100 = 12{,}000$

       $x = 12{,}000$ international units Fragmin

       PROOF

       $1 \times 12{,}000 = 12{,}000$

       $100 \times 120 = 12{,}000$

10. c. KNOW   WANT TO KNOW

    25,000 international units : 1 mL =

                    12,000 international units : x mL

    $25{,}000x = 12{,}000$

           $x = 0.48$ mL

    PROOF

    $1 \times 12{,}000 = 12{,}000$

    $25{,}000 \times 0.48 = 12{,}000$

CHAPTER 11 FINAL: ANTICOAGULANTS (page 402)

1. 0.6 mL

2. 0.25 mL

3. 0.2 mL using the 10,000 units per mL strength or 0.4 mL using the 5000 units per mL strength
Give 0.2 mL the smallest amount. Use the 10,000 units per mL vial

4. 0.35 mL using the 20,000 units per mL strength or 0.7 mL using the 10,000 units per mL strength or 1.4 mL using the 5,000 units per mL strength
Give 0.35 mL, the smallest amount.

5. 0.65 mL

6. 17.5 mL/hr or 18 mL/hr
27 hr, 46 min

7. 30 mL per hr
16 hr, 40 min

8. 42 mL per hr
1458 units per hr

9. 100 mL per hr via infusion device
10 hr to infuse

10. 42 mL per hr
1042 units per hr

Children's Dosages

Objectives
- Evaluate drug doses for safe dose range (SDR).
- Calculate doses in mcg per kg and mg per kg and square meters of body surface area (BSA).
- Calculate 24-hour drug doses and divided doses for specific weights for oral and parenteral medications.
- Identify medication-related safety precautions with pediatric patients.
- Analyze medication errors using critical thinking.

Introduction

The trend for increased safety in medication administration for pediatric patients is to provide pediatric customized doses and supplies. The usual medication doses and supplied amounts for adults have resulted in adverse drug events (ADE) for pediatric patients. Pediatric patients often receive very small (fractional) medication doses compared to an adult. Nurse competency for safe medication administration is essential to protect this at-risk population that cannot protect itself. Communication about the medications with the family caretaker(s) is also essential. Mentoring with an experienced, intuitive pediatric nurse is ideal during the clinical experience phase.

Vocabulary

Anaphylactic Shock: An extreme life-threatening inflammatory allergic reaction that can occur in any age group. Immediate medication is needed en route to emergency room. A few of the common offenders are medications such as penicillin, sulfa drugs, aspirin; foods such as tree nuts, shellfish, and eggs; and insect bites and bee stings. The patient's history—including prior mild allergic reactions—must be documented on the MAR and rechecked before each medication is administered.

Body Surface Area (BSA): Square meters (m^2) of external skin area used to calculate drug dosages for specific drugs and patient conditions.

Milligrams or Micrograms per kilogram (mg per kg; mcg per kg): Metric measurement of drug dose per body weight in kilograms (kg). Common units of measurement for medications for pediatric and adult patients, particularly for parenteral medications.

Nomogram: Graphic representation of numerical relationships.

Safe Dose Range (SDR): Minimum-to-maximum therapeutic dose range for a target population: adult, child, infant, neonate, and/or older adult. Prescription and administration of medications requires prior knowledge of the SDR to provide patient safety.

Square Meter (m²): Metric unit of area measurement, slightly more than a square yard (1 sq meter = 1.19 sq yd), used in measurement of body surface area for drug calculations. Doses are much smaller than weight-based doses.

Dosages Based on Body Weight and Surface Area

Infants and children have special medication needs because of their smaller size and weight as well as larger body surface area (BSA) per kilogram of body weight, which is larger than that of an adult. Pediatric patients have varying capabilities of drug absorption, digestion, distribution, metabolism, and excretion. It is very important for the nurse to check current references for pediatric medication orders and to verify safe dose ranges (SDRs) with current, reliable drug references or a pharmacist before administering the dose to prevent errors and injury. Minute doses that require scrupulous mathematics may be ordered. Pediatric and intensive care nurses use written pediatric drug guidelines and calculators to determine weights and verify SDRs.

Two methods currently used for calculating safe pediatric and adult doses are based on (1) *body weight* in milligrams per kilogram (mg per kg) or micrograms per kilogram (mcg per kg) and (2) *body surface area* in square meters (m²) using a scale called a *nomogram*.

mg per kg Method (Weight-Based Dosing)

The most *frequently* used calculation method for customized dosing is *mg per kg*. References usually state the safe amount of drug in mg per kg for a 24-hour period to be given in one or more divided doses. You may also see *mcg per kg* cited for therapeutic doses when very small amounts of medication are to be given.

Because kilograms are required for weight-based medications, the nurse does not usually have to convert pounds and ounces to kilograms. In the event that only a pound/ounce weight is available, the nurse needs to know how to convert pounds and ounces to kilograms.

Steps to Solving mg per kg Problems

Step 1 a. **Estimate** the weight in kilograms by dividing the pounds in half*; then *calculate* the weight in kilograms using 2.2 lb = 1 kg equivalency (divide pounds by 2.2). Use a calculator. Check your estimate with the answer.

b. If a weight is in *pounds* and *ounces,* convert the ounces to the nearest tenth of a pound and *add* this to the total pounds. Then convert the total pounds into kilograms to the nearest tenth (two-step calculation). (Refer to page 417 for kilogram-to-pound conversions and page 16 for rounding instructions.)

Step 2 **Calculate** the safe dose range (SDR) using a calculator and current safe dose recommendations found in current, reliable drug literature for this child's weight in mg per kg or mcg per kg.

Step 3 **Compare** and **evaluate** the 24-hr ordered dose with the recommended SDR. Be sure the comparisons are for the *same* dosing frequency!

Step 4 If safe, **calculate** the actual dose to be administered using written ratio and proportion. If the ordered dose is *less* than or *more* than the SDR, hold the medication and clarify the order promptly.

Shortcut Steps
1. Weight in kg to nearest tenth of a kilogram
2. SDR per 24 hours and per dose
3. Compare with order
4. Calculate whether or not dose is safe to give

---

*Estimation helps prevent major math errors; it must be followed by calculation and verification.

RULE All pediatric medication administration begins with an accurate kilogram weight (Step 1) and a calculation of the SDR (Step 2).

Example **Ordered:** erythromycin oral suspension 150 mg po q6h for an infant allergic to penicillin who has an infection. Patient weight: 15 lb, 6 oz today. The literature states that the SDR is 30 to 100 mg per kg per day in four divided doses for severe infections.

[Drug label: Erythromycin Ethylsuccinate Oral Suspension, USP. NDC 0074-3747-16. One Pint (473 mL). 200 mg Erythromycin Activity per 5 mL. Shake well before using. Store in refrigerator to preserve flavor. Refrigeration by patient is not required if used within 14 days. Dispense in a USP tight, light-resistant container. Usual dose: Children — 30-50 mg/kg/day in equally divided doses. See package enclosure for adult dose and full prescribing information. 02-8499-3/R5. Do not accept if band on cap is broken or missing. Rx only. Pediatric erythromycin ethylsuccinate. Each teaspoonful (5 mL) contains: erythromycin ethylsuccinate equivalent to 200 mg of erythromycin. Abbott Laboratories, North Chicago, IL 60064, U.S.A.]

Step 1 **Estimate** the infant's weight.
 a. *Pounds to kilograms:* 15 lb ÷ 2 = 7.5 kg
 Calculate the actual weight.
 b. **Two-step** conversion because ounces are involved.
   Ounces to pounds: 6 oz ÷ 16 = 0.37 lb. Add part of pound to total pounds. The infant thus weighs 15.4 lb.
   Pounds to kilograms: 15.4 lb ÷ 2.2 = 7 kg (close to estimate)

Step 2 The **SDR** recommended for children more than 1 month of age is 30 to 100 mg per kg per day po in four divided doses.
 Low-range calculation: 30 mg × 7 kg = 210 mg (low SDR) per day ÷ 4 = 52.5 mg per dose
 High-range calculation: 100 mg × 7 kg = 700 mg (high SDR) per day ÷ 4 = 175 mg per dose

Step 3 **Compare** and **evaluate:** The **SDR** recommended for this child's weight is 210 to 700 mg total q24h in four divided doses.
 Ordered: 150 mg q6h or 150 mg × 4 or 600 mg total in 24 hr.

Step 4 **Decision:** Give medication. Administering 600 mg for the day is within the SDR of 210 to 700 mg in four divided doses. Administer with an oral syringe.
 Calculate the individual dose (write out and prove).

KNOW	WANT TO KNOW	FRACTION CROSS PRODUCT
200 mg : 5 mL = 150 mg : x mL		$\dfrac{200}{5} = \dfrac{150}{x}$

$\dfrac{200}{200}x = \dfrac{750}{200}$ (5 × 150)

$x = 3.75$ mL

PROOF
200 × 3.75 = 750
5 × 150 = 750

ANSWER
Give 3.75 mL*

Hint Review and analyze the logic of these four steps.

⊙ CLINICAL ALERT!
 Avoid two potential errors when converting pounds and ounces to kilograms. First, ounces must be converted to part of a pound *before* converting total pounds to kilograms; for example, 6 oz does not convert to 0.6 lb. Second, 15.4 lb does not equal 15.4 kg.
 Do not forget the second step—convert the total pounds to kilograms.

---

*Use a 1-mL syringe to add 0.75 mL if the exact dose or calibrated dropper is not supplied by the pharmacy.

CHAPTER 12 Children's Dosages

Answers on page 442

WORKSHEET 12A | Calculator Practice

RULE Calculators are used in pediatric and adult care units for long division and multiplication problems. Dividing ounces by 16 will give the pound equivalent in the first step of two-step problems. Dividing or multiplying by 2.2 will give pound and kilogram equivalents. Note: Knowing your own weight in kilograms is a helpful reminder of the difference between pound and kilogram weight.

1. Estimate the weight conversions, then use a calculator to convert from pounds to kilograms or kilograms to pounds. Round to the *nearest tenth*. Double-check all work.

   a. 14 lb (1 or 2 steps?)
      Estimate:
      Actual:
   b. 12 lb, 2 oz (1 or 2 steps?)
      Estimate:
      Actual:
   c. 10 lb
      Estimate:
      Actual:
   d. 14 kg
      Estimate:
      Actual:
   e. 10 kg
      Estimate:
      Actual:

2. Calculate the 24-hr total dose in milligrams.
   a. 150 mg q8h
   b. 200 mg q6h
   c. 400 mcg q4h
   d. 50 mg tid
   e. 750 mcg q12h

3. Calculate the unit dose.
   a. 1 g in 4 equally divided doses
   b. 750 mg divided in 3 equal doses
   c. 2 g in 4 to 6 equally divided doses
   d. 16 g a day in 2 to 4 divided doses
   e. 500 mg in 4 divided doses

4. Calculate the SDR in milligrams for the following weights. Note that the answers will only be in milligrams or micrograms because *x*, the unknown, is a *dosage* measurement not a weight measurement. You want to know how many milligrams a day and milligrams per dose are safe for this patient. (2.2 lb = 1 kg)

   SDR per kg; Weight
   a. 10 mg per kg; weight is 5 kg
   b. 5 to 8 mg per kg; weight is 7.3 kg
   c. 6 to 8 mg per kg; weight is 8 lb
   d. 3 to 6 mg per kg; weight is 5 lb, 8 oz
   e. 200 to 400 mcg per kg; weight is 4 lb, 6 oz

   SDR for This Weight
   _____ Safe total mg per day
   _____ SDR for the day in mg
   _____ SDR for the day in mg
   _____ SDR for the day in mg
   _____ SDR for the day in mg

5. **Ordered:** Drug X, 50 mg tid. **SDR:** 2 to 3 mg per kg given in three divided doses. Patient weight: 18 kg.
   a. SDR for 24 hr
   b. SDR per dose
   c. Total ordered dose for day and per dose
   d. Evaluation and decision: Safe or unsafe to give? Why?

418 Drug Calculations: *Ratio and Proportion Problems for Clinical Practice*

WORKSHEET 12B | Safe Dose Range (SDR) Practice

Answers on page 443

For each problem, use a calculator to calculate the SDR, and compare it with the order. If the total dose for 24 hours is excessive, the unit dose is automatically excessive. Evaluate the order and make a decision.

1. Give medication (within SDR for unit dose and 24-hr dose).
2. Hold and clarify promptly (overdose or underdose).

1. Weight: 9.1 kg
   SDR in literature: 2 to 4 mg per kg per day
   Ordered: 50 mg daily
   a. SDR for this child:
   b. Dose ordered:
   c. Evaluation and decision:

2. Weight: 15 kg
   SDR in literature: 100 to 200 mcg per kg per day in divided doses
   Ordered: 0.5 mg tid
   a. SDR for this child:
   b. Dose ordered:
   c. Evaluation and decision:

3. Weight: 11.5 kg
   SDR in literature: 10 to 30 mg per kg per day in divided doses*
   Ordered: 100 mg tid
   a. SDR for this child:
   b. Dose ordered:
   c. Evaluation and decision:

4. Weight: 38.6 kg
   SDR: 10 to 15 mg per kg per day in 4 to 6 divided doses
   Ordered: 100 mg q6h
   a. SDR for this child:
   b. Dose ordered:
   c. Evaluation and decision:

5. Weight: 2.3 kg
   SDR: 10 to 20 mcg per kg per day
   Ordered: 0.03 mg four times daily
   a. SDR for this child:
   b. Dose ordered:
   c. Evaluation and decision:

---

*In divided doses, the total dose must be divided into two or more doses.

CHAPTER 12 Children's Dosages

BSA Method (mg per m²)

The term "body surface area" refers to the total external body area. The estimated BSA in square meters (m²) is derived from height and weight measurements by using a mathematical formula. It is considered the most reliable way to calculate therapeutic dosages.

This method may be used to calculate safe dosages of antineoplastic drugs, of new drugs, and of drugs for special populations such as infants, children, frail elderly patients, and patients with cancer.

Example Child weighs 33 lb (15 kg) and has a BSA of 0.55 m².

Ordered: 20 mg per kg	vs	**Ordered:** 20 mg per m²	vs	**Ordered:** 20 mg per lb
20 mg : 1 kg = x mg : 15 kg		20 mg : 1 m² = x mg : 0.55		20 mg : 1 lb = x mg : 33 lb
x = 20 × 15 = 300 mg		x = 20 × 0.55 = 11 mg		x = 20 × 33 = 660 mg

As seen, the doses calculated range from 11 mg to 660 mg and, depending on the unit of measurement, reflect extremely large differences. This illustrates the need to check not only the numbers but also the units of measurement.

The West nomogram in Figure 12-1 allows the user to plot the *estimated* square meters of BSA by using height and weight measurements.

FIGURE 12-1 West nomogram for estimation of body surface area (BSA). *A,* The estimated BSA in square meters for children of normal height for weight is determined by reading the m² at the alignment point with the child's weight in pounds in the highlighted column. The blue line denoted by the arrow reveals that an infant weighing 10 lb has an approximate BSA of 0.27 m². *B,* The BSA in square meters for children who are *under*weight or *over*weight (refer to pediatric standard growth charts and development grids for normal height and weight ranges for pediatric groups) is determined by connecting the child's plotted weight in the left column and plotted height in the right column with a straight line and reading the intersection point on the SA (surface area) column, as indicated by the arrow on the red line. This illustrates an estimated BSA of 0.28 m² for an infant of 60 cm height weighing 4.5 kg. Reading the SA column requires that height and weight be plotted in the same system of measurement—metric or pounds/inches. (From Kliegman RM, Stanton BF, St. Geme JW, et al: *Nelson textbook of pediatrics,* ed. 19, Philadelphia, 2011, Saunders.)

> **CLINICAL ALERT!**
>
> Nurses are not expected to calculate BSA. The pharmacy provides the BSA calculations. Nurses *do* have a critical responsibility to distinguish the difference in a medication order based on mg per **kg** of weight and an order based on mg per **m²** of BSA (e.g., 20 mg per kg vs 20 mg per m²).

Calculating BSA (m²) Using a Mathematical Formula

There are two formulas for calculating BSA (m²), and both use height and weight dimensions.
A. Formula using only metric system. B. Formula using only pounds and inches

$$\sqrt{\frac{\text{Weight (kg)} \times \text{Height (cm)}}{3600}} = m^2 \text{ BSA} \qquad \sqrt{\frac{\text{Weight (lb)} \times \text{Height (in)}}{3131}} = m^2 \text{ BSA}$$

Note the differences in the divisors. The formulas must be used exactly as shown.

Example Using a calculator and the metric formula, determine the BSA in square meters for a child with a weight of 20 kg and a height of 95 cm.

Step 1 Multiply the kilograms by centimeters first and *divide* the result by 3600 (20 × 95 = 900/3600 = 0.527)

Step 2 Obtain the *square root* of 0.527 by pushing the square root button. *Round* your answer to the *nearest* hundredth.

$$\frac{20 \times 95}{3600} = 0.527 \qquad \sqrt{0.527} = 0.725 = 0.73 \text{ m}^2$$

Compare this answer with the West nomogram (see Figure 12-1). Create a straight line between 20 kg and 95 cm and read the result in the surface area (SA) column on the nomogram. Take care to plot the height and weight on the metric graph—the outside columns. When reading the results (m²) columns, be sure to note the value of each calibrated line on the scale at the intersection point. The formula method is more accurate.

A square meter is slightly larger than a square yard. Visualize a square meter or a square yard of skin. As seen on the nomogram, a child of 90 lb has only about 1 square meter of BSA (1 m²). Use one of the formulas to calculate your own BSA.

Answers on page 443

WORKSHEET 12C | Comparing BSA-Based (mg per m²) Dosages With mg per lb and mg per kg Orders

Use the West nomogram (see Figure 12-1), highlighted section for children of normal height and weight, to obtain the BSA (m²) based on weight.

Calculate the dose to be given based on the mg per m² and dose ordered. Compare the doses to be given. All the weights are the same.

	Wt in lb	BSA in m²	Dose Ordered	Dose to be Given
1.	4 lb	0.15	10 mg per m²	10 × 0.15 = 1.5 mg
2.	6 lb	_____	15 mg per m²	_____
3.	10 lb	_____	5 mg per m²	_____

Calculate the dose to be given in mg per kg measurements. Divide lb by 2.2 to obtain kilogram weight.

	Wt in kg (to nearest tenth)	Dose Ordered	Dose to be Given
4.	4 lb = 1.8 kg	10 mg per kg	10 × 1.8 = 18 mg
5.	6 lb = _____ kg	2 mg per kg	_____
6.	20 lb = _____ kg	5 mg per kg	_____

Calculate the dose for the same-weight children in mg per lb measurements.

	Wt in lb	Dose Ordered	Dose to be Given
7.	4 lb	10 mg per lb	4 × 10 = 40 mg
8.	6 lb	15 mg per lb	_____
9.	20 lb	5 mg per lb	_____

10. Using the appropriate BSA formula on page 421, obtain the BSA in m^2 for a child who weighs 70 lb and is normal height for weight.

CLINICAL ALERT!

Consider the patient safety implications when mg per m^2, mg per lb, and mg per kg are erroneously interchanged. This mistake has resulted in serious errors. The nurse must understand the differences among these three terms and focus to ensure that the correct values are being used when calculating the dose.

Answers on page 443

WORKSHEET 12D | Additional Children's Safe Dose Range (SDR) Practice

Calculate SDRs and doses. Evaluate the order. If dose is within the SDR, calculate and prove the answer.

1. SDR: 1 to 2 g per day in 4 divided doses
Ordered: 500 mg q6h
  a. SDR for this child:
  b. Dose to be administered:
  c. Evaluation and decision:

2. Weight: 44 lb, normal weight for height
SDR: 5 to 8 mg per m^2* daily
Ordered: 4 mg daily
  a. SDR for this child:
  b. Dose ordered:
  c. Evaluation and decision:

3. Weight: 8.6 kg
SDR: 0.1 to 0.3 mg per kg per day in 2 divided doses
Ordered: 2500 mcg bid
  a. SDR for this child:
  b. Dose ordered:
  c. Evaluation and decision:

4. Weight: 4.1 kg
SDR 1 to 5 mcg per kg per day
Ordered: 0.01 mg daily
  a. SDR for this child:
  b. Dose ordered:
  c. Evaluation and decision:

5. Weight: 6.4 kg
SDR: 0.02 to 0.05 mg per kg per day
Ordered: 150 mcg bid
  a. SDR for this child:
  b. Dose ordered:
  c. Evaluation and decision:

---

*For BSA conversion, refer to West nomogram (see Figure 12-1).

CLINICAL ALERT!

Estimating the approximate dose of a medication before doing the actual calculation is a valuable safety check for calculation errors. Estimation can alert you to major math errors. Verify your estimate with calculations.

The trend is to supply the appropriate calibrated equipment with pediatric medications to reduce potential dosing errors caused by using household equipment (Figure 12-2).

FIGURE 12-2 **A,** Acceptable devices for measuring and administering oral medication to children (clockwise): measuring spoon, plastic syringes, calibrated nipple, plastic medicine cup, calibrated dropper, hollow-handled medicine spoon. **B,** Prefilled oral syringe. **C,** Calibrated droppers. **D,** Medibottle. (**A,** From Wong DL et al: *Wong's nursing care of infants and children,* ed 7, St. Louis, 2005, Mosby. **C,** From Macklin D, Chernecky C, Infortuna H: *Math for clinical practice,* ed 2, St. Louis, 2011, Mosby.)

Fluid Requirements

CLINICAL ALERT!

Volume needs for infants and children are very different from those of adults. Overhydration and dehydration can present grave risks to pediatric patients. The nurse must be aware of the fluid orders, including fluid restriction orders, in relation to the current intake and output when administering liquid medications. This is a critical responsibility. Infants have a higher fluid volume as a percentage of body weight than do older children and adults. They lose more water through the skin and a higher percentage of fluids from the lungs and excrete more urine, which is less concentrated.

Contrast the differences between the normal requirements of a healthy adult and a child (Table 12-1).

Table 12-1 Fluid Requirements of Healthy Children and Adults

Weight	Normal Fluid Volume Need	Sample Weight (kg)	Average Daily (mL)	Hourly (mL)
Neonate	90 mL per kg per 24 hr	3	270	11
Up to 10 kg	120 mL per kg per 24 hr after age 7 days	8	960	40
11-20 kg	1000 mL + 50 mL per kg over 10 kg	15	1250	52
Over 20 kg	1500 mL + 20 mL per kg over 20 kg	25	1600	67
Average adult	2-3 L per day	68	2000-3000	125

Note the differences in adult and pediatric safe dosages in Table 12-2.

Table 12-2 Drug Dosage Comparison by Age-Group

Drug Name	Dosage Comparison
▶ **Potassium chloride (KCl)***	SDR, **Adult,** individualized: IV 20-60 mEq q24h 200 mEq per 24 hr for hypokalemia is usually not exceeded. 40 mEq dilution per liter preferred. SDR, **Child,** individualized: IV 1-4 mEq per kg of body weight per 24 hr. or 10 mEq per hr, whichever is **less,** not to exceed 40 mEq per 24 hr. Must be at least 40 mEq dilution per liter. Monitor serum potassium levels. Contact prescriber if patient is fluid restricted. Monitor ECG for symptoms of hypokalemia and hyperkalemia. Pediatric: KCL must be infused on electronic infusion pump. Obtain written order for *each* infusion.
▶ **Morphine sulfate**	
Pain relief	**Adult,** IV: 2.5-15 mg q4h
Postoperative analgesia	**Child,** IV: 0.01-0.04 mg per kg per hr
	Neonate, IV: 015-0.02 mg per kg per hr†
Severe chronic cancer pain	**Child,** IV: 0.025-2.6 mg per kg per hr
Amoxicillin	**Adult,** PO: 250-500 mg q8h **Child,** PO: 25-50 mg per kg per day (max 60-80 per kg per day divided q8h)
▶ **Digoxin IV injection**	Initial loading (digitalizing) dose **Premature:** 15-25 mcg per kg **2-5 yr:** 25-35 mcg pr kg **Over 10 yr:** 8-12 mcg per kg

*All formulations of KCl must always be diluted and well mixed before administration and before placing it on an IV apparatus.

†A neonate refers to an infant in the first 4 weeks of life. Consult drug references for child age-related dosage guidelines; they vary.

Slashes (/) will be seen in printed drug references. Write out "per" for slashes to avoid misinterpretation and medication errors.

WORKSHEET 12E: Children's Oral Medications

Answers on page 444

These medications can be given to infants and children with a dropper or in an oral medication syringe. Small amounts may be given to an infant in a nipple.

For each problem, use a calculator to determine the child's weight in kilograms or pounds if required, calculate the SDR, and compare it with the order. Evaluate the order and make a decision:

1. Give medication (within SDR for unit dose and 24-hr dose).

2. Hold and clarify promptly (overdose or underdose).

⊙ CLINICAL ALERT!

If a nipple is used to deliver medication, rinse the nipple with water first so that the medicine will flow rather than stick to the nipple. Family may be very helpful with oral medication administration by holding the child or by giving the oral medication or something pleasant-tasting following the medication.

For decisions 1 and 2 only, calculate the medication amount to be administered using *written ratio and proportion*. Prove your work. Do *not* calculate overdose or underdose orders. Hold them and clarify promptly.

1. **Ordered:** acetaminophen children's oral suspension 160 mg po for a 4-year-old child who weighs 14 kg today.
   a. Estimated weight in lb:
   b. Actual weight in lb:
   c. SDR for this child:
   d. Dose ordered:
   e. Evaluation and decision:
   f. Amount to be given in mL if applicable:

Drug Facts (continued)
- use only enclosed dosing cup designed for use with this product. Do not use any other dosing device.
- if needed, repeat dose every 4 hours while symptoms last
- do not give more than 5 times in 24 hours
- do not give for more than 5 days unless directed by a doctor
- this product does not contain directions or complete warnings for adult use

Weight (lb)	Age (yr)	Dose (tsp or mL)
under 24	under 2 years	ask a doctor
24-35	2-3 years	1 tsp or 5 mL
36-47	4-5 years	1 1/2 tsp or 7.5 mL
48-59	6-8 years	2 tsp or 10 mL
60-71	9-10 years	2 1/2 tsp or 12.5 mL
72-95	11 years	3 tsp or 15 mL

Attention: use only enclosed dosing cup specifically designed for use with this product. Do not use any other dosing device.

Other information
- each teaspoon contains: sodium 3 mg
- store at 20°-25°C (68°-77°F)
- do not use if printed neckband is broken or missing

Inactive ingredients anhydrous citric acid, butylparaben, carboxymethylcellulose sodium, carrageenan, D&C red no. 33, FD&C blue no. 1, flavor, glycerin, high fructose corn syrup, hydroxyethyl cellulose, microcrystalline cellulose, propylene glycol, purified water, sodium benzoate, sorbitol solution

Questions? Call 1-800-910-6874

*This product is not manufactured or distributed by the Tylenol Company, owner of the registered trademark Tylenol®.

094 01 0137 ID209441
Distributed by Target Corporation
Minneapolis, MN 55403
© 2009 Target Brands, Inc.
All Rights Reserved Shop Target.com

NDC 11673-130-26

children's acetaminophen
oral suspension
80 mg per ½ teaspoon
(160 mg per 5 mL)
fever reducer/pain reliever

Compare to active ingredient in Children's Tylenol® Oral Suspension*

see new warnings information

alcohol free
ibuprofen free
aspirin free

up&up
grape flavor
AGE 2-11 YEARS

4 FL OZ (118 mL)

2. **Ordered:** Clindamycin HCl pediatric solution 300 mg q8h po. The child weighs 30 kg today. The SDR is 10 to 30 mg per kg per day in 3 to 4 divided doses. **Available:** Clindamycin palmitate pediatric oral solution 75 mg per 5 mL.
   a. SDR for this child:
   b. Dose ordered:
   c. Evaluation and decision:
   d. Amount to be given in mL if applicable:

> **CLINICAL ALERT!**
>
> Avoid mixing medicines in essential foods such as formula or milk. A changed taste may result in long-term refusal of that food. Gelatin, applesauce, or sherbet in small amounts may be used to mix the medications if the diet allows. The medicine may be followed immediately with formula, juice, or an ice pop as the diet permits. Keep in mind that if not all of the mixture is ingested, all of the medication will not be administered.

3. **Ordered:** Tegretol (carbamazepine) oral suspension 0.25 g po tid for a child with seizures. The SDR for maintenance in a child over 12 years of age is 400 to 800 mg per day in 3 to 4 divided doses. **Available:** carbamazepine 100 mg per 5 mL.
   a. SDR for this child:
   b. Dose ordered in mg:
   c. Evaluation and decision:
   d. Amount to be given if applicable:

4. **Ordered:** leucovorin calcium 5 mg q6h po. The child weighs 24 lb and has normal weight and height. The SDR according to the literature is 10 mg per m^2 q6h for 72 hr. For BSA calculation, refer to the West nomogram (see Figure 12-1). The BSA is determined by pounds, not kilograms. **Available:** leucovorin calcium tablets 5mg.
   a. SDR for this child:
   b. Dose ordered:
   c. Evaluation and decision:
   d. Amount to be given if applicable:

5. **Ordered:** Augmentin 200 mg q8h po for a child with an infection who weighs 12.3 kg. The SDR is 20 to 40 mg per kg per day in 3 divided doses. **Available:** Augmentin oral suspension 125 mg per 5 mL.
   a. SDR for this child:
   b. Dose ordered:
   c. Evaluation and decision:
   d. Amount to be given in mL if applicable:

> **CLINICAL ALERT!**
>
> Monitor for allergic-type reactions: rash, diarrhea, or increased respiratory difficulty.

Multiple subcutaneous and intramuscular injections are not preferred for pediatric patients because of limited sites and potential emotional and physical trauma. Nevertheless, some vaccines, analgesics, and single-dose medicines or daily hormones are given using this route. The technique must be practiced in a clinical laboratory setting under supervision.

- The vastus lateralis can be used from birth to adulthood but is a *preferred injection* site for IM injections for babies younger than 7 months (Figure 12-3).
- The ventrogluteal muscle is an *alternate site* for IM injections for children over 7 months and for adults (Figure 12-4).
- The deltoid site may be used for small-volume, nonirritating IM medications, 0.5 to 1 mL, in older children and adults with *well-developed* deltoid muscles (Figure 12-5).
- Needle lengths and gauges and fluid amounts are much smaller for pediatric patients.

FIGURE 12-3 Vastus lateralis intramuscular injection site. (From Wilson D, Hockenberry MJ: *Wong's clinical manual of pediatric nursing,* ed. 9, St. Louis, 2011, Mosby.)

FIGURE 12-4 Ventrogluteal intramuscular injection site. (From Wilson D, Hockenberry MJ: *Wong's clinical manual of pediatric nursing,* ed. 9, St. Louis, 2011, Mosby.)

FIGURE 12-5 Deltoid intramuscular injection site. (From Wilson D, Hockenberry MJ: *Wong's clinical manual of pediatric nursing,* ed. 9, St. Louis, 2011, Mosby.)

CLINICAL ALERT!

The dorsogluteal site is not a recommended injection site because of the dangers both in children and adults of damaging the sciatic nerve and striking blood vessels.

Subcutaneous injections are given in the anterolateral thigh (upper outer thigh portion) of infants up to age 1 and adults. The mid-lateral thigh can be used for children and adults with a sufficient fatty layer. The size of needle and angle of injection is adjusted for the depth of the fatty layer that can be pinched up. Parents are asked to comfort the child after the staff perform a painful procedure.

Answers on page 445

WORKSHEET 12F | Children's Subcutaneous and Intramuscular Medications

Subcut and IM injections are rarely ordered on a regular basis for pediatric patients. Calculate the SDR, and compare it with the order. Evaluate the order and make a decision:

1. Give medication (within SDR for unit dose and 24-hr dose).

2. Hold and clarify promptly (overdose or underdose).

For decisions 1 and 2 only, calculate the medication amount to be administered *using written ratio and proportion.* Double-check and prove your work. Do *not* calculate overdose orders.

1. **Ordered:** morphine sulfate 4 mg subcut stat to treat a child with pain (Figure 12-6) who weighs 25.2 kg. The SDR is 0.1 to 0.2 mg per kg per dose.
   a. SDR for this child:
   b. Dose ordered:
   c. Evaluation and decision:
   d. Volume to be administered if applicable:

Label: NDC 10019-176-44 Morphine Sulfate Inj., USP 5 mg/mL FOR SC, IM OR SLOW IV USE 1 mL DOSETTE Vial PROTECT FROM LIGHT DO NOT USE IF PRECIPITATED. Mfd. for an affiliate of Baxter Healthcare Corporation by: Elkins-Sinn Cherry Hill, NJ 08003 400-823-01

Asking children and adults to point with one finger where it hurts the most is helpful for localizing specific areas.

CLINICAL ALERT!
Do not confuse morphine with hydromorphone. Do not use the popular abbreviation MS for morphine sulfate or magnesium sulfate even if only one of the two is used in a specific clinical area. One can be misread for the other. Clarify any MS order with the prescriber.

0	1 or 2	2 or 4	3 or 6	4 or 8	5 or 10
No hurt	Hurts little bit	Hurts little more	Hurts even more	Hurts whole lot	Hurts worst

FIGURE 12-6 Wong-Baker FACES pain rating scale for children over 3 years of age and adults. (From Hockenberry MJ, Wilson D, Winkelstein ML: *Wong's essentials of pediatric nursing,* ed. 9, St Louis, 2013, Mosby.)

2. **Ordered:** atropine sulfate 0.2 mg subcutaneous preoperatively for a child who weighs 8.6 kg. The SDR for a child weighing 7 to 9 kg is 0.2 mg, 30 to 60 min before surgery.
   a. SDR for this child:
   b. Dose ordered:
   c. Evaluation and decision:
   d. Volume to be administered if applicable:

3. **Ordered:** ampicillin sodium 500 mg IM q12h for a 3.2-kg infant with septicemia. SDR is 100 to 200 mg per kg per day in 2 divided doses.
   a. SDR for this child:
   b. Dose ordered:
   c. Evaluation and decision:
   d. Volume to be administered if applicable:

4. **Ordered:** glycopyrrolate 0.16 mg IM 60 minutes before anesthesia induction. Patient's weight: 40 kg. SDR: 0.004 mg per kg IM.
   a. SDR for this child:
   b. Dose ordered:
   c. Evaluation and decision:
   d. Volume to be administered if applicable:

5. **Ordered:** EpiPen (adrenalin)* 2-pack subcut single-use autoinjector with trainer 0.3 mg for a child who is being discharged after an anaphylactic reaction. Patient's weight: 30 kg. SDR is 0.3 mg, 1:1000 for a patient weighing ≥30 kg. **Available:** EpiPen single-use autoinjectors 0.3 mg, 1:1000 and EpiPen 0.15 mg, 1:2000.
   a. What are the metric terms for the concentrations: 1:1000? 2:2000? (Hint: they are the same as for basic IV solutions taught in Chapter 7)
   b. How is an autoinjector different from other syringes?
   c. How many mg per mL are in a 1:1000 concentration?
   d. How many mg per mL are in a 1:2000 concentration?
   e. Is the dose ordered safe?

---

*Do not confuse EpiPen with Epifrin.

The pen must be kept near the child at all times and plans made with responsible people when the child is away from home. Nurses and family need to be very well informed on all aspects of this type of allergic reaction and how to use the pen, including practice with the trainer. Encourage the family to read all the literature and to have follow-up visits with the provider or referred allergist. Recommended reference for the nurse and family: https://www.epipen.com.

CLINICAL RELEVANCE
Only the **middle** of the autoinjector is held. It does not have a plunger. The ends are not to be touched.

The **orange end** contains the needle and is immediately pressed against the *middle of the upper outer* (anterolateral) *thigh*—NO OTHER LOCATION—*through clothing if necessary* for both children and adults. On contact with the skin, the autoinjector releases the hidden fine needle to the subcutaneous layer. The **blue end** is touched to deactivate the autoinjector after use.

CLINICAL RELEVANCE
Discharge planning needs to start when the EpiPen is ordered.

Children's IV Medications: Reconstitution, Dilution, and Flow Rate Information

Hospital pharmacies and pediatric drug references provide directions for dilution and rates of administration of IV medications for children. The volumes are smaller than those for adults. After determining that the ordered dose is within the SDR, the nurse may have to dilute the medication in a prescribed ratio, withdraw the ordered amount, then further dilute it using a compatible IV solution, and administer it directly or by an infusion pump in a volume-control device. Devices used to administer IV medications to children are shown in Figure 12-7. Volume-control devices help prevent fluid and/or drug overdoses.

FIGURE 12-7 A, Electronic infusion pump with volume-control device. **B,** Gravity infusion with microdrip tubing (60 gtt per mL delivered through a needle) and volume-control device. Electronic infusion devices with volume-control devices are preferred for the administration of IV fluids to infants and children. If one of these is not available, microdrip (60-drop factor) tubing should be used with a volume-control device to prevent fluid or drug overload. Small volumes to be delivered IV within a short period may be administered directly through a syringe or a syringe pump. **C,** Freedom 60-syringe infusion pump. This portable reusable manual infusion uses standard 60-mL syringes and can be filled from 1 to 60 mL. It offers flow rates with rate-controlled tubing from 0.5 to 1200 mL per hr. It does not permit free flow. (**C,** From A B Repro-Med Systems, Inc., Chester, N.Y.)

Example **Ordered:** Antibiotic 1 g q6h IV. Supplied: A powdered form of antibiotic that requires reconstitution. Pediatric directions from pharmacy: *Dilute to 100 mg per mL, withdraw ordered amount, then further dilute to 30 mL, and administer over 20 min.* The label reads 2 grams (2 g).

Step 1 Dilute to 100 mg per mL. The label reads 2 g. (Change to milligrams for dilution: 2 g = 2000 mg.)

KNOW   WANT TO KNOW

100 mg : 1 mL = 2000 mg : x mL

$$\left(\frac{100}{1} = \frac{2000}{x\ mL}\right) \quad \frac{Drug}{Volume} = \frac{Drug}{Volume}$$

$$\frac{100}{100}x = \frac{2000}{100}$$

$$x = 20\ mL$$

PROOF
100 × 20 = 2000
1 × 2000 = 2000

Reconstitute antibiotic with 20 mL compatible solution.*

Step 2 Withdraw ordered amount (1 g).

KNOW   WANT TO KNOW

2 g : 20 mL = 1 g : x mL $\left(\dfrac{2}{20} = \dfrac{1}{x}\right)$

$2x = 20$
$x = 10\ mL = 1\ g$

PROOF
2 × 10 = 20
20 × 1 = 20

ANSWER
10 mL

Step 3 Place the medication in a volume-control device, adding a compatible IV solution to 30 mL. Set the flow rate. Consult a procedure book for use of volume-control devices. Flow rate:

KNOW   WANT TO KNOW

30 mL : 20 min = x mL : 60 min $\left(\dfrac{30}{20} = \dfrac{x}{60}\right)$

$$\frac{20}{20}x = \frac{1800}{20}$$

$$x = 90\ mL\ per\ hour$$

PROOF
30 × 60 = 1800
20 × 90 = 1800

ANSWER
Set rate at 90 mL per hr for 20 min

RULE To *estimate* hourly IV flow rates for amounts to be delivered in less than 60 minutes by a pump: for **10** minutes, multiply the volume by 6 because there are six 10-minute periods in an hour; for **15** minutes, multiply the volume by 4; for **20** minutes, multiply the volume by 3; and for **30** minutes, multiply the volume by 2. This will work only for 10-, 15-, 20-, and 30-minute orders.

To *calculate* the setting for mL per hr on a pump for medications to be delivered in less than **1 hour,** set up a ratio and proportion of milliliters to minutes. The final dilution may be made with an existing IV solution if it is compatible with the medication.

Example To give 10 mL in 15 min with a pump, *estimate* (10 × 4 = 40 mL per hr). Calculate:

KNOW   WANT TO KNOW

10 mL : 15 min = x mL : 60 min $\left(\dfrac{10}{15} = \dfrac{x}{60}\right)$

$$\frac{15}{15}x = \frac{600}{15}$$

$$x = 40\ mL$$

PROOF
10 × 60 = 600
15 × 40 = 600

ANSWER
40 mL per hr

---

*For information and practice reconstituting medications, refer to Chapter 6.

Example **Ordered:** Antibiotic 250 mg q4h IV.
The label reads: *Mix (dilute) with 4.2 mL sterile water for injection to yield 5 mL of 100 mg per mL.*
Amount of ordered antibiotic to be withdrawn after mixing:

KNOW   WANT TO KNOW

100 mg : 1 mL = 250 mg : x mL

$$\left(\frac{100}{1} = \frac{250}{x}\right)$$

$$\frac{\cancel{100}}{\cancel{100}}x = \frac{250}{100}$$

$$x = 2.5 \text{ mL}$$

PROOF
100 × 2.5 = 250
1 × 250 = 250

ANSWER
2.5 mL

Directions for pediatric administration: *Further dilute to 25 mL and administer over 30 minutes.* Total volume to be administered: 25 mL.

Example Flow rate in volume-control device, estimate (2 × 25 = 50 mL per hr):

KNOW   WANT TO KNOW

25 mL : 30 min = x mL : 60 min

$$\left(\frac{\cancel{25}^{5}}{\cancel{30}_{6}} = \frac{x}{60}\right)$$

30x = 25 × 60 or 1500
x = 50 mL

PROOF
26 × 60 = 1500
30 × 50 = 1500

ANSWER
50 mL per hr

Answers on page 446

WORKSHEET 12G | Children's IV Medications

For each problem, use a calculator to determine the child's weight in kg if required, calculate the SDR, and compare it with the order. Round oz, lb, and kg to the nearest tenth. Evaluate the order and make a decision:

1. Give medication (within SDR for unit dose and 24-hr dose).

2. Hold and clarify promptly (overdose or underdose).

Calculate the medication amount to be administered based on the label provided. Use written ratio and proportion and prove your answer even if you use a calculator to verify it. Calculate the IV pump flow rate in mL per hr if medication is to be administered for more than 5 min. Round ounces and kilograms to the nearest tenth. Enter calculator data twice for verification.

🚩 **1. Ordered:** phenobarbital sodium 50 mg IV preoperative sedation.
Patient's weight: 28.2 kg. The SDR for sedation is 1 to 3 mg per kg,
1 to 1½ hr before procedure.
   a. SDR for this child:
   b. Dose ordered:
   c. Evaluation and decision:
   d. Dose in mL to the nearest hundredth to be withdrawn before dilution:

NDC 0641-0476-21
Phenobarbital Sodium Injection, USP IV
65 mg/mL ℞ only
FOR IM OR SLOW IV USE
1 mL Vial
Do not use if discolored or precipitated.
Manufactured by
WEST-WARD
462-349-02
(01)00306410476214
Lot:
Exp.:

432   Drug Calculations: *Ratio and Proportion Problems for Clinical Practice*

2. **Ordered:** Initial dose of furosemide 25 mg IV stat for a child with urinary retention. The SDR is 1 mg per kg to titrate gradually in 1 mg per kg increments to desired response, not to exceed 6 mg per kg. The child weighs 25 kg today.
   a. SDR for this child:
   b. Dose ordered:
   c. Evaluation and decision:
   d. Volume to be administered if applicable:

   4 mL Single-dose Vial   Rx only   NDC 0409-6102-04
   Furosemide Injection, USP
   Do not use if solution is discolored or contains particulate.   RL-3862
   Hospira, Inc.
   Lake Forest, IL 60045 USA
   40 mg/4 mL (10 mg/mL)
   INTRAVENOUS or INTRAMUSCULAR USE.
   Hospira

3. **Ordered:** Garamycin 15 mg IV q8h for a child with an infection. Patient weight: 6 kg today. The SDR is 2 to 2.5 mg per kg q8h. Directions from the pharmacy say to dilute *to* 50 mL with 0.9% NaCl and administer over 60 minutes. **Available:** Garamycin pediatric injectable 20 mg per 2 mL.
   a. SDR for this child:
   b. Dose ordered:
   c. Evaluation and decision:
   d. Amount withdrawn from vial:

> **CLINICAL ALERT!**
> Many of the generic antibiotics, particularly the cephalosporins, have very similar names, such as ceftizoxime, ceftriaxone, and cephradine. However, the uses and the SDRs are very different!

4. **Ordered:** digoxin 0.5 mg IV stat for a child with congestive heart failure. SDR: 0.015 to 0.35 mg per kg. Patient's weight: 11.1 kg. **Directions:** Administer IV over 5 minutes. Dilute each mL of drug in 4 mL SW to permit small amounts of drug to be infused over 5 minutes. Use a calculator to determine SDR.
   a. SDR for this child:
   b. Dose ordered:
   c. Evaluation and decision:
   d. How many mL of digoxin will you prepare before dilution?
   e. What flow rate per minute will you administer after dilution?

   NDC 0641-1410-35
   Digoxin Injection, USP
   500 mcg/2 mL
   Store at 20°-25°C (68°-77°F).
   Baxter Healthcare Corporation
   Deerfield, IL 60015 USA
   40 packs each containing 25 x 2 mL DOSETTE Ampuls
   475-523-00
   LOT/EXP
   (01) 5 03 10019 12345 0 (30) 0100

5. **Ordered:** Geopen (carbenicillin disodium) 2 g IV q6h for a child with an infection. The SDR is 50 to 500 mg per kg q24h in divided doses every 4 to 6 hr. Dilute to 200 mg per mL with compatible solution and administer at rate of 1 per 10 min. Patient weight: 11.8 kg.
   a. SDR for this child:
   b. Dose ordered:
   c. Evaluation and decision:
   d. Amount withdrawn after reconstitution:
   e. Flow rate in mL per hr if applicable:

➤ CLINICAL ALERT!

Pediatric IV flow rates carry a high potential for errors. Consult current, reliable pediatric IV drug references and the pharmacy for pediatric IV dilutions and rates of administration. Note that liquids added to solids result in a higher total volume than just the amount of liquid added. Instructions to dilute **with** x mL result in more volume than instructions to dilute **to** x mL. Dilute *to* limits a total volume for the mixture. Dilute **with** is just stating the amount of liquid to be added to the solid. When in any doubt about IV dilutions and flow rates, consult the pharmacy and document the verification. The prescriber may have to be contacted, too.

Answers on page 447

WORKSHEET 12H | Multiple-Choice Practice

For the following problems, estimate kilograms, then calculate kilograms to the *nearest* tenth when a pound-to-kilogram conversion is needed, and estimate the answers before solving each step.

1. A child weighs 50 lb. What is a rough estimate of the equivalent kg?
   a. 200
   b. 50
   c. 100
   d. 25

2. **Ordered:** methotrexate sodium 30 mg per m^2 po daily maintenance for a child with leukemia. The child's BSA is 1.20 m^2.* How much medication will you administer?
   a. 1.20 mg
   b. 30 mg
   c. 36 mg
   d. 30.12 mg

3. **Ordered:** 1.5 tsp of acetaminophen suspension liquid po stat for a child with fever. How many milliliters will you administer?
   a. 5 mL
   b. 7.5 mL
   c. 8 mL
   d. 10 mL

4. Which foods are best to administer with medications for infants and children?
   a. Their favorite fruit juices
   b. Formula or milk
   c. High-protein shakes
   d. Applesauce, sherbet, gelatin

5. Which of many instructions is accurate to give a parent of a child who is being discharged with a prescription for an EpiPen?
   a. Always keep the EpiPen in the refrigerator or a cooler.
   b. Have an unexpired EpiPen in a convenient location near the child at all times.
   c. If the EpiPen is not used before its expiration date, it will not be necessary to spend the money on another one.
   d. Use the EpiPen as a backup when you cannot transport the child to an emergency department.

6. Which IM route is not recommended for infants and children and patients with undeveloped gluteal muscles?
   a. Vastus lateralis
   b. Ventrogluteal
   c. Dorsogluteal
   d. Deltoid

---

*Note: Trailing zeros appear in BSA m^2 measurements. Delete them for math calculations.

434 Drug Calculations: *Ratio and Proportion Problems for Clinical Practice*

7. **Ordered:** Phenytoin oral suspension 15 mg bid po for a 6-kg child with seizures. The SDR is 5 mg per kg in 2 to 3 divided doses. Label reads: Dilantin pediatric suspension 30 mg per 5 mL. Your decision:
   a. Hold and clarify the order with the physician. It is an overdose.
   b. The order is safe. Give 2.5 mL.
   c. Clarify the order with an experienced supervisor.
   d. The order is safe. Give 15 mL.

8. Which muscle is recommended for IM injections for infants less than 7 months of age or for underweight infants?
   a. Vastus lateralis
   b. Ventrogluteal
   c. Dorsogluteal
   d. Deltoid

9. Which medication order would result in the largest dose?
   a. 20 mg
   b. 20 mg per kg
   c. 20 mg per m^2
   d. 20 mg per lb

10. In addition to distracting a young pediatric patient, how is it best to involve a parent when administering an injection?
    a. Have the parent assist with restraining the child to avoid movement during the injection.
    b. Ask the parent to comfort the child after the procedure.
    c. Have the parent(s) leave the room during the procedure.
    d. Ask the parent to visit children who do not have visitors until the child has calmed down.

Critical Thinking Exercises

Critical Thinking Exercises provide math and medication-related patient safety issues for student discussion. Answers are not provided.

Analyze the following scenarios.

1. Baby Louise is in your unit with a diagnosis of congestive heart failure secondary to a congenital heart defect. She weighs 8.4 kg at age 18 months. Her orders include lanoxin 0.05 mg po bid. The orders include temporary fluid restriction to 500 mL per 24-hr period. On hand is furosemide oral solution 10 mg per mL. Given this a.m. by the reporting nurse: 2 mL. During report, the nurse tells you that for the past 24 hours the intake exceeded 500 mL by 120 mL because the baby wouldn't take the medicine without a lot of juice.

   Is there a problem with mathematics?

   What error in concepts of arithmetic rounding might have led to an error?

   Which knowledge bases are insufficient?

   Medication error(s) and possible causes:

   Fluid intake error:

   Potential injuries:

   Nursing actions:

   Recommendations for the nurse and for patient safety if you were on a hospital committee studying this incident:

2. John, a 3-year-old boy weighing 20 kg, has an order for IV anticoagulation. Heparin *25 units per kg per hr* continuous infusion is ordered until the next laboratory checks. Pharmacy supplies a premixed drug concentration (12,500 International Units in 250 mL D5W). Pharmacy instruction is to infuse at 10 mL per hr. Nurse A has calculated that the child needs 500 units per hr, that 50 units per mL (12,500 per 250) are in the solution, and that the flow rate should be 50 mL per hr.

How many units per hr are needed based on John's kg weight? How many units of heparin per mL are there in the solution?

How many mL per hour should be infused? Who is correct, the pharmacist or the nurse?

Potential ADE/sentinel events:

What would you do if you were Nurse A?

Recommendations for the agency Safety Committee if you were on the committee:

Do you believe that nurses should also double-check the SDR for all drug orders?

3. A 10-kg child admitted with hyperglycemia, patient of Nurse A, has an order for Regular insulin 0.05 units per kg per hr. The agency requires a second independent nurse check for all high-risk drugs. Nurse A and Nurse B agree that the order is safe. Nurse B, the independent check nurse, leaves. Nurse A programs 0.5 units Regular insulin per kg per hr on the IV Smart Pump. An overdose alarm alert sounds. There is also an option on the pump to override the visual and auditory alert and administer the IV. Nurse A needs to decide whether to override or recheck.

How much of an error was programmed?

Why do you think this happened?

Potential ADE from this event?

Under what circumstances do you believe an agency should or should not permit an override of a pump alert?

What sort of procedure should a hospital have for an override?

Do you have any recommendations for Nurse B, the independent check nurse?

Web reference: www.ihi.org

CHAPTER 12 Final

Use a calculator to find the SDR for each child. Compare it with the order. Make a decision: Safe to give or hold and contact prescriber. If safe, calculate the dose.

1. **Ordered:** Cephalexin capsules* 2 g per day in 4 divided doses po q6h × 7 days for John, a 14-year-old with a respiratory infection. The SDR for adults and teenagers is 1000 to 4000 mg per day in divided doses.
   a. Dose ordered:
   b. SDR:
   c. Decision: Safe to give or hold and contact prescriber?
   d. If safe, how many capsules will you give?

2. **Ordered:** levothyroxine† sodium tablets 0.15 mg po daily to John's 16-year-old sister, who has hypothyroidism. The SDR for patients more than 12 years old, 2 to 3 mcg per kg. Patient's weight: 60 kg.
   a. SDR:
   b. Dose ordered:
   d. Decision: Safe to give or hold and contact prescriber? If unsafe, state reason.
   e. How many tablets will you give?

---

*Read the antibiotic labels that begin with *C* very carefully. Many of the generic versions look alike and sound alike (e.g., cefazolin, cefaclor, cefepime, cefotaxime, cefotetan) but have different purposes and dosing. For more information, visit www.ismp.org/tools/confused-drugnames.pdf.
†Do not confuse levothyroxine with levofloxacin, an antibiotic.

3. **Ordered:** Benadryl Allergy Liquid (diphenhydramine HCl) 25 mg po tid and at bedtime × 3 days for John's pruritus. Johnny is 8 years old. Read the label and make your decision.
   a. Safe daily dose maximum for this child:
   b. Dose ordered for 24 hr:
   c. Decision: Safe to give or hold and contact prescriber? If unsafe, state reason.
   d. Dose to be administered:

CLINICAL ALERT!

Approximately 15% of people, or 1 in 6 persons, with an allergy to penicillin will have an allergy to the cephalosporins.

4. Ordered amoxicillin clavulanate potassium* oral suspension 700 mg po q8h for Marissa, a 13-year-old with otitis media. Patient's weight: 35 kg. The SDR for children less than 40 kg is 20 to 40 mg per kg per day in divided doses q8h.
   a. SDR for this child:
   b. Dose ordered:
   c. Decision: Safe to give or hold and contact prescriber?
   d. If safe, how many mL will you give? If unsafe, state reason.

---

*Do not confuse amoxicillin with the compound drug amoxicillin clavulanate potassium or amoxipine. They are different drugs for different uses.

5. Karen, age 3, is admitted to the hospital with a compound fracture of the femur incurred during an automobile accident. **Ordered:** atropine sulfate 0.3 mg preop IM. The SDR for children weighing 12 to 16 kg is 0.3 mg 30 to 60 min before surgery. Karen weighs 35 lb.
   a. SDR for this child:
   b. Dose ordered:
   c. Decision: Safe to give or hold and contact prescriber?
   d. Dose to be administered:

6. **Ordered:** valproic acid* oral solution 0.1 g po bid for a child with a seizure disorder. The SDR for initial administration is 10 to 15 mg per kg per day in 2 or 3 divided doses. Patient's weight: 20 kg. *Directions:* immediately before use, dilute the medication with distilled water, acidified tap water, or juice.
   a. SDR for this child:
   b. Decision: Safe to give or hold and contact prescriber?
   c. If safe, how many mL will you give?

CLINICAL ALERT!

Check compatibility with the other medications ordered for the patient. Double-check the eMAR for orders for more than one antiseizure medication and clarify before administration. Usually a patient is on only one antiseizure medication. Note: Many antiseizure medications are incompatible with several other drugs.

7. **Ordered:** Nystatin 200,000 units 4 times a day for a 3-month-old infant with oral candidiasis (thrush). The SDR is 100,000 units to each side of the mouth 4 times a day. Directions: this suspension must be well mixed before administration. For children and adults, have the patient swish the solution around the inside of the mouth and retain in the mouth for several minutes if possible. For infants, paint the solution in recesses of the mouth, inside cheeks, and on the tongue.
   a. If the order is safe, how many milliliters will you place on each side of the mouth?
   b. Which device in Figure 12-2 would you use to administer this medication if a "brush" was not available to coat the inside of the mouth?

---

*The brand name equivalent of valproic acid is Depakote. Do not confuse Depakote with Depakene.

8. **Ordered:** epinephrine 0.01 mg per kg 1:1000* subcut stat (not to exceed 0.5 mg) for a child brought to an outpatient clinic with an anaphylactic reaction, bronchospasm/airway obstruction caused by an insect bite. May repeat in 20 minutes, not to exceed 0.5 mg for bronchospasm/airway obstruction. Patient weight: 20 kg. The patient has a history of eczema and asthma.
   a. 1:1000 solution = _____ mg per mL; 1:10,000 solution = _____ mg per mL
   b. What is the numerical difference between the solutions?
   c. How many milliliters will you administer subcut?
   d. What would be the difference in dose if the nurse prepared a 0.1 mg per kg instead of 0.01 mg because of misreading the order or a decimal calculation error?

CLINICAL ALERT!
Clarify any questions about the order or the supply with the most appropriate professional on the site.

CLINICAL RELEVANCE
Epinephrine orders vary depending on the use, the route of administration, and the age of the patient. Because there is less familiarity with these types of solutions, the nurse needs to take time to study the usual orders and labels of acute lifesaving medications so that when an emergency arises, the label and contents will be familiar.

CLINICAL ALERT!
Review agency policies for verbal orders. These occur with emergency situations. Repeating the order with the medication label in hand while facing the person who ordered the medication is very important.

9. **Ordered:** leucovorin calcium 0.01 g q6h po for a child with toxic effects resulting from an antineoplastic agent. The child weighs 70 lb and has normal height for weight. The SDR for children is up to 10 mg per m^2 q6h for 72 hr. Use the West nomogram* to determine the BSA for this child's weight.
   a. BSA in m^2:
   b. SDR for this child:
   c. Dose ordered:
   d. Evaluation and decision:
   e. Amount to be given if applicable:

*Refer to Figure 12-1 for the West nomogram.

10. **Ordered** for a child with hemophilia: a recommended dose of NovoSeven 90 mcg per kg, IV bolus, q3h until hemostasis is achieved or until the treatment has been judged to be inadequate. The child's weight is 22 kg. Directions: Administer over 2 to 5 minutes slow bolus. This bolus will be administered over 3 minutes with the syringe provided. These are single-dose vials that must be discarded 3 hours after reconstitution. Use a calculator for long division and multiplication.

   a. Dose in mcg ordered for this child:
   b. Equivalent dose in mg:
   c. Total mL to be administered:
   d. How many vials of medication will the nurse need?
   e. Total calibrations to be occupied by the volume (refer to syringe):
   f. mL per minute:
   g. Indicate the total dose with an arrow on the syringe.

   h. How many mL will remain after a. 1 minute; b. 2 minutes; c. 3 minutes?

CLINICAL ALERT!

Beware of medication orders for "T" and "t" and "tsp"—for example, 1 T daily or 1 tsp daily. Teaspoon and tablespoon abbreviations can easily be confused. Also, dosage strength may vary per teaspoon among infant, child, and adult preparations and may also vary among manufacturers. Call the physician and clarify the specific strength desired in milligrams, milliequivalents, or units.

evolve Refer to the Pediatric Calculations section of Drug Calculations Companion, version 5 on Evolve, for additional practice problems.

Answer Key

12 Children's Dosages

WORKSHEET 12A (page 418)

1. **a.** Estimate: 7 kg
      Actual: 6.4 kg
   b. Estimate: 6 kg
      Actual: 12.1 lb (2 steps)
      5.5 kg
   c. Estimate: 5 kg
      Actual: 4.5 kg
   d. Estimate: 28 lb
      Actual: 30.8 lb
   e. Estimate: 20 lb
      Actual: 22 lb

3. **a.** 1 g or 1000 mg ÷ 4 = 250 mg
   b. 750 mg ÷ 3 = 250 mg
   c. 2 g or 2000 mg ÷ 4 = 500 mg
      2 g or 2000 mg ÷ 6 = 333.3 mg
   d. 16 g a day ÷ 2 = 8 g
      16 g a day ÷ 4 = 4 g
   e. 500 mg ÷ 4 = 125 mg

2. **a.** 150 mg × 3 = 450 mg
   b. 200 mg × 4 = 800 mg
   c. 400 mcg × 6 = 2400 mcg or 2.4 mg
   d. 50 mg × 3 = 150 mg
   e. 750 mcg × 2 = 1500 mcg or 1.5 mg

4. **a.** 10 × 5 = 50 mg
   b. 5 × 7.3 = 36.5 mg (low dose)
      8 × 7.3 = 58.4 mg (high dose)
      SDR is 36.5 to 58.4 mg.
   c. 8 lb = approximately 4 kg estimated
      Step 1: 8 lb = 3.6 kg actual
      Step 2: Low dose: 6 × 3.6 = 21.6 mg
           High dose: 8 × 3.6 = 28.8 mg
      SDR is 21.6 to 28.8 mg.
   d. 5 lb, 8 oz = approximately 2.5 kg
      Step 1: *oz to lb:* 8 oz/16 = 0.5 lb
      Step 2: *lb to kg:* 5.5 lb ÷ 2.2 = 2.5 kg
      Step 3: Low dose: 3 × 2.5 = 7.5 mg
           High dose: 6 × 2.5 = 15 mg
      SDR is 7.5 to 15 mg.
   e. 4 lb, 6 oz = approximately 2 kg
      Step 1: *oz to lb:* 6 oz/16 = 0.37 rounded to 0.4 lb
      Step 2: *lb to kg:* 4.4 lb ÷ 2.2 = 2 kg
      Step 3: Low dose: 200 mcg × 2 = 400 mcg
           or 0.4 mg
           High dose: 400 mcg × 2 = 800 mcg
           or 0.8 mg
      SDR is 400 to 800 mcg or 0.4 to 0.8 mg.

5. a. 36 to 54 mg (2 × 18 = 36)
      (3 × 18 = 54)
   b. 12 to 18 mg (36 ÷ 3)
      (54 ÷ 3)
   c. 150 mg per day; 50 mg per dose
      (50 × 3)   (150 ÷ 3)
   d. Unsafe to give. Overdose ordered. Hold and clarify promptly with the physician.

WORKSHEET 12B (page 419)

1. a. SDR for this child: 18.2 to 36.4 mg per day
      2 × 9.1 = 18.2 mg
      4 × 9.1 = 36.4 mg
   b. Dose ordered: 50 mg daily
   c. Evaluation and decision: Hold and clarify promptly (overdose)

2. a. SDR for this child: 1500 to 3000 mcg per day or 1.5 to 3 mg per day
      15 × 100 mcg = 1500 mcg or 1.5 mg
      15 × 200 mcg = 3000 mcg or 3 mg
   b. Dose ordered: 0.5 mg tid or 1.5 mg per day
   c. Evaluation and decision: Safe to give

3. a. SDR for this child: 115 to 345 mg per day
      10 × 11.5 = 115 mg
      30 × 11.5 = 345 mg
   b. Dose ordered: 100 mg tid or 300 mg per day
   c. Evaluation and decision: Safe to give

4. a. SDR for this child: 386 mg to 579 mg per day in divided doses
   b. Dose ordered: 100 mg q6h or
      100 × 4 = 400 mg per day
   c. Evaluation and decision: Safe to give

5. a. SDR for this child: 23 to 46 mcg per day
      10 × 2.3 = 23 mcg
      20 × 2.3 = 46 mcg
   b. Dose ordered: 0.03 mg × 4 = 0.12 mg per day or 120 mcg per day
   c. Evaluation and decision: Hold and clarify promptly (overdose)

WORKSHEET 12C (page 421)

1. 0.15 m^2
   10 × 0.15 = 1.5 mg

2. 0.20 m^2*
   15 × 0.2 = 3 mg

3. 0.27 m^2
   5 × 0.27 = 1.35 mg

4. 10 × 1.8 = 18 mg

5. 2.72 kg
   2 × 2.7 = 5.4 mg

6. 5 × 9.1 = 45.5 mg

7. 4 × 10 = 40 mg

8. 15 × 6 = 90 mg

9. 20 × 5 = 100 mg

10. 1.10 m^2

WORKSHEET 12D (page 422)

1. a. SDR: 1000 to 2000 mg in 4 divided doses
   b. Dose ordered: 500 mg × 4 or 2000 mg
   c. Evaluation and decision: Safe to give
      Total dose is divided by 4.

2. a. SDR for this child: 4.0 to 6.4 mg 4 times daily
      $5 × 0.8 \text{ m}^2 = 4.0$ mg (low safe dose)
      $8 × 0.8 \text{ m}^2 = 6.4$ mg (high safe dose)
   b. Dose ordered: 4 mg daily
   c. Evaluation and decision: Safe to give

---

*Note: Trailing zeros are seen in BSA square meters. Delete them for math calculations.

3. **a.** SDR for this child: 0.9 to 2.6 mg in 2 divided doses or 860 to 2600 mcg in 2 divided doses
   $0.1 \times 8.6 = 0.86$ mg rounded to 0.9 mg (low safe dose)
   $0.3 \times 8.6 = 2.58$ rounded to 2.6 mg (high safe dose)
   b. Dose ordered: 2500 mcg bid or 2.5 mg $\times$ 2 = 5 mg per day
   c. Evaluation and decision: Hold and clarify promptly (overdose)

5. **a.** SDR for this child: 0.13 to 0.32 mg per day
   $0.02 \times 6.4 = 0.128$ mg (low safe dose)
   $0.05 \times 6.4 = 0.32$ mg (high safe dose)
   b. Dose ordered: 150 mcg $\times$ 2 = 300 mcg per day or 0.3 mg per day
   c. Evaluation and decision: Safe to give

4. **a.** SDR for this child: 4.1 to 20.5 mcg per day
   $1 \times 4.1 = 4.1$ mcg
   $5 \times 4.1 = 20.5$ mcg
   b. Dose ordered: 0.01 mg or 10 mcg daily
   c. Evaluation and decision: Safe to give

WORKSHEET 12E (page 425)

1. **a.** Estimated wt in lb: 14 $\times$ 2 or 28 lb
   b. Actual wt in lb: 30.8 lb
   c. SDR for this child: For 24 to 35 lb, 1 tsp
   d. Dose ordered: 160 mg
   e. Evaluation and decision: Safe to give
   f. Give: 1 tsp or 5 mL (80 mg per ½ tsp)

2. **a.** SDR for this child: 300 to 900 mg per day in 3 to 4 doses
   $10 \times 30 = 300$ mg (low safe daily dose)
   $30 \times 30 = 900$ mg (maximum safe daily dose)
   b. Dose ordered: 300 $\times$ 3 = 900 mg per day.
   c. Evaluation and decision: Safe to give
   d. Give
   HAVE   WANT TO HAVE
   75 mg : 5 mL = 300 mg : x mL
   $\dfrac{\cancel{75}}{\cancel{75}}x = \dfrac{1500}{75}$
   $x = 20$ mL
   PROOF
   $75 \times 20 = 1500$
   $1 \times 1500 = 1500$

3. **a.** SDR for this child: 400 to 800 mg per day in 3 to 4 doses
   b. Dose ordered in mg:
   0.25 g = 250 mg $\times$ 3 = 750 mg per day
   HAVE   WANT TO HAVE
   1 g : 1000 mg = 0.25 g : x mg
   $x = 1000 \times 0.25$ or 250 mg
   PROOF
   $1 \times 250 = 250$
   $1000 \times 0.25 = 250$
   c. Evaluation and decision: Safe to give
   d. Give 12.5 mL
   HAVE   WANT TO HAVE
   100 mg : 5 mL = 250 mg : x mL
   $\dfrac{\cancel{100}}{\cancel{100}}x = \dfrac{\cancel{1250}}{\cancel{100}}$ (5 $\times$ 250)
   $x = 12.5$ mL
   PROOF
   $100 \times 12.5 = 1250$
   $5 \times 250 = 1250$

4. **a.** SDR for this child:
   $10 \times 0.5 \times 4 = 20$ mg per day
   b. Dose ordered: 5 mg four times a day.
   c. Evaluation and decision: Safe to give
   d. Give 1 tab

5. a. SDR for this child: 246 mg to 492 mg per day
   b. Dose ordered: 200 mg per dose × 3 = 600 mg per day
   c. Overdose. Hold and clarify promptly with prescriber.
   d. N/A

WORKSHEET 12F (page 428)

1. a. SDR for this child: 2.52 to 5.04 mg q4h-6h
   $0.1 \times 25.2 = 2.52$ mg
   $0.2 \times 25.2 = 5.04$ mg
   b. Dose ordered: 4 mg subcut
   c. Evaluation and decision: Safe to give
   d. Give 0.8 mL

   HAVE   WANT TO HAVE
   5 mg : 1 mL = 4 mg : x mL

   $$\frac{5x}{5} = \frac{4}{5}$$

   $x = 0.8$ mL

   PROOF
   $5 \times 0.8 = 4$
   $1 \times 4 = 4$

2. a. SDR for a child between 7 and 9 kg: 0.2 mg
   b. Dose ordered: 0.2 mg
   c. Evaluation and decision: Safe to give
   d. Give 0.5 mL

   HAVE   WANT TO HAVE
   0.4 mg : 1 mL = 0.2 mg : x mL

   $$\frac{0.4}{0.4}x = \frac{0.2}{0.4}$$

   $x = 0.5$ mL

   PROOF
   $0.4 \times 0.5 = 0.2$
   $1 \times 0.2 = 0.2$

3. a. SDR for this child: 320 to 640 mg per day (based on 3.2 kg wt)
   b. Dose ordered: 1000 mg per day
   c. Evaluation and decision: Overdose. Hold and clarify promptly. Also ask whether IV route is preferred.
   d. Not applicable.

4. a. SDR: 0.004×40 kg = 0.16 mg
   b. 0.16 mg
   c. Safe to give
   d. HAVE   WANT TO HAVE
   0.2 mg : 1 mL = 0.16 mg : x mL

   $$\frac{0.2}{0.2}x = \frac{0.16}{0.2}$$

   $x = 0.8$ mL

   PROOF
   $0.2 \times 0.8 = 0.16$
   $1 \times 0.16 = 0.16$

5. a. 1 gram: 1000 mL; 2 grams per 2000 mL
   b. There is no plunger. It injects a hidden needle upon contact.
   c. 1 mg per mL (1000 mg = 1 g; 1000 mg : 1000 mL = 1 : 1)
   d. 2 mg per mL
   e. Safe to give

WORKSHEET 12G (page 432)

1. a. SDR for this child: 28.2 to 84.6 mg q24h
   b. Dose ordered: 50 mg IV
   c. Evaluation and decision: Safe to give
   d. Dose withdrawn from vial: 0.5 mL
      65 mg : 1 mL = 50 mg : x mL
      65x = 50
      x = 0.769 rounded to 0.77 mL
      PROOF
      65 × 0.769 = 49.9
      1 × 50 = 50

2. a. SDR for this child: 25 to 150 mg
      (1 to 6 mg per kg)
      1 × 25 = 25
      6 × 25 = 150
   b. Dose ordered: 25 mg IV stat
   c. Evaluation and decision: Safe to give
      (The initial dose for this drug must not exceed the lowest dose in the SDR.)
   d. Give 2.5 mL
      HAVE   WANT TO HAVE
      40 mg : 4 mL = 25 mg : x mL
$$\frac{\cancel{40}}{\cancel{40}}x = \frac{\cancel{100}}{\cancel{40}} \ (4 \times 25)$$
      x = 2.5 mL
      PROOF
      40 × 2.5 = 100
      4 × 25 = 100

3. a. SDR for this child: 12 to 15 mg q8h
      2 mg × 6 kg = 12 mg
      2.5 mg × 6 kg = 15 mg
   b. Dose ordered: 15 mg q8h
   c. Evaluation and decision: Safe to give
   d. Amount withdrawn from vial: Give 1.5 mL
      HAVE   WANT TO HAVE
      20 mg : 2 mL = 15 mg : x mL $\left(\frac{10}{1} = \frac{15}{x}\right)$
$$\frac{\cancel{20}}{\cancel{20}}x = \frac{30}{20}$$
      x = 1.5 mL
   e. The 50 mL can be administered with a syringe pump or a volume-control device. Monitor urinary output hourly and during visits to bedside.*

4. a. SDR IV for this child: 0.17 mg to 3.9 mg per day
      0.015 × 11.1 = 0.166 rounded to 0.17 mg per day
      0.35 × 11.1 = 3.88 rounded to 3.9 mg per day
   b. 0.5 mg IV
   c. Safe to give. 0.5 mg is within the SDR
   d. 2 mL (0.5 mg = 500 mcg) Label states 0.5 mg per 2 mL
   e. Infuse at 1.6 mL per minute for 5 minutes
      HAVE   WANT TO HAVE
      8 mL : 5 minutes = x mL : 1 minute
      5x = 8 $\left(\frac{8 \text{ mL}}{5 \text{ minutes}} = \frac{x \text{ mL}}{1 \text{ minute}}\right)$
      x = 1.6 mL
      PROOF
      5 × 1.6 = 8
      8 × 1 = 8

5. a. SDR for this child: 590 to 5900 mg
      divided into 4 doses = 1475 mg
      maximum unit dose
      50 × 11.8 = 590
      500 × 11.8 = 5900
   b. Dose ordered: 2 g or 2000 mg q6h
   c. Evaluation and decision: Hold and clarify promptly (overdose)
   d. Not applicable
   e. Not applicable

---

*Dilute "to" is interpreted as, "Add diluent to the prepared medicine to make 50 mL total volume."
Dilution "with" a substance adds to the volume. Dilution "to" an amount does not add to the volume.

WORKSHEET 12H (page 434)

1. d 25 kg (lb ÷ 2 = rough estimate of kg)

2. c
30 mg : 1 m² = x mg : 1.20 m²
x = 30 × 1.20 or 36 mg

PROOF
30 × 1.2 = 36
1 × 36 = 36

3. b
5 mL = 1 tsp
5 mL : 1 tsp = x mL : 1.5 tsp
x = 7.5 mL
Measure 7.5 mL

PROOF
5 × 1.5 = 7.5
1 × 7.5 = 7.5

4. d If the taste is unpleasant or unfamiliar, the child may refuse the essential food.

5. b Administer the EpiPen first, then call 911; consult provider for any questions about use, how long to retain, and read the accompanying information and practice with the trainer.

6. c The sciatic nerve and blood vessels are close together in undeveloped gluteal muscles. Occasionally they may also be located in a different quadrant than the upper outer.

7. b
SDR
5 mg : 1 kg = x mg : 6 kg
x = 5 × 6 or 30 mg
Compare the SDR with the order. 30 mg ÷ 2 = 15 mg bid. The order is 15 mg bid. The order is safe.
Step 3: Calculate the unit dose.
30 mg : 5 mL = 15 mg : x mL
30x = 75 × 2.5 mL
Give 2.5 mL using a syringe to measure, if necessary.

PROOF
5 × 6 = 30
1 × 30 = 30

PROOF
30 × 2.5 = 75
5 × 15 = 75

8. a Vastus lateralis is the largest developed muscle at that age.

9. d 20 mg per pound. Refer to the examples on page 420.

10. b The child associates the parent with the inflicted pain.

CHAPTER 12 FINAL: CHILDREN'S DOSAGES (page 437)

1. a. Ordered: 2 g per day = 2000 mg in 4 divided doses of 500 mg each
   b. SDR: 1000 to 4000 mg per day in divided doses
   c. Safe to give
   d. 2 capsules four times a day

2. a. SDR: 120 to 180 mcg daily
   b. Ordered: 0.15 mg daily
   c. Safe to give, 0.15 mg = 150 mcg
   d. 3 tablets

3. a. SDR for this child: 150 mg maximum (6 × 25 mg) in 24 hr in 4 to 6 divided doses
   b. Dose ordered: 25 mg × 4 or 100 mg per day
   c. Evaluation and decision: Safe to give
   d. Dose to be administered: 2 tsp or 25 mg per dose

4. a. SDR: 233.3 to 466.76 mg per dose every 8 hr
   b. Ordered: 700 mg q8h
   c. Overdose; contact prescriber promptly
   d. Not applicable

5. a. SDR for this child: 0.3 mg (for 12- to 26-kg child)
   b. Dose ordered: 0.3 mg
   c. Safe to give (35 lb = 15.9 kg)
   d. Give 0.75 mL in anterolateral thigh.

6. a. SDR: 200 to 300 mg ÷ 2 = 100 mg to 175 mg per dose
   b. Safe to give
   c. 2 mL = 100 mg per dose at 50 mg per mL

7. a. 100,000 units (1 mL) each side of mouth
   b. the dropper; flow could be controlled and directed to desired areas more easily than the other devices, permitting a couple of applications over a few minutes

8. a. 1 : 1000 = 1 mg per mL (1 g per 1000 mL) = (1000 mg per 1000 mL), commonly ordered IM or subcut for allergic reactions; 1 : 10,000 = 0.1 mg per mL (1 g per 10,000 mL) = (1000 mg per 10,000 mL), more commonly order IV (more dilute)*
   b. Ten times difference
   c. 0.2 mL = 0.2 mg dose ordered (0.01 mg × 20 kg)
   d. Child would receive 10 times the ordered dose

9. a. BSA in m^2: 1.10 m^2
   b. SDR for this child: Up to 44 mg per day
      1.10 × 10 × 4 = 44
   c. Dose ordered: 40 mg per day
   d. Evaluation and decision: Safe to give.
   e. Give 2 tab.

10. a. 1980 mcg (90 mcg × 22 kg)
    b. 1.98 mg rounded to 2 mg

       KNOW   WANT TO KNOW
       $$\frac{1000}{1000} x = \frac{1980}{1000}$$
       x = 1.98 mg rounded to 2 mg
    c. 2.2 mL
       1 mg : 1.1 mL = 2 mg : x mL
       x = 2.2 mL
    d. 2 vials
    e. 11 calibrations
    f. 0.7 mL per minute
       2.2 mL : 3 minutes = x mL : 1 minute
       2.2x = 3
       x = 0.73 mL per minute or approximately 0.7 mL per minute

    g.

    h. a. 1.5 mL; b. 0.8 ml; c. 0

*Only use commercially prepared correct dilutions.

Multiple-Choice Final

Estimate reasonable answers when possible. Round kg to the nearest tenth. Round liquid oral and injection doses to the nearest tenth of a mL. Round IV flow rates to the nearest whole mL. Answers can be found on page 458.

1. **Ordered:** cimetidine 0.4 g tablet po daily for a patient with a gastric ulcer.
   Available: cimetidine 200 mg tablets. **Give:**
   a. 0.5 tablet
   b. 1 tablet
   c. 2 tablets
   d. 4 tablets

2. **Ordered:** Klonopin (clonazepam) 1 mg tablet po stat for a patient who has seizures.
   Available: Klonopin (clonazepam) 0.5 mg tablets. **Give:**
   a. 0.5 tablet
   b. 1 tablet
   c. 2 tablets
   d. 4 tablets

3. **Ordered:** lanoxin 0.25 mg tablet po daily in the a.m. for a patient with heart failure.
   Available: lanoxin 0.125 mg tablets, scored. **Give:**
   a. 2 tablets
   b. 1 tablet
   c. 0.5 tablet
   d. 0.25 tablet

4. What is the purpose of the Tall-Man Lettering promoted by the FDA, TJC, ISMP, and Clinical Pharmacology Organizations?*
   a. All prescription drug names are to be written legibly in tall letters so that pharmacy can input the correct orders on the EMAR.
   b. Drugs that have similar names need adjacent sections of letters that are written in uppercase to reduce confusion and errors.
   c. PRN drug orders must be written in capital letters to distinguish them from scheduled drugs.
   d. Patients who are over 6 feet tall must have their identification distinguished by Tall Man letters.

5. **Ordered:** naloxone HCl 600 mcg IM stat to reverse effects of a narcotic overdose.
   Available: naloxone 400 mcg per mL. How many mL will you administer?
   a. 0.8 mL
   b. 1.1 mL
   c. 1.3 mL
   d. 1.5 mL

---

*Refer to http://ismp.org/tools/tallmanletters.pdf.

6. **Ordered:** Cipro (ciprofloxacin) 1.5 g tablets po bid for a patient with an infection.
   Available: Cipro (ciprofloxacin HCl) 750 mg tablets. **Give:**
   a. 0.5 tablet
   b. 1 tablet
   c. 2 tablets
   d. 3 tablets

7. **Ordered:** morphine sulfate 8 mg IM q4h prn for a patient with severe pain. **Give:**

   a. 0.6 mL
   b. 0.8 mL
   c. 1 mL
   d. 1.2 mL

8. **Ordered:** glycopyrrolate 0.3 mg IM at 8 a.m. preoperatively to reduce excessive pharyngeal secretions and protect the heart from vagal stimulation. **Available:** glycopyrrolate injection 0.2 mg per mL. Will you give more or less than the available unit dose? **Give:**
   a. 0.5 mL
   b. 0.7 mL
   c. 1.5 mL
   d. 2 mL

9. The nurse is trying to interpret a prescriber order that is illegible. What is the best action to take?
   a. Ask a staff nurse who works regularly on the floor.
   b. Check to see if something similar has been given before to the patient.
   c. Call the pharmacy.
   d. Call the prescriber.

10. **Ordered:** promethazine 20 mg IM stat for a patient with nausea. **Available:** promethazine HCl injection 50 mg per mL. **Give:**
    a. 0.4 mL
    b. 0.5 mL
    c. 0.8 mL
    d. 1.2 mL

11. **Ordered:** Ativan (lorazepam) 5 mg IM stat for an agitated patient. **Give** (to the nearest tenth of a milliliter):

   a. 0.8 mL
   b. 1.2 mL
   c. 1.3 mL
   d. 1.4 mL

12. **Ordered:** oxacillin sodium 300 mg IM q6h for a patient with an upper respiratory infection. After reconstituting with sterile water for injection, what is the strength of the medication?

   a. 250 mg per mL
   b. 500 mg per mL
   c. 2.7 mg per mL
   d. 250 mg per 1.5 ML

   How many milliliters will you administer?

   a. 2.1 mL
   b. 2.0 mL
   c. 1.2 mL
   d. 1.8 mL

13. **Ordered:** ampicillin 400 mg IM q6h for a patient with an infected leg ulcer. After reconstituting with the accompanying diluent, how many milliliters will you administer?

   a. 1.6 mL
   b. 2.0 mL
   c. 1.5 mL
   d. 3.5 mL

   What is the shelf life of the medication?

   a. 24 hours
   b. 1 week, refrigerated
   c. 1 hour
   d. 48 hours

Multiple-Choice Final   451

14. Ordered: penicillin G potassium 300,000 units IM q6h for a patient with tonsillitis. Available: Pfizerpen 1 million units for reconstitution for injection. If you add 4.0 mL of diluent, how many milliliters of medication will you give?

   a. 2.0 mL
   b. 2.4 mL
   c. 1.2 mL
   d. 0.5 mL

15. The IV is infusing at 30 gtt per minute. The drop factor is 20 gtt per mL. The IV label reads 500 mL 5% dextrose and 0.45% sodium chloride. The IV had been infusing for 1½ hours when you came on duty. How much longer does the IV have to infuse?

   a. 4 hours
   b. 50 minutes
   c. 3 hours
   d. 3½ hours

16. **Ordered:** Monocid 600 mg IM. **Available:** cefonicid 1 g for reconstitution. How many milliliters will you administer?

   a. 1.8 mL
   b. 0.7 mL
   c. 1.3 mL
   d. 1.5 mL

17. **Ordered:** 1000 mL D5W IV to infuse at 125 mL per hr on admission. The drop factor is 20. How many gtt per min will you set the IV to infuse?

   a. 12 gtt per min
   b. 22 gtt per min
   c. 20 gtt per min
   d. 42 gtt per min

18. **Ordered:** ampicillin 1 g IV bid. **Available:** ampicillin 1 g for IV use. **Directions:** Add 4.5 mL of sodium chloride diluent to yield 5 mL. Dilute with normal saline to 50 mL and infuse in 30 minutes. On hand you have a microdrip infusion set. At how many drops per min will you set the IV?

   a. 100 drops per minute
   b. 150 drops per minute
   c. 200 drops per minute
   d. 250 drops per minute

   At how many mL per hr will you set the IV?
   a. 100 mL per hr
   b. 150 mL per hr
   c. 200 mL per hr
   d. 250 mL per hr

▶19. The pharmacy standard insulin drip is 100 units of Humulin Regular in 250 mL of normal saline. 1 unit = 2.5 mL. The patient's blood glucose level is 218 mg per dL. Use the following chart to determine the correct insulin rate for the IV. How many units per hr should the patient receive?

Blood Glucose (BG) per dL	Standard Rate in units per hr
101-140	1.0
141-180	1.5
181-220	2.0
221-260	2.5
261-300	3.0

   a. 1.5 units per hr
   b. 2.5 units per hr
   c. 2.0 units per hr
   d. 3.0 units per hr

   At what rate will you set the IV infusion device?
   a. 3 mL per hr
   b. 4 mL per hr
   c. 5 mL per hr
   d. 6 mL per hr

20. Ordered: Novolin R insulin 15 units per hr IV for a patient having surgery. **Available:** 250 mL of sodium chloride 0.9% with 100 units of Humulin R insulin. At how many mL per hr will you need to set the electronic infusion device?

a. 56 mL per hr
b. 38 mL per hr
c. 33 mL per hr
d. 58 mL per hr

How many hours will it take to infuse the 250 mL?
a. 5 hr 30 min
b. 6 hr 36 min
c. 9 hr 40 min
d. 8 hr

21. Ordered: heparin sodium 10,000 units IV in 15 hr for a patient after hip surgery.
Available: pharmacy has sent 1000 mL of normal saline solution with 10,000 units of heparin sodium. At how many mL per hr will you set the IV infusion device?
a. 67 mL per hr
b. 125 mL per hr
c. 83 mL per hr
d. 100 mL per hr

If the IV described above was started at 2000 hr on 10/21, when should it be finished?
a. 10/22 at 0900 hr
b. 10/23 at 0200 hr
c. 10/23 at 1000 hr
d. 10/22 at 1100 hr

22. Ordered: Fragmin 18,000 units subcutaneous for a patient with a deep venous thrombosis (DVT). **Available:** Fragmin in 9.5-mL multidose vial. The label reads: 1 mL = 10,000 units. How many milliliters will you give?

10,000 international units/mL
9.5 mL multidose vial
NDC 0013-2436-06

(Used with permission from Pfizer, Inc.)

a. 1.8 mL
b. 2 mL
c. 1.5 mL
d. 1.2 mL

23. A blood glucose level (BGL) of 120 mg per dL is desired. **Ordered:** give 1 unit Regular insulin for every 8 mg above 120 mg per dL; give 1 unit of Regular insulin for each 8 g of CHO consumed. The BGL is 160 mg per dL. The amount of CHO consumed is 64 g. How many total units of insulin will the patient receive?

  a. 10 units
  b. 13 units
  c. 24 units
  d. 28 units

24. Ordered: IV heparin to infuse at 20 units per kg per hr. **Available:** 1000 mL D5W with 25,000 units of heparin sodium. Patient's weight: 80 kg. How many units per hour will the patient receive on the electronic infusion device?
  a. 160 units
  b. 1600 units
  c. 1620 units
  d. 1640 units

At how many mL per hr will you set the infusion device?
  a. 58 mL per hr
  b. 48 mL per hr
  c. 66 mL per hr
  d. 64 mL per hr

25. Ordered: 90 units per kg of heparin for a loading dose. Set the infusion to run at 1200 units per hr. **Available:** 500 mL NS with 25,000 units of heparin. Patient's weight: 177 lb. How many units will you give as the loading dose?
  a. 5700 units
  b. 6900 units
  c. 7000 units
  d. 7240 units

At how many mL per hr will you set the infusion device?
  a. 84 mL per hr
  b. 60 mL per hr
  c. 64 mL per hr
  d. 24 mL per hr

26. The patient has a TPN solution for nutritional therapy with 8.5% amino acids in 375 mL. The total volume (TV) is 1500 mL. How many grams of protein will the patient receive? Use the following formula for calculating the amino acids.
Step 1: % × mL = g per L
Step 2: g per L × TV per L = g per bag
  a. 8.5 g per bag
  b. 47.8 g per bag
  c. 478 g per bag
  d. 31.8 g per bag

27. **Ordered:** A maintenance dose of methotrexate 30 mg per m² po for a child with lymphocytic leukemia. Patient's weight: 30 lb, which is equivalent to a BSA of 0.6 m². **Give:**
    a. 12 mg
    b. 15 mg
    c. 18 mg
    d. 20 mg

28. **Ordered:** Dobutrex HCl to be infused at 4 mcg per kg per minute for a patient with cardiac decompensation. Patient's weight: 50 kg. **Available:** Dobutrex solution (dobutamine HCl solution) 500 mg in 250 mL (2 mg per mL). Given the total drug in mg to total solution ratio, how many mL per hr should be infused?
    a. 12 mL per hr
    b. 10 mL per hr
    c. 8 mL per hr
    d. 6 mL per hr

29. **Ordered:** morphine sulfate 5 mg IV push for a patient in severe pain. **Directions:** Dilute to 5 mL with NS or sterile water for injection and administer over 5 minutes. Identify the correct total dose and mL per minute to inject.
    a. Administer 5 mL at 1 mL per minute
    b. Administer 5 mL at 0.4 mL per minute
    c. Administer 6 mL at 0.4 mL per minute
    d. Administer 8 mL at 0.03 mL per minute

NDC 10019-179-63

Morphine Sulfate Inj., USP C II

15 mg/mL R only
FOR SC, IM OR
SLOW IV USE
NOT FOR EPIDURAL OR
INTRATHECAL USE
20 mL
Multiple Dose Vial

Baxter ESILEDERLE™
Mfd. for an affiliate of
Baxter Healthcare Corporation
Deerfield, IL 60015 USA
by: Elkins-Sinn
Cherry Hill, NJ 08003

30. **Ordered:** A diuretic, furosemide 15 mg IV stat for a child with edema. Dosing is based on weight in kilograms; patient's weight: 14 kg. SDR: 1 to 2 mg per kg per dose IV every 6 to 12 hours. Your decision:
    a. Give 15 mg. The order is within the safe dose range.
    b. Hold. Contact the physician promptly and clarify. The order is an underdose.
    c. Hold. Contact the physician promptly and clarify. The order is an overdose.
    d. Hold. The order is unclear.

Answer Key

Multiple-Choice Final

1. c
2. c
3. a
4. b
5. d
6. c
7. b
8. More; c
9. d
10. a
11. c
12. d; d
13. a; c
14. c
15. a
16. a
17. d
18. a; a
19. c; c
20. b; b
21. a; d
22. a
23. b
24. b; d
25. d; d
26. d
27. c
28. d
29. a
30. a

Comprehensive Final

Estimate answers and then solve the following problems. Prove your answers. Answers can be found on page 470.

1. **Ordered:** Nitrostat 600 mcg SL tablets every 5 minutes × 3, prn angina (chest pain). Call MD if relief not obtained with 3 tablets.
   a. What is the dose in milligrams?
   b. What route is ordered?

2. **Ordered:** Septra DS 80/400 tab PO daily for a urinary tract infection.
   a. How many tablets will you give?
   b. How is DS different from abbreviations such as E-R, X-L, S-R, D-R, and so forth?

459

3. **Ordered:** carbamazepine chewable tablet 0.2 g daily for a patient with seizures. **Available:** carbamazepine 100 mg chewable tablets. How many tablets will you give?

4. **Ordered:** diltiazem HCl 0.24 g at bedtime daily for a patient with high blood pressure. How many tablets will you give?

5. **Ordered as a discharge prescription:** zidovudine syrup 0.2 g po bid for a patient who is HIV positive. **Available:** zidovudine syrup 50 mg per 5 mL.
   a. How many mL will you instruct the patient to take?
   b. What kind of equipment should the patient use to measure the medication?

6. **Ordered:** isoniazid 0.6 g po daily for 9 months as preventive therapy for an adult patient with a positive test result for latent tuberculosis infection (LTBI); patient has positive test results for presence of TB bacteria without any active signs and symptoms. Patient weighs 120 kg. SDR for patients with LTBI ages 11 to adult is 5 mg per kg daily for 9 months. **Available:** isoniazid tablets 300 mg.
   a. Is the ordered dosage safe?
   b. How many tablets will you give?

7. **Ordered:** fluoxetine hydrochloride (Prozac) oral solution 30 mg po for a patient with anxiety. **Available:** Prozac oral solution 20 mg per 5 mL. How many mL will you administer? Shade in the medicine cup with the nearest measurable dose. Mark the syringe provided with the additional amount needed to the nearest measurable dose.

8. **Ordered:** butorphanol tartrate 0.6 mg IM stat for a patient with a severe migraine headache.
   Available: butorphanol tartrate 2 mg per mL.
   a. Would you give *more* or *less* than 1 mL?
   b. How many mL (to the nearest measurable amount) will be needed? Indicate the amount on the syringe.

9. **Ordered:** morphine sulfate, an opioid narcotic, 10 mg IM q4h prn pain; last administered by Nurse A, according to the MAR, at 0800 hr.
   Given: Morphine 10 mg IM at 0845 hr by Nurse B, a busy staff nurse who covered Nurse A's patient during Nurse A's break.
   Error:
   Potential complications:
   Nurse actions:
   How could this error have occurred? What are some ways it might have been prevented?

10. **Ordered:** haloperidol decanoate LA 60 mg IM every 28 days for an adult patient with schizophrenia. SDR for monthly dosing not to exceed 100 mg. **Available:** haloperidol decanoate LA inj 50 mg per mL. How many mL will you give?

11. **Ordered:** atropine sulfate 0.6 mg IV for a patient with bradycardia, an apical pulse 40 beats per minute. **Available:** atropine sulfate inj 0.4 mg per mL. How many mL (to the nearest tenth of a mL) will you administer?

12. **Ordered:** ceftriaxone 300 mg IM q4h for a patient with pelvic inflammatory disease. **Available:** ceftriaxone 500 mg for reconstitution. How many milliliters will you give? Shade in the amount on the syringe.

13. **Ordered:** Cefadyl 500 mg IM q8h for a patient with cellulitis. **Available:** Cefadyl 1 g for reconstitution.
    a. How much diluent will you add?
    b. How many milliliters will you give per dose? Shade in the syringe.

14. **Ordered:** MethylPREDNISolone 20 mg IM daily for 7 days for a patient with lumbar pain.
    Available: MethylPREDNISolone sodium 40 mg for reconstitution.
    a. How many milliliters of bacteriostatic water will you use to reconstitute?
    c. How many milliliters will you give?

MethylPREDNISolone Sodium Succinate for Injection, USP
NDC 55390-209-10 Single Dose Vial
Reconstitute with 1.2 mL of Bacteriostatic Water for Injection with benzyl alcohol.
FOR IM OR IV USE
*Each 1 mL (when mixed) contains: Methylprednisolone sodium succinate equiv. to 40 mg methylprednisolone.
40 mg*
Lyophilized in container.
Protect from light.
Rx ONLY
Recommended Diluent Contains Benzyl Alcohol as a Preservative.
Manufactured for: Bedford Laboratories™
Bedford, OH 44146   MPNL-V01

15. **Ordered:** 2000 mL D5/Ringer's lactate solution to be infused in 24 hr for hydration. The drop factor is 10.
    a. How many gtt per min will be infused via gravity infusion?
    b. How many mL per hr will be infused by an electronic device?

16. **Ordered:** Gentamicin 60 mg in 50 mL, IVPB for pneumonitis. Infuse in 40 minutes.
    a. At how many mL per hr will you set the electronic infusion device?
    b. How many gtt per min will be infused by a microdrip set?

17. **Ordered:** 1000 mL D5NS followed by 1000 mL D5W, then 500 mL NS to infuse in 24 hr for hydration. The drop factor is 15.
    a. At how many mL per hr will you set the electronic infusion device to deliver 2500 mL in 24 hr?
    b. At how many gtt per min will you regulate the IV?

18. The patient's blood glucose level (BGL) at 0600 hr is 176 mg per dL. According to the titration schedule, Lantus will be increased to how many units per day? Shade in the amount on the insulin syringe.

Effective Diabetes Management

Logical titration schedule helps achieve tight control, with low incidence of severe hypoglycemia

Self-monitored FPG (mg/dL) for 2 consecutive days with no episodes of severe hypoglycemia or PG ≤72 mg/dL	Increase in insulin dose (international units/day)
100-120 mg/dL	2
120-140 mg/dL	4
140-180 mg/dL	6
≥180 mg/dL	8

Treat-to-Target FPG ≤100 mg/dL

Small decreases (2-4 international units/day per adjustment) in dose are allowed in the instance of self-monitored plasma glucose below 56 mg/dL or in the occurrence of a severe hypoglycemic episode.

19. Ordered: Humulin R insulin 50 units in 500 mL of 0.9% NS IV to infuse at 4 units per hr. At what rate will you set the IV infusion device?

20. Ordered: The patient consumed 22 g CHO for breakfast, 90 g CHO for lunch, and 25 g CHO for dinner. Patient weight: 110 kg. How many total units of R has the patient received based on the units-to-CHO ratio chart?

Insulin Units Required Based on CHO Intake and Weight

Weight in Pounds	Weight in Kg	Unit: grams of CHO
100-109	45.5-49.5	1:16
110-129	50-58.6	1:15
130-139	59-63.2	1:14
140-149	63.6-67.7	1:13
150-159	68.2-72.3	1:12
160-169	72.7-76.8	1:11
170-179	77.3-81.4	1:10
180-189	81.8-85.9	1:9
190-198	86.4-90	1:8
200-239	90.9-108.6	1:7
240+	109.1+	1:6

21. Ordered: Regular Humulin insulin to infuse at 3 units per hr. **Available:** 250 mL NS with 40 units of Humulin R insulin.
   a. At how many mL per hr will you set the electronic infusion device?
   b. The IV was started at 0830. At what hour will the IV be complete?

22. Ordered: Fragmin injection 6000 units subcutaneous q12h before surgery. **Available:** A multidose vial of Fragmin (dalteparin sodium injection). How many milliliters will you give? Shade in the amount on the syringe.

10,000 international units/mL
9.5 mL multidose vial
NDC 0013-2436-06

(Used with permission from Pfizer, Inc.)

23. **Ordered:** heparin sodium 1000 units per hr IV. The pharmacy sent 1000 mL of 0.9% sodium chloride with 20,000 units of heparin sodium for a patient with a DVT.
    a. At what rate will you set the infusion device?
    b. What is the antidote for heparin?

```
LOT                    EXP
                            2B1324
                            NDC 0338-0049-04
                            DIN 00060208

0.9% Sodium
Chloride
Injection USP
Heparin Sodium 20,000 units
1000 mL
EACH 100 mL CONTAINS  900 mg SODIUM CHLORIDE USP
pH 5.0 (4.5 TO 7.0)  mEq/L  SODIUM 154  CHLORIDE 154
OSMOLARITY     308 mOsmol/L (CALC)     STERILE
NONPYROGENIC  SINGLE DOSE CONTAINER  ADDITIVES MAY BE
INCOMPATIBLE  CONSULT WITH PHARMACIST IF AVAILABLE  WHEN
INTRODUCING ADDITIVES USE ASEPTIC TECHNIQUE  MIX
THOROUGHLY  DO NOT STORE  DOSAGE  INTRAVENOUSLY AS
DIRECTED BY A PHYSICIAN  SEE DIRECTIONS  CAUTIONS
SQUEEZE AND INSPECT INNER BAG WHICH MAINTAINS PRODUCT
STERILITY  DISCARD IF LEAKS ARE FOUND  MUST NOT BE USED
IN SERIES CONNECTIONS  DO NOT USE UNLESS SOLUTION IS
CLEAR  FEDERAL (USA) LAW PROHIBITS DISPENSING WITHOUT
PRESCRIPTION  STORE UNIT IN MOISTURE BARRIER OVERWRAP AT
ROOM TEMPERATURE (25°C/77°F) UNTIL READY TO USE  AVOID
EXCESSIVE HEAT  SEE INSERT

Baxter
BAXTER HEALTHCARE CORPORATION
DEERFIELD IL 60015 USA
MADE IN USA                  Viaflex® CONTAINER
DISTRIBUTED IN CANADA BY     PL 146® PLASTIC
BAXTER CORPORATION           FOR PRODUCT INFORMATION
TORONTO ONTARIO CANADA       CALL 1-800-933-0303
```

24. **Ordered:** Loading dose of IV heparin at 82 units per kg per min. Set infusion to run at 18 units per kg per hr. **Available:** 500 mL D5W with 20,000 units of heparin. The patient weighs 160 lb.
    a. How many units of heparin will you give for the bolus loading dose?
    b. How many units per hr will infuse?
    c. How many hours will it take to infuse?
    d. At what rate will you set the infusion device to deliver 18 units per kg per hr?

25. Calculate the grams of amino acids, dextrose, and lipids per bag the patient on nutritional therapy will receive. Use the following formulas on the TPN label below. The total volume is 1158 mL.
    Step 1: % × mL = g per L
    Step 2: g per L × TV per L = g per bag
    TPN Label
    a. **Ordered:** amino acids 5.5% in 300 mL for a patient needing hyperalimentation.
    b. **Ordered:** dextrose 10% in 250 mL for a patient needing hyperalimentation.
    c. **Ordered:** lipids 15% in 125 mL for a patient needing hyperalimentation.

26. Using the answers from Problem 25, how many total kilocalories will the patient receive?

27. The pharmacy has supplied potassium chloride (KCl) 15 mEq in an IV of 500 mL D5W.
   a. How many mEq per mL are there on the available label for concentrated KCl?
   b. How many mg per mL are there on the available label?
   c. How many mL of the concentrated KCl would the pharmacy have added to prepare the IV solution?

28. Ordered: Thorazine 2 mg IV push for an agitated patient. **Directions:** Dilute each 25 mg (1 mL) with 24 mL of sterile NS for injection. Each mL will contain 1 mg. Give at slow rate of 1 mg per min.

   a. Total milliliters to be injected
   b. Total time in *seconds* to be injected
   c. mL per min to be injected for how many minutes
   d. Seconds to be injected per calibration

29. Ordered: Leucovorin calcium tablets 0.01 g po for a child who has delayed excretion of the anticancer drug methotrexate. The SDR is 10 mg/m². Patient weight: 70 lb with a BSA of 1.10 m². **Available:** Leucovorin calcium tablets 5 mg.
   a. How many tablets (to the nearest whole number) will you give?
   b. Which of the following orders would yield the lowest dose? mg per m², mg per lb, or mg per kg?

30. Ordered: DOPAmine IV infusion 5 mcg per kg per min for an adult with cardiac decompensation. The dopamine is infusing at 30 mL per hr on an infusion pump with an IV container of 200 mg per 250 mL D5W. Patient weight: 80 kg.
   a. How many mcg per hr are ordered?
   b. How many mg per hr are ordered?
   c. How many mg per mL are in the solution (to the nearest tenth of a mg)?
   d. Is the flow rate correct?

Answer Key

Comprehensive Final

1. **a.** 0.6 mg
   b. sublingual (SL) (under the tongue)

2. **a.** Give ½ tablet
   b. DS only refers to double strength/concentration compared to the regular strength. Note that DS medication is released *as soon as it is dissolved.* Extended-release medications are *released slowly (extended)* over a *longer* period of time and often are characterized by separate small, coated sprinkles. Extended-release formulation reduces the number of medications the patient has to take each day. Delayed-release medications are coated to avoid gastric irritation and are released *as soon as the coating dissolves.* Underdosing and overdosing ADE have been made because of confusion about these abbreviations.

3. 2 tablets

4. None. The order called for regular-strength tablets. Extended-release tablets were supplied. Reconfirm the order and contact pharmacy if there is a mismatch.

5. **a.** 20 mL.
   b. Instruct the patient to use a metric-calibrated medicine cup and to rinse it after use.

6. **a.** The ordered dose is safe.
   b. Give 2 tablets; emphasize adherence.

7. 7.5 mL

8. Give 0.3 mL

9. Error: 0845 Dose given 45 minutes after prior dose. Order stated q4h intervals prn.
   Current Actions: Prescribe complete bed rest for patient, assess mental status and vital signs, notify supervising nurse or charge nurse and physician immediately, and obtain orders for medication to reverse.
   Establish a patent IV line according to hospital policy in case emergency care may be needed.
   Have crash cart close at hand. Document the error and to whom reported, patient evaluations, and all interventions, and continue to make the above assessments and evaluate. Fill out incident report. Continue to assess and evaluate patient every 5 to 15 minutes until patient is stabilized, then gradually extend assessment time.
   Prevention: prn and stat medications must be charted as soon as possible after administration. Nurse A needed to report to Nurse B orally when her patients were due for their next prn medications. Nurse B needed to state she was too busy to care for additional patients beyond her own caseload. Nurse B needed to check record carefully to see when last medication for pain was given. Nurse B needed to ask patient when last medication for pain was received. (This is a recommended double-check but is not always reliable. The accuracy of response depends on the patient's mental status.) Refer to Hand-off Communication Report, Appendix A.

10. 1.2 mL

11. 1.5 mL

12. a. Give 0.9 mL

13. a. Add 2 mL of diluent
   b. Give 1.2 mL per dose

14. a. 1.2 mL sterile water for injection
   b. Give 0.5 mL.

15. a. 14 drops per min
   b. 83 mL per hr on infusion device

16. a. 75 mL per hr
   b. 75 gtt per min

17. a. 104 mL per hr
   b. 26 gtt per min

18. 6 units of Lantus

19. 40 mL per hr

20. 23 units of R insulin

21. a. Set infusion rate at 19 mL per hr
   b. IV will be completed at 2139 hours

22. 0.6 mL Fragmin

23. a. 50 mL per hr
   b. 20 hr to infuse

24. a. Give 5986 units of heparin for the bolus dose.
   b. 1314 units per hr will infuse
   c. 15 hr 36 min
   d. 33 mL per hr

25. a. 19 g per bag amino acids
   b. 29 g per bag carbohydrates
   c. 22 g per bag lipids

26. a. 76 protein kilocalories
   b. 116 carbohydrate kilocalories
   c. 198 fat kilocalories
   d. Total kilocalories = 390

27. a. 2 mEq per mL
   b. 149 mg per mL
   c. 7.5 mL

28. a. 2 mL
   b. 120 seconds
   c. 1 mL per min for 2 min
   d. 6 seconds per calibration

29. 10 mg; 2 tablets (based on approximate BSA of 1.10 m^2

30. a. 24,000 mcg per hr (5 mcg × 80 kg × 60 min)
  b. 24 mg per hr
  c. 0.8 mg per mL (200 mg ÷ 250 mL)
  d. Flow rate is correct

Note: Based on national agencies including TJC and ISMP recommendations to reduce medication errors with KCL administration, the pharmacy now supplies KCL premixed solutions. The nurse still needs to check the pharmacy label with the order to be sure the correct amount has been added.

Note: Many EID devices can deliver tenths of a mL per hr.

APPENDIX A

Institute for Safe Medication Practices (ISMP)
ISMP List of *High-Alert* Medications in Acute Care Settings

High-alert medications are drugs that bear a heightened risk of causing significant patient harm when they are used in error. Although mistakes may or may not be more common with these drugs, the consequences of an error are clearly more devastating to patients. We hope you will use this list to determine which medications require special safeguards to reduce the risk of errors. This may include strategies such as standardizing the ordering, storage, preparation, and administration of these products; improving access to information about these drugs; limiting access to high-alert medications; using auxiliary labels and automated alerts; and employing redundancies such as automated or independent double-checks when necessary. (Note: manual independent double-checks are not always the optimal error-reduction strategy and may not be practical for all of the medications on the list.)

Classes/Categories of Medications

- adrenergic agonists, IV (e.g., **EPINEPH**rine, phenylephrine, norepinephrine)
- adrenergic antagonists, IV (e.g., propranolol, metoprolol, labetalol)
- anesthetic agents, general, inhaled and IV (e.g., propofol, ketamine)
- antiarrhythmics, IV (e.g., lidocaine, amiodarone)
- antithrombotic agents, including:
  - anticoagulants (e.g., warfarin, low molecular weight heparin, IV unfractionated heparin)
  - Factor Xa inhibitors (e.g., fondaparinux, apixaban, rivaroxaban)
  - direct thrombin inhibitors (e.g., argatroban, bivalirudin, dabigatran etexilate)
  - thrombolytics (e.g., alteplase, reteplase, tenecteplase)
  - glycoprotein IIb/IIIa inhibitors (e.g., eptifibatide)
- cardioplegic solutions
- chemotherapeutic agents, parenteral and oral
- dextrose, hypertonic, 20% or greater
- dialysis solutions, peritoneal and hemodialysis
- epidural or intrathecal medications
- hypoglycemics, oral
- inotropic medications, IV (e.g., digoxin, milrinone)
- insulin, subcutaneous and IV
- liposomal forms of drugs (e.g., liposomal amphotericin B) and conventional counterparts (e.g., amphotericin B desoxycholate)
- moderate sedation agents, IV (e.g., dexmedetomidine, midazolam)
- moderate sedation agents, oral, for children (e.g., chloral hydrate)
- narcotics/opioids
  - IV
  - transdermal
  - oral (including liquid concentrates, immediate and sustained-release formulations)
- neuromuscular blocking agents (e.g., succinylcholine, rocuronium, vecuronium)
- parenteral nutrition preparations
- radiocontrast agents, IV
- sterile water for injection, inhalation, and irrigation (excluding pour bottles) in containers of 100 mL or more
- sodium chloride for injection, hypertonic, greater than 0.9% concentration

Specific Medications

- **EPINEPH**rine, subcutaneous
- epoprostenol (Flolan), IV
- insulin U-500 (special emphasis)*
- magnesium sulfate injection
- methotrexate, oral, non-oncologic use
- opium tincture
- oxytocin, IV
- nitroprusside sodium for injection
- potassium chloride for injection concentrate
- potassium phosphates injection
- promethazine, IV
- vasopressin, IV or intraosseous

*All forms of insulin, subcutaneous and IV, are considered a class of high-alert medications. Insulin U-500 has been singled out for special emphasis to bring attention to the need for distinct strategies to prevent the types of errors that occur with this concentrated form of insulin.

Background

Based on error reports submitted to the ISMP National Medication Errors Reporting Program, reports of harmful errors in the literature, studies that identify the drugs most often involved in harmful errors, and input from practitioners and safety experts, ISMP created and periodically updates a list of potential high-alert medications. During May and June 2014, practitioners responded to an ISMP survey designed to identify which medications were most frequently considered high-alert drugs by individuals and organizations. Further, to assure relevance and completeness, the clinical staff at ISMP, members of the ISMP advisory board, and safety experts throughout the US were asked to review the potential list. This list of drugs and drug categories reflects the collective thinking of all who provided input.

© ISMP 2014. Permission is granted to reproduce material with proper attribution for internal use within healthcare organizations. Other reproduction is prohibited without written permission from ISMP. Report actual and potential medication errors to the ISMP National Medication Errors Reporting Program (ISMP MERP) via the website (www.ismp.org) or by calling 1-800-FAIL-SAF(E).

ISMP
INSTITUTE FOR SAFE MEDICATION PRACTICES
www.ismp.org

APPENDIX B

Institute for Safe Medication Practices

ISMP's List of *Error-Prone Abbreviations, Symbols,* and *Dose Designations*

The abbreviations, symbols, and dose designations found in this table have been reported to ISMP through the ISMP National Medication Errors Reporting Program (ISMP MERP) as being frequently misinterpreted and involved in harmful medication errors. They should **NEVER** be used when communicating medical information. This includes internal communications, telephone/verbal prescriptions, computer-generated labels, labels for drug storage bins, medication administration records, as well as pharmacy and prescriber computer order entry screens.

Abbreviations	Intended Meaning	Misinterpretation	Correction
μg	Microgram	Mistaken as "mg"	Use "mcg"
AD, AS, AU	Right ear, left ear, each ear	Mistaken as OD, OS, OU (right eye, left eye, each eye)	Use "right ear," "left ear," or "each ear"
OD, OS, OU	Right eye, left eye, each eye	Mistaken as AD, AS, AU (right ear, left ear, each ear)	Use "right eye," "left eye," or "each eye"
BT	Bedtime	Mistaken as "BID" (twice daily)	Use "bedtime"
cc	Cubic centimeters	Mistaken as "u" (units)	Use "mL"
D/C	Discharge or discontinue	Premature discontinuation of medications if D/C (intended to mean "discharge") has been misinterpreted as "discontinued" when followed by a list of discharge medications	Use "discharge" and "discontinue"
IJ	Injection	Mistaken as "IV" or "intrajugular"	Use "injection"
IN	Intranasal	Mistaken as "IM" or "IV"	Use "intranasal" or "NAS"
HS	Half-strength	Mistaken as bedtime	Use "half-strength" or "bedtime"
hs	At bedtime, hours of sleep	Mistaken as half-strength	
IU**	International unit	Mistaken as IV (intravenous) or 10 (ten)	Use "units"
o.d. or OD	Once daily	Mistaken as "right eye" (OD-oculus dexter), leading to oral liquid medications administered in the eye	Use "daily"
OJ	Orange juice	Mistaken as OD or OS (right or left eye); drugs meant to be diluted in orange juice may be given in the eye	Use "orange juice"
Per os	By mouth, orally	The "os" can be mistaken as "left eye" (OS-oculus sinister)	Use "PO," "by mouth," or "orally"
q.d. or QD**	Every day	Mistaken as q.i.d., especially if the period after the "q" or the tail of the "q" is misunderstood as an "i"	Use "daily"
qhs	Nightly at bedtime	Mistaken as "qhr" or every hour	Use "nightly"
qn	Nightly or at bedtime	Mistaken as "qh" (every hour)	Use "nightly" or "at bedtime"
q.o.d. or QOD**	Every other day	Mistaken as "q.d." (daily) or "q.i.d." (four times daily) if the "o" is poorly written	Use "every other day"
q1d	Daily	Mistaken as q.i.d. (four times daily)	Use "daily"
q6PM, etc.	Every evening at 6 PM	Mistaken as every 6 hours	Use "daily at 6 PM" or "6 PM daily"
SC, SQ, sub q	Subcutaneous	SC mistaken as SL (sublingual); SQ mistaken as "5 every"; the "q" in "sub q" has been mistaken as "every" (e.g., a heparin dose ordered "sub q 2 hours before surgery" misunderstood as every 2 hours before surgery)	Use "subcut" or "subcutaneously"
ss	Sliding scale (insulin) or ½ (apothecary)	Mistaken as "55"	Spell out "sliding scale"; use "one-half" or "½"
SSRI	Sliding scale regular insulin	Mistaken as selective-serotonin reuptake inhibitor	Spell out "sliding scale (insulin)"
SSI	Sliding scale insulin	Mistaken as Strong Solution of Iodine (Lugol's)	
i/d	One daily	Mistaken as "tid"	Use "1 daily"
TIW or tiw	3 times a week	Mistaken as "3 times a day" or "twice in a week"	Use "3 times weekly"
U or u**	Unit	Mistaken as the number 0 or 4, causing a 10-fold overdose or greater (e.g., 4U seen as "40" or 4u seen as "44"); mistaken as "cc" so dose given in volume instead of units (e.g., 4u seen as 4cc)	Use "unit"
UD	As directed ("ut dictum")	Mistaken as unit dose (e.g., diltiazem 125 mg IV infusion "UD" misinterpreted as meaning to give the entire infusion as a unit [bolus] dose)	Use "as directed"

Dose Designations and Other Information	Intended Meaning	Misinterpretation	Correction
Trailing zero after decimal point (e.g., 1.0 mg)**	1 mg	Mistaken as 10 mg if the decimal point is not seen	Do not use trailing zeros for doses expressed in whole numbers
"Naked" decimal point (e.g., .5 mg)**	0.5 mg	Mistaken as 5 mg if the decimal point is not seen	Use zero before a decimal point when the dose is less than a whole unit
Abbreviations such as mg. or mL. with a period following the abbreviation	mg mL	The period is unnecessary and could be mistaken as the number 1 if written poorly	Use mg, mL, etc. without a terminal period

Institute for Safe Medication Practices

ISMP's List of *Error-Prone Abbreviations, Symbols,* and *Dose Designations* (continued)

Dose Designations and Other Information	Intended Meaning	Misinterpretation	Correction
Drug name and dose run together (especially problematic for drug names that end in "l" such as Inderal40 mg; Tegretol300 mg)	Inderal 40 mg Tegretol 300 mg	Mistaken as Inderal 140 mg Mistaken as Tegretol 1300 mg	Place adequate space between the drug name, dose, and unit of measure
Numerical dose and unit of measure run together (e.g., 10mg, 100mL)	10 mg 100 mL	The "m" is sometimes mistaken as a zero or two zeros, risking a 10- to 100-fold overdose	Place adequate space between the dose and unit of measure
Large doses without properly placed commas (e.g., 100000 units; 1000000 units)	100,000 units 1,000,000 units	100000 has been mistaken as 10,000 or 1,000,000; 1000000 has been mistaken as 100,000	Use commas for dosing units at or above 1,000, or use words such as 100 "thousand" or 1 "million" to improve readability

Drug Name Abbreviations	Intended Meaning	Misinterpretation	Correction
To avoid confusion, do not abbreviate drug names when communicating medical information. Examples of drug name abbreviations involved in medication errors include:			
APAP	acetaminophen	Not recognized as acetaminophen	Use complete drug name
ARA A	vidarabine	Mistaken as cytarabine (ARA C)	Use complete drug name
AZT	zidovudine (Retrovir)	Mistaken as azathioprine or aztreonam	Use complete drug name
CPZ	Compazine (prochlorperazine)	Mistaken as chlorpromazine	Use complete drug name
DPT	Demerol-Phenergan-Thorazine	Mistaken as diphtheria-pertussis-tetanus (vaccine)	Use complete drug name
DTO	Diluted tincture of opium, or deodorized tincture of opium (Paregoric)	Mistaken as tincture of opium	Use complete drug name
HCl	hydrochloric acid or hydrochloride	Mistaken as potassium chloride (The "H" is misinterpreted as "K")	Use complete drug name unless expressed as a salt of a drug
HCT	hydrocortisone	Mistaken as hydrochlorothiazide	Use complete drug name
HCTZ	hydrochlorothiazide	Mistaken as hydrocortisone (seen as HCT250 mg)	Use complete drug name
MgSO4**	magnesium sulfate	Mistaken as morphine sulfate	Use complete drug name
MS, MSO4**	morphine sulfate	Mistaken as magnesium sulfate	Use complete drug name
MTX	methotrexate	Mistaken as mitoxantrone	Use complete drug name
PCA	procainamide	Mistaken as patient-controlled analgesia	Use complete drug name
PTU	propylthiouracil	Mistaken as mercaptopurine	Use complete drug name
T3	Tylenol with codeine No. 3	Mistaken as liothyronine	Use complete drug name
TAC	triamcinolone	Mistaken as tetracaine, Adrenalin, cocaine	Use complete drug name
TNK	TNKase	Mistaken as "TPA"	Use complete drug name
ZnSO4	zinc sulfate	Mistaken as morphine sulfate	Use complete drug name

Stemmed Drug Names	Intended Meaning	Misinterpretation	Correction
"Nitro" drip	nitroglycerin infusion	Mistaken as sodium nitroprusside infusion	Use complete drug name
"Norflox"	norfloxacin	Mistaken as Norflex	Use complete drug name
"IV Vanc"	intravenous vancomycin	Mistaken as Invanz	Use complete drug name

Symbols	Intended Meaning	Misinterpretation	Correction
ʒ	Dram	Symbol for dram mistaken as "3"	Use the metric system
♏	Minim	Symbol for minim mistaken as "mL"	
x3d	For three days	Mistaken as "3 doses"	Use "for three days"
> and <	Greater than and less than	Mistaken as opposite of intended; mistakenly use incorrect symbol; "< 10" mistaken as "40"	Use "greater than" or "less than"
/ (slash mark)	Separates two doses or indicates "per"	Mistaken as the number 1 (e.g., "25 units/10 units" misread as "25 units and 110" units)	Use "per" rather than a slash mark to separate doses
@	At	Mistaken as "2"	Use "at"
&	And	Mistaken as "2"	Use "and"
+	Plus or and	Mistaken as "4"	Use "and"
°	Hour	Mistaken as a zero (e.g., q2° seen as q 20)	Use "hr," "h," or "hour"
Ø or ∅	zero, null sign	Mistaken as numerals 4, 6, 8, and 9	Use 0 or zero, or describe intent using whole words

**These abbreviations are included on The Joint Commission's "minimum list" of dangerous abbreviations, acronyms, and symbols that must be included on an organization's "Do Not Use" list, effective January 1, 2004. Visit www.jointcommission.org for more information about this Joint Commission requirement.

© ISMP 2013. Permission is granted to reproduce material with proper attribution for internal use within health care organizations. Other reproduction is prohibited without written permission from ISMP. Report actual and potential medication errors to the ISMP National Medication Errors Reporting Program (ISMP MERP) via the Web at www.ismp.org or by calling 1-800-FAIL-SAF(E).

ISMP — INSTITUTE FOR SAFE MEDICATION PRACTICES

www.ismp.org

APPENDIX C
Sample Medication Administration Errors With Potential Clinical Outcomes

Medication errors may be made in each step of the process, including a prescription order error; pharmacy misinterpretation; pharmacy preparation, labeling, and dispensing; and finally, nurse interpretation, calculation, and administration. The nurse who administers the medication is the last protector of the patient. The nurse must review the order, patient allergies, and idiosyncrasies, followed by a check for drug interactions, before preparing and administering the medication. Each of the processes mentioned, including checking safe dose range, is necessary to protect the patient from an adverse drug event (ADE). Failure to do so not only may harm the patient but may result in disciplinary actions by the agency and/or the State Board of Nursing. There may be additional legal implications should an injury occur.

Sample Order	Error	Type of Error and Comments	Potential Outcomes
Morphine SO$_4$ 10–20 mg q4h IM prn severe pain	Morphine SO$_4$ (10 mg per mL supplied in CarboJet) 20 mg given for initial dose	Lack of knowledge: initial dose should be lowest of the range Failure to monitor for side effects	Respiratory depression Coma Death
Blood administration	Administered with dextrose solution instead of normal saline Dextrose solution also administered through same line after transfusion	Lack of knowledge Failure to check the solutions for compatibility Failure to change line after transfusion	Hemolytic reaction (jaundice) and coagulation of blood in infusion line because of dextrose
Ordered: Furosemide, a diuretic, 0.05 mg per kg per hr, initial dose for a continuous IV for a 25-kg child	Programmed: Furosemide, 0.5 mg per kg per hr The nurse overrode the dose limit alarm on the smart pump, which resulted in a tenfold dosage error.	Lack of knowledge of initial safe dosage range and failure to focus Failure to double check the order and safe dosage range for this weight of child when the alarm sounded	Diuresis Dehydration Electrolyte imbalances Nephrocalcinosis Death
IV potassium chloride solution (KCl)	Administered undiluted or improperly diluted by nurse who obtained concentrated KCl 20 mEq per mL from pharmacy cabinet after hours per agency policy	Lack of knowledge related to potassium dilution and administration procedures when adding to IV solutions to ensure dilution is achieved	Burning pain Damage to the lining of the vein Arrhythmias Cardiac arrest
Gabapentin (Neurontin) for seizures	Two doses omitted because patient was nauseated Recorded on MAR Discovered by Pharmacy when medication cart returned and checked	Lack of knowledge of actions and dangers of omitted drugs Failure to report promptly to prescriber	Seizures Status epilepticus (continuous seizures) Prolonged hospitalization
Risperdal (risperidone) 4 mg bid po, an antipsychotic to treat a patient with schizophrenia Supplied: Requip (ropinirole) 2 mg tid po	Given: Requip (ropinirole) two 2-mg tablets A sound-alike/look-alike drug An antiparkinsonian drug also used for restless legs syndrome	Lack of knowledge regarding patient and drug: inappropriate medication Failure to check medication with prescriber order	Some side effects of Requip: Nausea Vomiting Low blood pressure Dizziness Relapse of psychotic behavior because of missed dose of Risperdal

Consequences depend on the history of errors; type of error; severity of error; whether corrective measures were sought and/or instituted promptly and by whom; patient outcome; and perceptions of those evaluating the incident, including the patient and family.

Action may be taken by the employing agency, the State Board of Nursing, and legal representatives of the patient. The actions can include a discussion; a letter of reprimand; required course(s) of study; probation with or without clinical supervision followed by reinstatement if probation period reflects competence; loss of employment; suspension of license; revocation of license; and lack of renewal of malpractice insurance. A civil and/or criminal lawsuit by the patient may be brought against the employee and the employer regardless of the previously mentioned actions.

Nurses should carry their own private malpractice insurance for personal representation, even if the employer "covers malpractice insurance." There may be occasional conflicts of interest when the nurse depends on the employer's insurance.

APPENDIX D
5-Minute Sample Verbal Communication From Nurses to Subsequent Caregivers

A hand-off report is the transfer and acceptance of critical patient information through effective communication between caregivers at shift change or for transfer between units or agencies, or when patients are discharged to home to ensure patient safety. Many errors, *including medication errors,* have been attributed to inadequate hand-off communication. The highlighted areas in the sample report presented here pertain to key medication-related information. Additional information would be given for discharge communication to home, including accompanying written materials about all medications and treatments and when to make appointments for checkups. Whereas only major medication issues are verbally reported for a shift change, complete medication resolution must be provided in writing for all physical patient transfers. Check agency procedures and forms for hand-off communication and medication resolution.

Nurse giving report to next caregiver at shift change on a medical–surgical unit

(Sex, Age, Mental/Emotional Status, Main Diagnoses, Dates of Admission and Transfers, Additional Diagnoses, Allergies)

Mr. G. is a 73-year-old, moderately hard-of-hearing, alert, oriented (to person, time, and place) cooperative, English-speaking male in no acute distress admitted to ICU with uncontrolled hypertension and acute bronchitis on the 3rd of October and transferred to our unit on the 6th. He also has chronic prostatitis, mild anemia, and an artificial hip replacement as of a year ago that requires use of a cane for stability. He has occasional asthmatic episodes controlled with an inhaler. He is allergic to penicillin and aspirin, reacting with hives and wheezing as well as diarrhea from penicillin, and is a fairly reliable historian. He lives with his daughter, so it is best to include her in all teaching, particularly because of the hearing loss.

(Vital Signs)

His vital signs are all stable today.

(Medications: Medication Changes, Medications Due, Related Orders)

He had a central line removed before transfer here. His main medications are: an intravenous antibiotic piggyback (IVPB) every 6 hr for 24 more hr for his bronchitis. His next one is due soon at 1700 hr. He is on digoxin every morning and two new blood pressure meds; one is a diuretic in the morning and the other is an ACE inhibitor in the evening. His blood pressure needs to be recorded each shift and after any complaint of weakness or extreme fatigue. Notify the attending physician if the systolic pressure exceeds 170. Make sure his inhaler is within reach and record his use.

(Labs)

His white blood count is still elevated at 13,000 but has been improving steadily. He is NPO after midnight for fasting blood work and also has a lung function test scheduled in the morning. His other labs are within normal limits. Hold the diuretic in the morning until the labs are completed.

(Treatments)

The discontinued central line site needs to be assessed once a day. He is receiving respiratory therapy every morning beween 0800 and 0900 and wants to bathe before the therapist arrives.

(Nutrition/Intake and Output)

He is now tolerating a regular diet well but needs encouragement to drink more fluids. Since he started on the diuretic, he self-limits fluids to try to reduce urination. The fluid intake and urinary output are to be recorded until discharge. Notify the attending physician if the intake or output drops below 1000 mL per day.

(Activity Level: Mobility)

He needs assistance and encouragement getting in and out of bed but does not need assistance walking as long as he has the cane. The doctor wants him to be out of bed most of the day if possible. Bedrails are up at bedtime and a urinal within reach at all times because of the diuretic and urinary frequency.

(Other Needs/Discharge Planning)

His discharge is tentatively planned for next Monday, so special emphasis needs to be given to teaching Mr. G about the new medication regimen and the need for fluids and activity. He lives with his daughter, who visits after work daily. Be sure to include her in all teaching and discharge planning because day shift does not see her often. A main issue is that he is unhappy about having to take "new pills," so we have already started reinforcing the importance of compliance with him and his daughter. Be sure to get feedback because he does not always mention that he did not hear everything.

Note: Although this seems like a lot of information, the nurse who cares for the patient for a full shift and who has established a sequential format for reporting information can communicate this information verbally on each assigned patient with ease. It helps to keep a checklist on hand with abbreviated cues (see the sample boldfaced subheadings) to ensure that the verbal hand-off report covers all the major areas. The receiving nurse refers to the written record for further details. There are many potential variations for reporting; for example, fasting could be included under Nutrition/Intake and Output instead of Labs.

Index

A
AA (amino acids or protein), 353
abbreviations, 57
   avoiding errors with, 104
   Clinical Alerts for, 96
   for common IV solutions, 239
   for drug forms, 66
   error-prone, 59, 61f–62f
   for measurement, 68–69
   for medication administration, 60–63, 60t, 61f–62f, 97–98
   in metric system, 100
   for milliliters, 108
   potential for confusion with, 101
   for safe drug routes, 59
   as source of medication errors, 312
   for time and routes, 68
   writing, 102
acetaminophen, compared with aspirin products, 73
acetylsalicylic acid (aspirin), 73, 398
activated partial thromboplastin time (aPTT), 379
addition
   of decimals, 19
   of fractions and mixed numbers, 10–11
ADD-Vantage system, 251–253, 251f, 252f
adverse drug event (ADE), 57
   with medication administration routes, 67
   for pediatric patients, 415
Afrezza insulin, 308t, 309
alarms, with high-tech infusion devices, 286, 286f
alerts. *see* Clinical Alerts
amino acids or protein (AA), 353
ampules, 157, 157f
anaphylactic shock, 415
antibiotics
   allergic reaction to, 192
   sound-alike, 191
anticoagulants, 116, 379
   IV flushes for, 390
   and polypharmacy, 390
   vocabulary for, 379–380
anticoagulants, injectable, 380–383
   low molecular weight heparin (LMWH), 381
   subcutaneous heparin injections, 383–384
anticoagulants, oral
   new class of, 398
   warfarin, 396–398
antiinfectives, Clinical Alert for, 199
antiplatelet agents, 398
anti-Xa assay, 379
Apidra insulin, 308t, 309
apothecary system, 99
aqueous suspensions, 64
Arixtra (fondaparinux), 382, 383, 383f
aspirin, 73, 398
atrial fibrillation (AF), warfarin for, 398
automatic dose calculators, for TPN, 359, 359f

B
basal rates, 305, 340, 340t
Baxter Mini-Bag Plus system, 251, 251f
bedside monitor blood glucose (BMBG), 305
bleb, formation of, 158f
blood-borne illnesses, and needlestick injuries, 152
blood glucose (BG)
   insulin dosage based on, 337
   logbook for recording, 337f
blood glucose level (BGL)
   defined, 305
   insulin dose based on, 338
blood glucose level (BGL) tracker, 334f
blood transfusions, 254, 254f
body surface area (BSA), 415, 416
   for children, 420, 420f
   estimated, 420
   mathematical formula for, 421
bolus IV administration, 229, 274–277, 275f–277f, 305
brand/trade name, 69, 70
Broviac catheter, 355f
buccal administration, 67
Byetta pens, 312, 313f

C
CADD-Prizm infusion pumps, 253, 253f
calculation process, 99. *see also* Dose calculations
calibration, 145
caplets, 63–64, 64f
capsules, 64, 64f
   administering, 64
   delayed release (DR), 64, 64f
carbohydrate (CHO) intake
   insulin dosage based on, 334–335, 334f, 336, 338
   logbook for recording, 337f
carbohydrate (CHO) ratio technique, 334
Carpuject syringe holder, 148, 149f
cc (abbreviation), 145
centimeter scale, 109, 109f
central lines, 358, 358f
central parenteral nutrition (CPN), 353, 355, 356, 368f
cephalosporins, allergy to, 438
chemical name, 69
children
   diabetes in, 306
   fluid requirements for, 423, 424t
   subcutaneous and intramuscular medications for, 428–430, 428f

---

Page references with *f* indicate figures; those with a *t*, tables.

children's doses
  based on body weight and surface area, 416
  Clinical Alerts for, 422, 423
  contrasted with adult, 424, 424t
  for IV medications, 430–432, 430f
  for oral medications, 425
  safe injection volumes for, 428
  vocabulary for, 415–416
  weight-based, 416–419
CHO (dextrose or sugar), 353. *see also* Carbohydrate intake
Clinical Alerts
  for abbreviation confusion, 96, 101, 108
  for allergy to penicillin, 438
  for antibiotic names, 433
  for antiinfectives, 199
  for antiseizure medications, 439
  for aspirin *vs.* acetaminophen products, 73
  for blood transfusions, 254
  for BSA calculations, 421
  for changing IV solutions, 291
  checking ability to swallow, 118
  for checking IV rates, 236
  for checking orders, 121
  for children's doses, 422, 423, 425, 426, 427
  on compound drugs, 74–75
  for controlled substances, 128
  converting to kilograms, 417
  for decimal fractions, 16
  for dilution directions, 274, 298
  for documentation, 59
  on DS (double-strength), 113
  for EIDs, 257
  for filter needles, 157
  for heparin, 382, 387, 388, 389, 390, 393
  for high-alert medications, 286–288, 287t, 291, 294
  for IM medications, 190, 202
  for incident reports, 85
  for infusion devices/pumps, 253
  for injectable medications, 169, 194
  for insulin administration, 310, 315, 316
  insulin *vs.* tuberculin syringes, 384
  for intermittent IV medications, 231
  for IV insulin, 327, 327f
  for IV push medications, 275, 277
  for MARs, 78, 79
  for medication administration, 59, 64, 66, 67, 83
  for medication errors, 60
  for medication orders, 76, 441
  for medication reconciliation, 85, 86
  for metric equivalents, 104
  for metric system, 104
  micrograms *vs.* milligrams, 285
  for mixing insulins, 322f, 323
  for morphine sulfate (MS) orders, 428
  for multidose containers, 95
  for needlestick injuries, 152, 153
  for oral syringe use, 118
  patient safety issue, 289
  for pediatric IV flow rates, 434
  for peripheral lines, 358
  for potassium chloride, 257
  preparing medications, 121
  problem solving, 111
  for recapping of needles, 152, 152f
  for reconstituted medications, 182, 187, 189
  rounding decimals, 16
  for syringes, 146, 150
  for TPN, 355, 360, 363
  for unit-dose *vs.* multidose containers, 72
  for units of medication *vs.* milligrams, 197
  for using original labeled containers, 116

Clinical Alerts (*continued*)
  for using unit measure, 122
  for verbal orders, 440
clock time, 76–78, 77f
clopidogrel (Plavix), 398
colons, using grammatical, 103, 110, 123
common denominators, 8–9
compatibility, checking for, 231
compound drugs, Clinical Alerts for, 74–75
computerized physician order entry (CPOE) systems, 63, 75
continuous glucose monitoring (CGM) system device, 333, 333f
continuous IV infusion, 229
controlled substances, Clinical Alert for, 128
CPN. *see* Central parenteral infusion
critical thinking
  about anticoagulants, 400–401
  about checking IVs, 259–260
  about children's doses, 435–436
  exercises in, 130–131
  for high-alert medications, 295
  for insulin administration, 342–343
  about parenteral nutrition, 371–372
  for reconstituted medications, 206
  about safety issues, 89–90
cubic centimeter (cc) abbreviation, 108

D

decimal fractions
  Clinical Alert for, 16
  definition of, 15
  reading, 15
decimal point, 15
decimals
  addition of, 19
  avoiding errors with, 18
  changing common fractions to, 23
  changing to fractions, 22–23
  changing to percentages, 24
  Clinical Alerts with, 16, 17
  comparison of, 15
  converting to percentage, 24
  division of, 20–22
  with metric equivalents, 105
  multiplication of, 20
  rounding of, 16–17, 18
  self-assessment for, 2
  subtraction of, 19–20
  value of, 15, 17
deep vein thrombosis (DVT), 379, 380
dehydration, in pediatric patients, 423
delivery sets, IV, 234–236, 234f–236f
  needleless systems, 234, 234f
  primary set, 234, 234f
deltoid site, 159f
denominators, 6
  definition of, 5
  finding common, 8–9
dextrose solutions, 240f, 242f
diabetes
  complications of, 311
  non-insulin injectables for, 309t
  type 2, 306, 354
diabetes flow sheet, 330
diabetes medications, oral, 331. *see also* Insulin
diabetes mellitus (DM), 306, 353
  type 1, 306, 354
  type 2, 306, 354
diabetic ketoacidosis (DKA), 306, 353
Dial-a-Flo tubing and extension set, 233, 233f
dibasic sodium, reconstituting medications with, 189
diluents (solvents), 179, 189

dilutions, 180, 434
dilution solution labels, 174
direct intravenous (IV) bolus, 274–277, 275f–277f
displacement, 180
disseminated intravascular coagulation (DIC), 380
division
    of decimals, 20–22
    of fractions and mixed numbers, 14–15
documentation
    Clinical Alert for, 59
    electronic, 59
    and patient rights, 59
"Do Not Use" List (abbreviations), of TJC, 60, 60t, 63
dose calculations, 71
    avoiding errors in, 124
    errors in, 114
    for injectable medications, 163–164
    kilograms used for, 107
    for liquid medications, 116, 116f, 119–121
    and medication labels, 71, 72
    for oral medications, 116
        liquids, 117–121, 117f, 118f
        solids, 111–113, 114
    and patient rights, 59
    ratio and proportion methods
        one-step, 102
        two-step, 123
dose designations, error-prone, 59, 61f–62f
dosing guidelines for (DVT-PE) treatment chart, 395, 395t
drop factor (DF), 229, 232, 232f
droppers, medicine, 65f
    calibrated, 116, 116f, 126
    for children's doses, 423f
drops per minute
    calculating, 235, 235f
    by manufacturer, 234
drug concentration (strength), 57
drug forms, abbreviations for, 66
drug names, types of, 69
DS medication, double checking, 74, 113

E

electronic infusion devices (EIDs), 229, 253, 253f, 257, 288, 359
electronic infusion pump, for children, 430, 430f
electronic medication administration records (EMARs), 78, 80f–81f
elixirs, 64
embolus, 379
emulsions, 64
epidural administration, 67
Epipen, 148, 149f, 429, 430
    discharge planning for, 430
    using, 430
equivalent fractions, 8, 9, 10
errors, medication. see Medication errors
estimates, compared with proofs, 45
estimation, 99
extracts, 64

F

filter needles, 157, 157f
Flowmeter tape, 236, 236f
flow rates, 273, 434
fluid extracts, 64
flushes
    with high-tech infusion devices, 286, 286f
    ranges for, 358, 358t
    SAS, 274
    SASH, 274
    solutions for, 275f
Food and Drug Administration (FDA), 57, 70

fraction cross-product set up, using, 103, 110, 123
fractions
    adding/subtracting, 8–9
    addition of, 10–11
    change to percentage to make solutions, 25–26
    changing to decimals, 22–23
    changing to higher terms, 10
    changing to percentage, 24
    decimals
        addition of, 19
        avoiding errors with, 18
        changing common fractions to, 23
        comparison of, 15
    definition of, 5, 15
    division of, 14–15, 20–22
    equivalent, 8, 9
    improper, 7
    multiplication of, 13–14, 20
    percent numbers for, 23
    ratio as, 41–42
    reading, 15
    reducing to lowest terms, 10
    reduction of, 5–6
    rounding of, 16–17
    self-assessment for, 1
    subtraction of, 12–13, 19–20
    value of, 6
    whole number for, 6
Fragmin (dalteparin), 382
free-flow, 230

G

gastric administration, 67
gel, delayed-release, 64
generic drugs, 70–73
    forms of, 71–73
    information about, 70–71
    labels for, 70
generic name, 69
glucagon, 306, 353
glucagon injection, emergency kits for, 306, 307f
glucose gel, 306
glucose tablets, 306
gram (g), 99
    abbreviation for, 100
    English system equivalent for, 100
    medications in, 106–107
granules, extended-release, 64, 64f
gravity infusions, 230
    for children, 430, 430f
    drop factor for, 232–234, 232f, 233f
    limits of, 359
    piggyback, 250, 250f
gravity tubing
    extension set for, 233, 233f
    indications for, 233
    using Flowmeter tape with, 236, 236f
Groshong catheter, 355f

H

half-life, 273
hand-off report, 488
hard alert, 286, 286f
heparin, 379
    antidote for, 393
    Clinical Alerts for, 382, 387, 388, 389
    as continuous IV drip, 382
    fractionalized vs. unfractionated, 380–381
    injection sites for, 381, 381f, 384
    low molecular weight, 380–381
    MAR for, 381, 381f

Index **487**

heparin (continued)
    multidose vials for, 385
    subcutaneous injections of, 383–384
heparin, intravenous (IV), 390–391
    dosing guidelines for, 395–396
    symptoms associated with, 391
    titrated to kilograms, 393
heparin flushes, 380, 390
heparin-induced thrombocytopenia and thrombosis (HITT), 380
heparin-induced thrombocytopenia (HIT), 380–381
heparin lock, 230f, 231, 379
heparin resistance, 389
heparin sodium injection, USP, indications for, 380
heparin therapy, Clinical Alert for, 393
hep/heparin lock, 230f, 231, 379
Hickman catheter, 355f
Hickman catheter site, 357f
high-alert drugs, ISMP-identified, 127
higher terms (fractions), 10
home parenteral nutrition (HPN), 353
Hospira ADD-Vantage system, 251–253, 251f, 252f
household equivalents, using approximate, 115–116
household measurements, compared with metric, 99, 106, 107–108
Humalog insulin, 308t, 309
human insulin, 312, 313f
hyperglycemia, 306, 354
hyperglycemia protocol, 338
hypertonic solution, 230
hypodermic, 146
hypoglycemia, 306, 354
    causes of, 306
    protocol for, 339
    treatments for, 306
hypothyroidism, testing for, 105
hypotonic solution, 230

I

improper fractions, 7–8
incident reports, medication, 83, 84f, 85
    Clinical Alerts for, 85
    example of, 84f
incretin, 309
incretin mimetics
    action of, 309
    defined, 306
infants
    estimating weight of, 417
    fluid requirements for, 423, 424t
Information Management Standards, 63
infusion devices/pumps
    ambulatory, 256
    Clinical Alert for, 253
    electronic, 257
    high-tech, 286, 286f
    insulin, 333, 333f
    pressure-flow, 256
    with safety features, 277, 277f
infusion pumps
    for children, 430, 430f
    for parenteral nutrition, 356
infusion syringe pumps, Freedom 60, 280f
inhalant administration, 67
injectable medication calculations, vocabulary for, 305–306
injectable medications, 145
    Clinical Alerts for, 169, 194
    dose calculation for, 163–164
    label interpretation for, 160–163
    parenteral, 158
    unit-dose, 145
    vocabulary for, 145–146

Innohep (tinzaparin), 382
INR (international normalized ratio), 380, 396
Institute for Safe Medication Practices (ISMP), 255, 384, 479–480
    high-alert medications of, 286–288, 287t
    List of Error-Prone Abbreviations, Symbols, and Dose Designations of, 59, 61f–62f, 479–480
    National Medication Errors Reporting Program of, 477
insulin, 306
    AM/PM shot record for, 318
    based on carbohydrate intake, 333–334, 333f, 336f
    labels for, 314–316
    logbook for recording, 337f
    mixed insulins, 315
    mixing, 322–323, 322f
    tactile measuring devices for, 310
    types of, 312–314, 313f, 314f
insulin, intravenous (IV), 327–328, 328f
insulin administration, injection sites for, 307, 307f
insulin comparison chart, 308t
insulin dose
    based on blood glucose and CHO intake, 338
    based on carbohydrate intake, 334–335, 336
    insulin-to-carbohydrate ratio for, 340, 340t
    logbook for recording, 337f
    sliding-scale calculations for, 339
insulin dose calculations, 305–306
insulin infusion chart, standard, 328f
insulin infusion devices, 333, 333f
insulin orders, 311
insulin pens, 309, 312, 313f
insulin resistance, 306
insulin shock, 306, 354
insulin syringes, 309–311, 310f, 311f
insulin therapy, complications of, 306
insulin-to-carbohydrate ratio, estimating, 339, 339t
insulin vials, 314, 314f
InterLink System Continu-Flo solution set, 232, 232f
international normalized ratio (INR), 380, 396
intradermal (ID) administration, 67
intradermal (ID) injections, 158, 158f, 159f
intramuscular (IM) administration, 67
intramuscular (IM) injections, 158, 158f, 159f, 230
    for babies, 426, 427f
    for children, 426, 427f
intramuscular (IM) medications
    for children, 428–430, 428f
    Clinical Alerts for, 190, 202
intrathecal administration, 67
intravenous (IV) administration, 67, 230–231
    blood transfusions, 254
    delivery sets for, 234–236, 234f–236f
    direct IV in, 274–277, 275f–277f
    with EIDs, 253, 253f
    injection port for, 230
    of insulin, 327–328, 388f
    MAR for, 249, 249f
    medication errors with, 294–295
    PCA, 255
    piggyback infusions, 256–257
    preparation for, 274
    pressure-flow infusion devices, 256
    vocabulary for, 229–230
intravenous (IV) calculations, 229
    determining mL per hr, 231
    drop factor, 232–234, 232f, 233f
    drops per minute by manufacturer, 232, 233, 234
    drops per minute in, 232, 233, 235, 235f
    with FloMeter tape, 236, 236f
    for hourly drug rate, 281–282
    for hourly volume rate, 281–282
    for insulin, 328, 328f

intravenous (IV) calculations (*continued*)
   for medication orders, 283
   microdrip, 234
   for obstetrics, 292–293
   for piggyback infusions, 256–257
   two steps in, 231
   vocabulary for, 273
intravenous (IV) flushes, 273, 390
intravenous (IV) infusions, 230. *see also* Infusion devices/pumps
intravenous (IV) lines
   flushing intermittent access locks for, 358, 358*t*
   types of, 356–360, 357*f*–359*f*, 358*t*
intravenous (IV) lock, intermittent, 230*f*, 231
intravenous (IV) medications
   charting of, 249, 249*f*
   for children, 430
intravenous (IV) push medications, 274–277, 275*f*–277*f*
   piggyback, 276, 276*f*
   procedure, 275, 275*f*, 276, 276*f*
   timing, 277–279
intravenous (IV) solutions, 243–244, 244*t*
   abbreviations for, 239
   osmolarity of, 243–244, 244*t*
intravenous piggyback (IVPB) infusions, 229, 230, 256–257
   gravity, 250, 250*f*
   nurse-activated, 251–253, 251*f*, 252*f*
   ports for, 234, 234*f*
   with premixed IVs, 250–251, 251*f*
   working with, 250
intravenous solutions
   examples of, 239*f*–242*f*
   osmolarity of, 243–244, 244*t*
   percentage of solute in, 242–243
isotonic solution, 230

J

The Joint Commission, 59
   "Do Not Use" list of, 60, 60*t*, 63
   on medication reconciliation, 85
Joint Commission on Accreditation of Healthcare Organizations (JCAHO), 255
Jordan Medical Count-a-Dose, 310

K

Kcal, 354
ketoacidosis, 333
kilograms, converting pounds to, 418

L

labels
   for central parenteral nutrition (CPN) (sample), 368*f*
   for heparin sodium injection, 383*f*
   oral antidiabetic, 331*f*, 332*f*
   for PPN, 369*f*
   TPN, 360–361, 360*f*, 361*f*
   for warfarin (Coumadin), 396*f*
labels, medication, 69–75
   brand name on, 70
   and dose calculation, 71, 72
   drug names on, 69
   for generic drugs, 70–73
   for injectable medications, 160–163
   interpreting, 73–75
   reading carefully, 173
   for reconstituted medications, 182
   types of print on, 71–72
labels, U-100 insulin
   immediate-acting, 315
   intermediate-acting, 315
   intermediate- and rapid-acting mixtures, 316
   for intermediate- and rapid-acting mixtures, 316

labels, U-100 insulin (*continued*)
   long-acting, 316
   for rapid-acting, 315
   short-acting, 314–315
lactated ringer's solutions, 241*f*
Lantus insulin, 316
latex allergy, checking for, 157
length, household *vs.* metric measurements for, 108
lidocaine, reconstituting medications with, 189
lipids
   delivery of, 356, 356*f*
   infusion of, 359, 359*f*
   order for, 356*f*
Liposyn, 354
liquid medications
   administration of, 65, 65*f*
   calculating dosage for, 119–121
   forms of, 64–66, 65*f*, 66*f*
   household and metric measurements for, 115
   measuring, 117–121, 117*f*, 118*f*, 180–181, 181*f*
   metric-calibrated equipment for, 66
   from multidose bottle, 66, 66*f*
   parenteral forms of, 65*f*
   rounding of, 116
liquids, measuring volume of, 107–108
liter (L), 99, 107
   abbreviation for, 100
   English system equivalent for, 100
Lovenox (enoxaparin), 382
lowest terms
   expressing ratios in, 42
   reducing fractions to, 10
low molecular weight anticoagulants, indications for, 382
low molecular weight heparin (LMWH), 380–381
Luer-Lok syringe tips, 153, 153*f*

M

Magni-Guide, for insulin syringes, 310, 310*f*
measurement systems
   household, 99
   units and milliequivalents, 122
measurements, abbreviations for, 68–69
measuring cups, oral, 180, 181*f*
measuring teaspoon, 65*f*
MedFlo postoperative pain management system, 256*f*
Medibottle, for children's doses, 423*f*
medical terminology, 57
medication administration, 82–83, 82*f*, 83*f*
   abbreviations for, 60–63, 60*t*, 61*f*–62*f*, 97–98
   Clinical Alerts for, 59, 64, 66, 67, 83
   of enteric-coated, 64
   and medication errors, 60
   prioritizing, 83, 84*f*, 85
   and right to refuse, 59
   routes of, 67, 68
   safe, 57
medication administration records (MARs), 76, 78
   Clinical Alerts for, 78
   example of, 192
   for heparin, 381, 381*f*
   interpreting, 81
   for IV therapy, 249, 249*f*
   pharmacy-generated, 79
   for PRN orders, 80*f*
   sample, 78, 79*f*
   for TPN, 365*f*
medication administration routes, abbreviations for, 68
medication carts, 82, 82*f*, 83, 83*f*
medication errors
   abbreviations as source of, 312
   attributed to inadequate communication, 483

medication errors (*continued*)
  Clinical Alerts for, 60
  IV, 294–295
  with labels, 72
  nursing responsibility for, 481–482
medication forms, 63
  abbreviations for, 66
  liquid medications, 64–66, 65*f*, 66*f*
  solid oral medications, 63–64, 64*f*
medication orders, 75–76, 75*f*
  identifying incomplete, 76
  IV calculations for, 283
medication reconciliation, 85
  calculations for, 86
  Clinical Alerts for, 85, 86
  failure to perform, 85
  interpretation of, 85
  and medication administration, 86
  preparation for, 85–86
medications, high-alert, 273, 379. *see also* Anticoagulants
  in acute care settings, 477
  ISMP-identified, 286–288, 287*t*
medicine cups, 65*f*, 115
  for children's doses, 423*f*
  measuring with, 117, 117*f*
  unit-dose packaged, 116, 116*f*
mediport, with central line, 358*f*
meniscus, 66, 66*f*, 180, 181*f*
meter (m), 99
  abbreviation for, 100
  English system equivalent for, 100
metric dose calculation, 110
metric equivalent chart, 100
metric equivalents, 106
  calculation setup for, 102–103
  compared with household, 106–109
  and household equivalents, 107
  memorizing, 106, 107, 108
  moving decimals for, 105
  using approximate, 115–116
  using ratio and proportion to find, 103–104
  for volume, 108
  for weight, 106, 108
metric measurements
  base units of, 99
  values and meanings for, 101, 101*t*
metric system, 99
  avoiding errors with, 106
  base units of, 100
  definition of, 100
  notation review for, 104
  prefixes in, 101, 101*t*
  understanding clinical relevance of, 105
metric units, writing, 102
Metric Units Number Line, 101
mg per kg calculation method, 416
microdrops, 232, 232*f*
micrograms
  medications in, 106–107
  potential confusion with, 110
micrograms per kilogram, 415
milliequivalent, 122
milliequivalent per liter, 122
milliequivalent per milliliter, 122
milligrams
  confusion with, 197
  medications in, 106–107
  potential confusion with, 110
milligrams per kilogram, 415
milliliters, 107
millimeter and centimeter scale, 109, 109*f*

milliunits, 122
minimal effective analgesic concentration (MEAC), 255
mixed numbers, 7
  addition of, 11
  changing improper fractions to, 7
  changing to improper fractions, 7–8
  division of, 14–15
  multiplication of, 13–14
  subtraction of, 12–13
mix-o-vial directions, 191, 191*f*
multidose containers
  Clinical Alerts for, 95
  vs. unit-dose containers, 72
multiplication
  of decimals, 20
  of fractions and mixed numbers, 13–14

N

nasogastric (NG) administration, 67
national drug code (NDC) number, 70
National Formulary (NF), 70
National Medication Errors Reporting Program (ISMP MERP), 477–480
National Patient Safety Goal #3, 85
needleless equipment, 153, 153*f*
needleless infusion system, for intermittent medications, 231, 231*f*
needles
  disposing of, 152, 152*f*
  filter, 157, 157*f*
  insertion of, 159*f*
  length and gauge for, 150*f*
  parts of, 150*f*
  recapping of, 152, 152*f*
  selection of, 150–157
  sizes for, 150, 150*f*
needlestick injuries
  avoiding, 152
  Clinical Alerts for, 152, 153
neonate, drug doses for, 424*t*
nomograms, 415, 416, 420, 421
nonparenteral (noninjectables) administration, 67
normal saline solution, 239, 239*f*, 240*f*
Novolog insulin, 308*t*, 309
numerators, 5, 6

O

obstetrics, IV calculations for, 292–293
Omnicell Savvy Mobile Medication System, 83*f*
oral diabetes medications (ODMs), 331
oral medications
  for children, 425
  rounding doses for, 116
  and swallowing ability, 118
oral (PO) administration, 67
ordering and dispensing system, computer-controlled, 82, 82*f*
osmol, 243
osmolarity, 230, 243–244, 244*t*
overhydration, in pediatric patients, 423
over-the-counter (OTC) medications, 85, 390

P

pain rating scale, Wong-Baker FACES, 428
parenteral administration (injectables), 67
parenteral infusion
  central (venous), 353
  peripheral (venous), 354
parenteral nutrition
  central, 355, 356
  home, 353
  peripheral, 355, 356
  protocol for, 353

parenteral nutrition (*continued*)
    total, 354–356, 354*f*–356*f*
    vocabulary for, 353–354
parenteral route, 146
partial thromboplastin time (PTT), 382, 390
patents, 70
patient-controlled analgesia (PCA), 230, 253
    protocol for, 255
    pumps for, 255*f*
patient identifiers, for medication administration, 83, 83*f*
peak and trough levels, 274
pediatric patients, 415. *see also* Children's doses
    IM injections for, 426, 427*f*
    medication administration for, 417
percentages
    changing to fraction, 24
    converting to decimal, 24
    definition of, 23
    finding, 25
    to make solutions, 25–26
    self-assessment for, 2
peripheral lines, 356
peripherally inserted central catheter (PICC), 354, 356, 357*f*
peripheral parenteral infusion, 354
peripheral parenteral nutrition (PPN), 355, 356, 369*f*
petechiae, 380
PICC line. *see* Peripherally inserted central catheter
piggyback infusions. *see* Intravenous piggyback infusions
pill splitter, 65*f*
platelet count, 380
polypharmacy, and anticoagulants, 390
postprandial, 306
potassium chloride, IV infusion of, 257
powders, 64, 64*f*
prefixes, metric, 101, 101*t*
preprandial, 306
prescription abuse, 127
PRN orders, MAR for, 80*f*
proofs, compared with estimates, 45
proportions
    definition of, 42
    proving correct, 42
    setting up, 45–48
    solving problems of, 43–44
protamine sulfate, 380, 390–391, 393
prothrombin time (PT or Pro Time), 380, 396
pulmonary embolus (PE), 380
pumps. *see also* Infusion devices/pumps
    infusion syringe, 280*f*
    insulin, 331

Q

Quality and Safety Education for Nurses (QSEN), 288
QSEN Institute Patient Goal No. 4, 288

R

ratio and proportion calculation method, 110, 111
ratios
    definition of, 41
    as fractions, 41–42
    setting up, 45–48
recombinant DNA insulins, 312
reconstituted medications, 179
    Clinical Alerts for, 182, 189, 191
    cost effectiveness of, 180
    labels for, 182
    measuring liquid medications for, 180–181, 181*f*
    for parenteral use, 188
    with prefilled vials and syringes, 191
    shelf life of, 179
    sound-alike, 191

reconstituted medications (*continued*)
    two-vial reconstitution method for, 189–190, 190*f*
    types of diluents used with, 189
    vocabulary for, 179–180
reconstitution, 180
red flag, 127
refuse, right to, 59
registration symbol ®, 70
respiratory administration, 67
rounding
    of decimals, 16–17, 18
    for oral medication doses, 116
    self-assessment for, 3
rubber latex stoppers, 157

S

safe dose ranges (SDRs), 86, 416
    calculating, 416, 417, 419
    for children, 416, 417
    determining, 290
safety practices, for medication administration, 57. *see also* Clinical Alerts
saline, administer [medication], saline, heparin (SASH), 274
saline, administer [medication], saline (SAS), 274
saline/heparin lock, 230, 230*f*
saline lock, 230*f*, 231
saline lock adapter, 276*f*
scheduled medications
    measuring, 127, 127*f*
    potential for use of, 127–128
scored-medication orders, 116
sensor glucose (SG) readings, 333
sepsis, 274
sharps container, 152, 152*f*
"shelf life," 180
shift report, 483–484
Sigma Spectrum Infusion Smart Pump, 286*f*
single-unit-dose package, 65*f*
skin lesions, estimating size of, 109
sliding scale, insulin administered on, 339
"smart pumps," 286, 286*f*
soft alert, 286, 286*f*
solid medications, rounding calculations for, 116
solid oral medications, administration of, 64, 65*f*
solutes, 180
    tonicity of, 244, 244*t*
    weight measurement (g) for, 243
solutions, 180
    preparing, 25–26
    using fractions to change percentage to make, 25–26
    vs. aqueous suspensions, 64
solvent, 179
square meter (m^2), 416
subcutaneous (subcut) injections, 67, 158, 158*f*, 159*f*
    for children, 428–430, 428*f*
    sites for, 159*f*
sublingual (SL) administration, 67
subtraction
    of decimals, 19–20
    of fractions and mixed numbers, 12–13
swallowing ability, checking, 118
symbols, error-prone, 59, 61*f*–62*f*
syringe pump, 276*f*
syringes
    for bolus injections, 277
    calibrations on, 147, 147*f*
    checking for blood return with, 147
    for children's doses, 423*f*
    Clinical Alerts for, 146, 150
    comparison of, 146*f*
    disposing of, 152, 152*f*

syringes (continued)
   5-mL, 148, 148f
   for flushing peripheral IV lines, 358
   holders for, 148, 149f
   insulin, 309–311, 309f, 311f
   with Luer-Lok tips, 153, 153f
   needleless, 153f
   parts of, 147f
   prefilled, 192
      auto-injector, 148, 149f, 150
      reconstituting with, 191, 191f
   reading and measuring with, 147
   reading measurements for, 154
   safety, 153f
   selection of, 146–150
   3-mL, 147, 147f
   tuberculin, 148, 148f, 310
   U-100 insulin, 310, 310f
syringes, oral, 65f, 118, 118f, 150, 150f, 180, 181f
   for children's doses, 423f
   measuring with, 117, 117f
   prefilled, 65f, 116
   tubing with, 118
   using, 127, 127f

T

tablet crushing system, 65f
tablets
   enteric-coated, 64, 64f
   extended-release, 64, 64f
   forms of, 63–64, 64f
   scored, 63–64, 64f, 65f, 74
target-specific oral anticoagulants (TSOACs), new class of, 398, 398t
terminology, medical, 57
thrombocytopenia
   defined, 380
   heparin-induced, 383
thrombolytic agent, 380
times, medication
   abbreviations for, 68
   traditional, 98
titration, 274
titration orders, 291
tonicity, 230, 243, 244, 244t
topical administration, 67
topical prescription ointments, measurements for, 109, 109f
total parenteral nutrition (TPN), 354–356, 354f–356f
   amino acids, dextrose and lipids in, 362
   Clinical Alerts for, 363
   contents of, 355
   kilocalories per bag, 363
   medication administration record for, 365f
   mL per hour to set pump, 362
   percentage of additives in, 362
   physician's order for, 364f, 367f
   physician's order form for, 360, 361f
   protocol for, 363

total parenteral nutrition (TPN) (continued)
   total grams per bag, 362
   validation of label for, 360–361, 360f, 361f
transdermal (skin) administration, 67
tuberculin syringes, 310
Tubex syringe holder, 148, 149f
tunneled catheter, for TPN, 359, 359f
24-hour clock, 76–78, 77f, 98

U

unfractionated heparin (UFH), 380–381
unit-dose containers, vs. multidose containers, 72
United States Pharmacopeia (USP), 70, 384
units, 146
   definition of, 122
   use of term, 122

V

vascular access device (VAD), 274, 275
vascular access port, implantable, 357f
vastus lateralis site, 159f
ventrogluteal site, 159f
verification, 99
vials, 157, 157f
   dissolving medications in, 192
   reconstituting with prefilled, 191, 191f
Victoza pen, 312
viscosity
   defined, 146
   and syringe selection, 147
vitamin K, 380, 396
volume
   equivalent measures for, 108
   household vs. metric measurements for, 107–108

W

warfarin (Coumadin), 396–398
   antidote for, 396
   blood-testing regimen for, 397, 397f
   compared with target-specific oral anticoagulants (TSOACs), 398t
   discharging patient on, 397, 397f, 398
   dosing for, 396, 396f
   drugs affecting efficacy of, 398
   indications for, 382
   labels for, 396f
   missed doses of, 398
weight
   equivalent measures for, 106, 108
   household vs. metric measurements for, 106
   solving mg per kg problems, 416
weight reporting, kilogram used for, 107
West nomogram, 420, 421
whole numbers, 7
Wong-Baker FACES pain rating scale, for children, 428

Y

young adults, diabetes in, 306

Metric Equivalents

Weight	Length
1000 mcg (microgram) = 1 mg (milligram)	10 mm (millimeter) = 1 cm (centimeter)
1000 mg = 1 g (gram)	100 cm = 1 m (meter)
1000 g = 1 kg (kilogram)	1000 mm = 1 m (meter)
Pound to Kilogram Conversion	1000 m = 1 km (kilometer)
2.2 lb = 1 kg (kilogram)	**Volume**
Household to Metric Length Equivalent	1000 mL (milliliter) = 1 L (liter)
1 inch = 2.54 cm (centimeter)	**Miscellaneous**
39.37 inches = 1 m (meter)	1000 milliunits = 1 Unit (U)

Approximate Equivalents of Metric and Household Measures*

Metric	Household	
5 mL	1 teaspoon (tsp)	
15 mL	1 tablespoon (Tbs),† 3 teaspoons (tsp)	½ ounce
30 mL	2 tablespoons (Tbs)	1 ounce
240 mL	1 measuring cup	8 ounces
500 mL	1 pint	1 pint or 16 ounces
1000 mL (1 liter)	1 quart	1 quart or 32 ounces
4 liters	1 gallon (gal) or 4 quarts	1 gallon (gal) or 4 quarts

*Household equipment and apothecary measurements are not a substitute for metric measurements. The volume capacity of household equipment varies greatly. The apothecary measurements are imprecise and not equal to the metric measurements. **Use Metric**. Clarify unfamiliar abbreviations with the prescriber.
†Capitalizing T for Tablespoons abbreviation helps avoid confusion with tsp (teaspoon).

Body Surface Area (BSA) Formulas

A. Formula using only metric system

$$BSA = \sqrt{\frac{weight\ (kg) \times height\ (cm)}{3600}}$$

B. Formula using only pounds and inches

$$BSA = \sqrt{\frac{weight\ (lb) \times height\ (in)}{3131}}$$